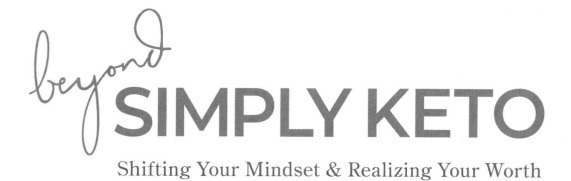

beyond SIMPLY KETO

Shifting Your Mindset & Realizing Your Worth

Suzanne Ryan

Victory Belt Publishing Inc
Las Vegas

First published in 2020 by Victory Belt Publishing Inc.

ISBN-13: 978-1-628603-71-2

The author is not a licensed practitioner, physician, or medical professional and offers no medical diagnoses, treatments, suggestions, or counseling. The information presented herein has not been evaluated by the U.S. Food and Drug Administration, and it is not intended to diagnose, treat, cure, or prevent any disease. Full medical clearance from a licensed physician should be obtained before beginning or modifying any diet, exercise, or lifestyle program, and physicians should be informed of all nutritional changes.

The author/owner claims no responsibility to any person or entity for any liability, loss, or damage caused or alleged to be caused directly or indirectly as a result of the use, application, or interpretation of the information presented herein.

Cover design by Chelsea B. Foster

Front cover photography by Jennifer Skog

Back cover photography by Bill Staley and Hayley Mason

Interior design by Yordan Terziev and Boryana Yordanova

Interior illustrations by Colleen Pugh

Recipe development by Suzanne Ryan and Jessica Morgan

Food styling by Betsy Haley, assisted by Jessie Bloom

Food photography by Suzanne Ryan

TC 0120

This book is dedicated to anyone who has ever struggled with not feeling good enough, and to the people battling anxiety, depression, or low self-esteem.

Our strength and beauty are not born on easy roads, but emerge from the battlegrounds of struggle, pain, vulnerability, and perseverance.

You are not alone.
You are strong.
You are enough.

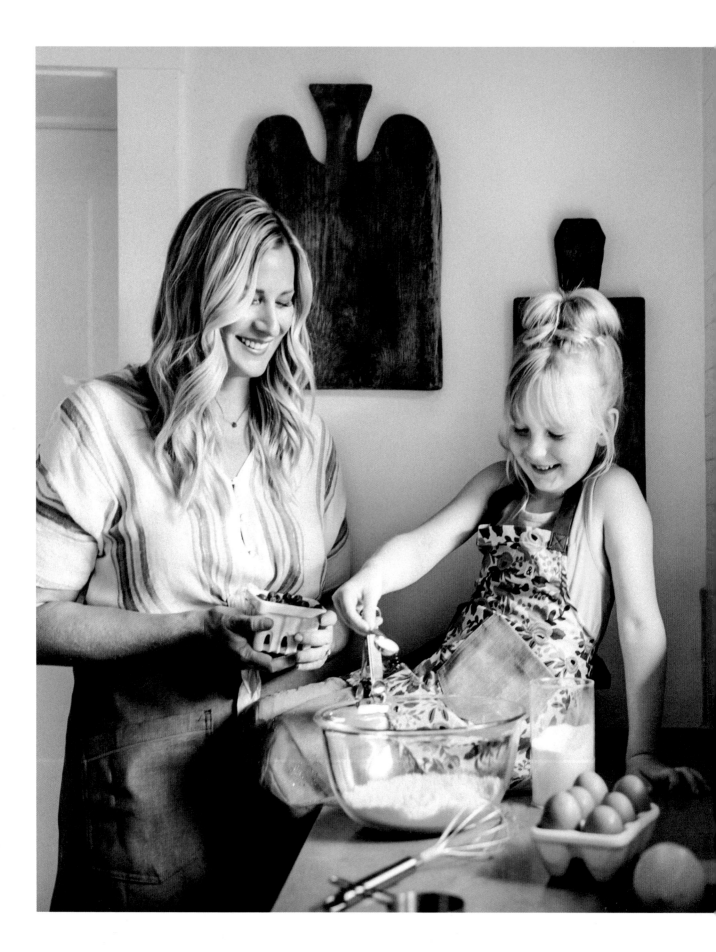

contents

LETTER TO READERS

To my readers:

Over the past five years, since starting my keto weight loss journey, I've been honored to connect with so many amazing people in the keto, low-carb, and various other health and wellness communities. So many of you have sent me thoughtful, vulnerable, and inspiring messages and emails. I've had the pleasure of meeting many of you on book tour stops, and even while I'm out shopping, around town, and traveling. You've been so real and raw, sharing your stories, triumphs, struggles, pain, and perseverance. Each message, interaction, smile, and hug has made an impact on my life, and for that I'm forever thankful. I truly believe that we all have important stories to share and that our stories connect us, which further shows us that we are all deeply valuable, seen, and never alone.

With each step on my journey, I have felt every emotion and have learned valuable lessons that have shaped me along the way. I've come to realize that there is no finish line when it comes to weight loss, personal growth, healing, or self-improvement. The road can be bumpy and scary, and sometimes you take a few steps back before taking a few steps forward, and then come the unexpected twists and turns. And this is the way it goes for most of us. The fact that the path isn't straight and narrow in no way means that we aren't good enough or dedicated enough to the effort of reaching our destination; it only shows that we are perfectly imperfect. Ultimately, we should all aim to always be works in progress, giving ourselves grace but also being open and committed to becoming everything that we envision for our life, our goals, and our legacy.

I think it's safe to say that the majority of the people I've met or messaged with have opened my eyes to a deeper realization for my own life and struggles with weight in this diet culture world. We are all so focused on the "fix" that we often overlook the "cause." We pour millions of dollars into an industry that tells us we need to buy things or to be thin to be happy, which couldn't be further from the truth.

Often the very first thing people ask me about when they find out about my story or the work I do is all focused on keto: What is keto, and how does it work? Wait, can I still eat oatmeal? Did you just say I can't eat bread? Or rice? Or potatoes? Hmm. What about quinoa? That's healthy, right?

Next, people almost always share about their own struggles with weight or body image and how they've tried many different things to lose weight, yet nothing seems to stick. You name it, they have tried it; and either it doesn't work or they quit, and the weight ends up coming back. At this point in the conversation, I'm usually nodding my head because I know that feeling so deeply in my soul—that feeling of wanting so badly to change, yet not knowing how the heck to do it.

Next comes the part that truly hits me the most. Often this is the point where people open up and begin to speak from a place of vulnerability. Diet and weight are often sectioned off and set aside as people begin to talk about their battles with mental or emotional health. I've heard stories of people growing up in abusive homes, or in homes in which they didn't feel valued or prioritized, or in homes in which they faced insanely high expectations and immense pressure from parents or other family members. I've heard stories of people losing loved ones, struggling with infertility or multiple miscarriages, battling illness or health crises, and fighting through anxiety, depression, or both. I've heard stories of people feeling a lack of self-esteem from being teased as children, feeling not good enough, and never feeling a sense of belonging. The list goes on and on, but these experiences place us in a common space of pain, sadness, struggle, and defeat. At this point, my eyes are usually welling up because we are connecting on a much deeper level. Beyond diet. Beyond weight. Beyond trying to reach a certain number on a scale. And I'm so deeply in tune with the truth that so many of us face in our ongoing struggle with feeling broken or not good enough.

The truth is that a lot of us are hurting, and a lot of us numb that pain with food. Emotional eating is pretty common, and it has a deceiving way of feeling like home, like comfort, or like a steadfast companion of sorts. Is this the case for everyone? No, but I can tell you that many people, myself included, have realized this important connection between trauma or stress and emotional eating. So many times, we view our mind and body as separate entities, but they are truly so deeply interconnected.

After losing 120 pounds with the ketogenic diet, I had a lot of ideas about what life as a thin person would be like. And while I want this book to have an overall happy and positive message, we all go through some tough things that I think need to be shared and normalized. My goal for this book is to encourage you to take a step beyond diet and to hold space for the much needed and often overlooked element that is so important in addition to your keto lifestyle, or whatever lifestyle you choose: your mindset, mental health, healing, and self-worth.

In this book, I'll be sharing with you the next steps of my journey, as well as a comprehensive yet simple guide to the ketogenic diet. I'll also be sharing the three biggest steps that have led to massive change and healing in my life and mental health. And last but not least, I've included over 100 all-new and delicious low-carb recipes!

So let's dive deeper, shall we?

Lots of love,

Suzanne

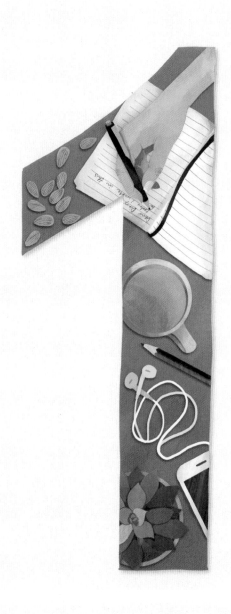

chapter 1:

BEYOND KETO

Keto is all the rage these days, and I have to admit that it's been exciting to see this healthy lifestyle spread all over the world. In a matter of a few years, we went from "What is keto?" to keto being all over the news and popular restaurants offering keto options on their menus.

While I'm happy to see this focus on whole foods and healthy fats, and to see the truth about sugar revealed, there is a much deeper topic that is often overlooked or under-discussed in the world of dieting and weight loss. In this chapter, I want to talk about going beyond keto, beyond dieting, and beyond the number you see on the scale. After chasing "thin" for most of my life, I've realized that this milestone was truly only the tip of the iceberg of much deeper work that needed to be done.

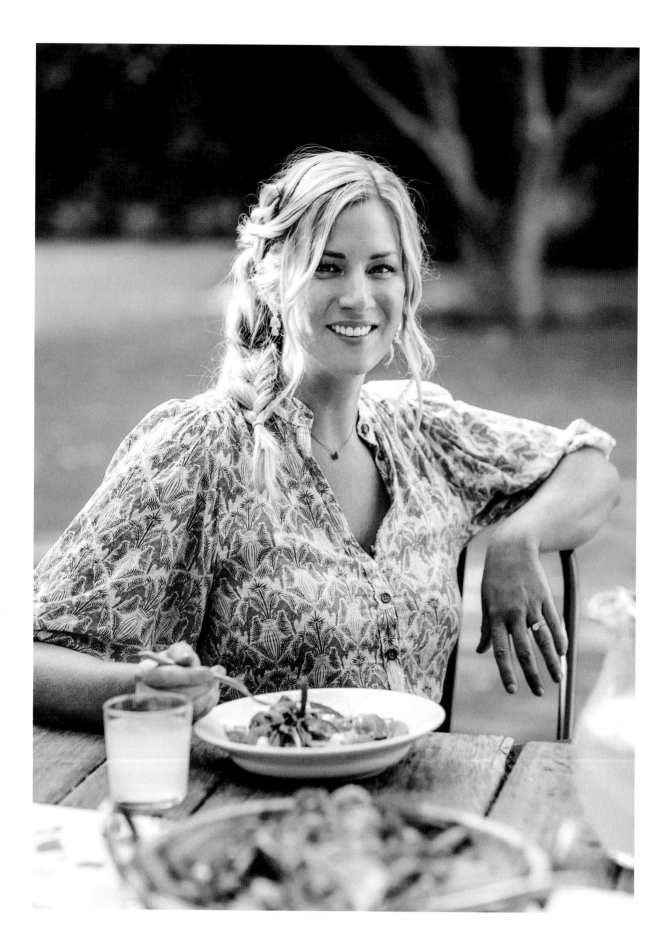

MY STORY, CONTINUED

As you may know from my first book, *Simply Keto,* I lost a total of 120 pounds in a little over a year with the ketogenic diet. And while I still thrive on a ketogenic lifestyle, along the way I came to a much deeper realization with regard to my weight, self-esteem, and mental health. In order to understand all that led to this discovery, I want to take you back through many pivotal years in my life that have shaped and changed my relationship with myself, and with food.

I was born in South Carolina in 1984 and completed my family of four. From the outside, I'm sure we seemed like the perfect family, the "American dream," but under the surface, things were falling apart.

We moved to Florida when I was in second grade to help take care of my aging grandparents. At first, it was a welcome change with a promise of new beginnings. But not long afterward, the fighting between my parents ramped up again, and the tension became palpable. I remember feeling sick to my stomach a lot as I struggled to understand what was going on and how to handle the chaos.

My parents ultimately ended their marriage in a bitter divorce that tore our family apart. Initially, my brother and I stayed with our mom and spent every other weekend with our dad. I remember feeling anxious and unsettled as we were passed back and forth between two parents who could barely communicate due to anger and resentment.

As a child, I took my parents' behaviors very personally. It took me many years to process these complex emotions, which I'll expand on later. At times, when tensions ran high, it was not uncommon for my brother and me to be told to pack our things as we were abruptly sent to live with the other parent. These actions reinforced the feeling that if and when I messed up, my stability could be left hanging in the balance. Eventually, I moved in with my dad, visiting my mom every other weekend. At such a pivotal time in my development, I felt cast aside and disregarded; it's not surprising that I struggled deeply with my own self-worth. However, I came to realize that although their actions were at times hurtful, it wasn't about me, but rather their own personal struggles during an extremely difficult time. Thankfully, as an adult and a parent, I can look back now through a more sympathetic lens and understand that we all make mistakes, even with the people we love the most.

One unintended consequence of the divorce was the difficulty of growing up in the crossfire of two hostile parents with vastly different expectations and households. With all the instability during this time, I often found myself coping with food. I remember going out for pizza or ice cream with my dad to shake off a bad day, or celebrating the passing of a test with a candy bar. When my mom would take me to see her therapist, I enjoyed the temporary escape provided by the three-layer vanilla ice cream and cookie dough parfait that had become my routine reward for each visit. Food was my constant, and it quickly became my steadfast comfort and friend.

In addition to developing emotional eating habits, the majority of the food I was eating was processed and very high in sugar and carbs, which was compounded by that era of fat-free everything. I was a big fan of soda, and I drank cola or ginger ale with almost every meal, including breakfast. In the morning, I usually ate cereal (often two bowls) or muffins, or I picked up a breakfast sandwich from the bagel shop on the way to school. I often bought lunch at school, and I generally picked nachos, pizza, or chicken tenders with fries, again paired with a soda. My dad would cook dinner on occasion, but his cooking experience was limited. Often, after working all day, he would just grab a pizza, subs, or takeout on his way home.

Naturally, these unhealthy eating patterns led me down a path of overeating, and as I put on weight, I began to feel uncomfortable with my body. My first attempt at dieting was in middle school, which is when my weight became noticeably higher from my peers', and boy, did they let me know. At school, I was referred to as the fat girl, the ugly girl, the Jolly Green Giant, a beached whale, and a fat-ass. Ultimately, I became the girl who felt really alone, broken, and inadequate, with complex struggles happening simultaneously at home. I often felt like there was no place where I was completely accepted or good enough.

The bullying continued through high school, and when I would get home, a box of cookies or a peanut butter and jelly sandwich with a tall glass of milk would seemingly make it all go away for a little while. I started and stopped numerous diets only to gain more weight with each passing year. Little by little, I began to feel like I wasn't worthy of friends, boyfriends, connection, or happiness, and on the really bad days, I felt unworthy of my life. I guess it's no surprise that due to these weight-focused attacks, I began to daydream about being thin and about how amazing my life would be if I could just lose weight. I just knew that once I was thin, things would be better. I could finally be normal, blend in, and be accepted.

Through my early twenties, I continued to struggle with my weight. By this point I had tried ten to fifteen diets with little to no lasting success. In 2005, when I was twenty-one, my world was flipped upside down when I suddenly faced an extremely hurtful and life-changing betrayal by two core people in my life. I felt so alone, and I began to question my ability to love or trust anyone ever again. I pulled back from any spark of life that I had left, and I mostly stayed at home in my room eating and sleeping. I had truly lost my will to live. I didn't have the desire or the energy to fight anymore. I was so depressed, and this time it seemed impossible to dig my way out.

A few weeks before everything fell apart, I had met Mick, who is now my husband. I still reflect on this moment and am reminded that even when the whole world feels like it's caving in, one person, one action, or one day can change everything. Mick stepped into my life and soon became the most amazing support system for me. I never expected it, and I certainly didn't feel worthy of it at the time. We would talk for hours, and he truly helped me pick up the pieces of my life as I battled my way through depression and mourned the loss of two people who had once meant everything to me. My life was different from this point forward, but looking back, I can see now that I needed to close some doors before I could grow and develop into a more independent and stronger version of myself.

Between 2009 and 2013, a lot of positive changes were happening in my life. Mick and I got married, moved across the country to California, and had our daughter, Olivia. As much as I love being a mom, it also added to my waves of anxiety and depression. I found myself obsessing over Olivia's health. I often checked to see if she was breathing and constantly felt anxious about her well-being. After all, she was the most important thing in my life, and I had never felt a love this strong and unconditional before.

Fast-forward to late 2014. Olivia was one, and I was struggling to keep up with her never-ending energy. I woke up feeling tired even after sleeping well each night, and I was so frustrated by my inability to change. My weight had reached over 300 pounds, my body ached, and I felt uncomfortable in my skin. Having tried so many ways to lose weight without success, I felt hopeless. Then one day, I received the devastating news that a dear friend's baby son, James, had been diagnosed with a terminal disease. This forever changed the way I view my health and the gift of life. Until that point, I was taking my life and health for granted. When James passed, I promised myself that I would fight in his honor to turn my life and health around.

I knew I needed a game plan, but I had already tried more than twenty diets, and none of them had worked. I researched weight loss surgery, but that didn't seem like the right choice for me. After much thought, I came to terms with the fact that I was an emotional eater, and I needed to make some serious lifestyle changes to address both what and why I was eating.

One day, I was randomly browsing on Reddit and discovered the ketogenic diet. I felt amazed and hopeful as I scrolled through countless transformation pictures. The fact that these people had lost weight without having to pay for any crazy programs, shakes, or pills really drew me in. The diet was sustainable, the food looked amazing, and I knew I had to give it a try.

I did some research and decided to try keto for my annual new year's resolution to lose weight. I just knew this would finally be the time that I wouldn't give up. But deep down, I also knew that I had told myself "this time I'm serious" many, many times before. Due to a blend of being unprepared with a side of self-sabotage and a lack of self-control, January first came and went, and I started and stopped keto that same day.

Two weeks later, I was sitting in my room, feeling miserable and trapped in my body yet knowing that this was all my own doing. I had no one to blame but myself, and in that moment, I decided it was time to buckle down and fight for my life. I went to the store, stocked up on lots of healthy food, and restarted the ketogenic diet. After ten weeks, I had lost 37 pounds, and my relationship with food had shifted in unexpected ways. I found myself less hungry, more satisfied with my meals, and not obsessing about food, and I started working on mindful eating instead of numbing my feelings with food.

For the first few weeks, I kept pretty quiet about trying keto. After all, I was the girl who had cried wolf with every single diet known to man, so I wanted to invest some time and walk the walk without the pressure of anyone watching and asking. But after eight or nine weeks, I decided that I really wanted to share my journey in hopes of helping and connecting with others. With Mick's help, in my tenth week of keto, I launched my YouTube and social media channels, Keto Karma. I was beyond excited to share about keto, and I just knew that this way of eating could help so many people, just like it was helping me. Each week I filmed an update, and right before my eyes, a tribe developed around me. I'd never had a support system like that before, and it truly changed my life. I will never forget or be able to repay the keto community for the endless love and support that I felt, and still feel. It was so healing to finally be vulnerable and to share each step along the way.

A year later, I had lost 100 pounds. Even more important, I had regained my health, my energy, and my passion for life, all while taking small steps toward working on my mental health. I started seeing a therapist, and little by little I began to realize that I had a lot of deep-rooted issues with feeling abandoned, rejected, betrayed, and worthless.

Even though my health was now my primary focus, I still had so many unrealistic expectations of what my life and self-esteem would be like once I was thin. I just knew that I would finally love my body, enjoy shopping for new clothes that actually fit, and rock a bikini every chance I could. I found myself at what I thought was the end—the finish line of losing 120 pounds—and much to my surprise, I was still struggling with anxiety, waves of depression, low self-esteem, and body dysmorphia. I sometimes found myself even more critical of my body than ever before. On top of that, I still despised clothes shopping with the dreaded dressing room mirrors, and when I wore a bikini, I would pick apart my thighs, stretch marks, and loose skin. In a moment of clarity but also a moment of "crap, what now?" I realized that losing the weight wasn't the fix-all solution I had built it up to be. And while I found myself with a "new" body shape, my mind remained almost the same. I was still my own worst critic, tearing myself apart, lacking self-worth, and never feeling good enough.

I think this is a pivotal point when a lot of people end up regaining weight—when you just know that the grass has to be greener on the other side, but then you get there only to find that the pain, struggles, and hard work of healing your mind and body are just sitting there patiently waiting for you. Looking back now, I see how easily it happened: I had been hurt, and I felt abandoned, made fun of, and betrayed. It was way easier to think that being overweight was my biggest hurdle, or the source of all my issues with self-worth, when in reality, one of my biggest battles had only just begun.

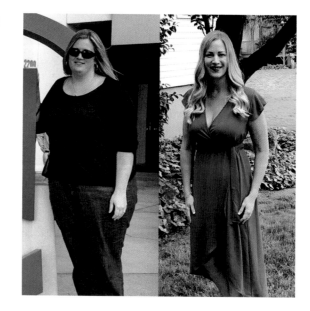

> "The grass isn't greener on the other side.
> It's greener where you water it."
>
> —NEIL BARRINGHAM

Amidst all the talk about self-love, I often felt stuck between understanding the concepts and importance yet not knowing how to really live it and truly love myself—you know, walking the walk. Losing weight absolutely changed my health for the better, but at the end of the day, I still found myself facing down that same unreasonably harsh inner critic, with waves of anxiety and depression. I decided it was time to dig deep to figure out how to break this vicious cycle, and I moved my therapy sessions to every week. At this point in my journey, I realized the very important but often overlooked element of mindset and mental health.

People often say, "Don't look back, you're not going that way," but I discovered that I needed to go back: to understand, to forgive, and to work on letting go of the thoughts and fears that weren't serving me anymore (and never had!). This led me to take off the armor that I had carried around my whole life. It was time to go beyond the diet, beyond food, and beyond weight loss to heal from the inside out.

Week after week, my therapist and I unpacked my life. We uncovered so many moments that had built up over a lifetime—experiences that had made me feel broken, discarded, and not good enough. Often, when we talked about my childhood, I was amazed to discover how even at a young age, when my ability to fully understand or process things was limited, I had built emotional walls for protection and formed beliefs about myself that stemmed from being hurt or afraid, and that those issues still revealed themselves in my life as an adult. I could also see that many of my issues with low self-esteem, anxiety, and fear were generational patterns that my parents, grandparents, and great-grandparents had experienced or learned as a result of their own struggles and hardships. We worked through a lot of painful moments in my life, and I learned pretty quickly not to wear mascara to my appointments. Truthfully, I needed to cry, I needed to process the hurt, and I needed to face it all to let some things go or process tough situations in a healthier way.

One of the most valuable outcomes of these discoveries was the shift in my outlook and mindset. Instead of seeing myself as less than, as unworthy, or as a victim, I began to see my parents, other people, and situations that had hurt me with a new perspective, and I could view them with compassion. I realized that while many people's hurtful actions felt extremely personal, they generally had nothing to do with me or my worth, and instead were largely due to their own sadness or struggles. Often, hurt people hurt people, and whether it's intentional or not, there is healing that needs to take place to let it go and move forward. As for my parents, I learned to look at them with empathy and grace—to see them as people: people who made mistakes, people who were going through battles of their own, but ultimately people who loved and cared for me all along. It was time for me to break the cycle and move forward by living my life from a place of gratitude, mindfulness, and empathy, not only for others, but for myself, too.

Ultimately, I came to the realization that there is so much more to this journey to health than losing weight or being thin. I had a lot of issues to work through and a lot of healing to do. It dawned on me that there is no finish line. Being the best version of yourself is a lifelong journey, and it was time to end the self-sabotage and lean into my inherent worth and capabilities. You have to redefine your struggles and failures to truly see that they aren't signs of weakness; they are expected factors in growth, in chasing your dreams, and in living a vulnerable life. Anticipate them and push forward. Remind yourself of your strength and your ability to get back up. Your mindset is critical in digging deep to accomplish everything you want for your life. Know that you don't have to choose between self-love and growth. You can have both, loving yourself through every step, setback, and comeback while continuing to push yourself to be the best version of yourself.

The way you think, the way you speak to yourself, and your day-to-day actions and mindset will dictate your outcomes. What you do and think heavily influences what you become. So, if you tear yourself down and tell yourself that things are too hard, that you're not good enough, or that you can't succeed, be prepared to see those thoughts manifest themselves. But I'm here to tell you that you were meant for more than drifting through life. You are strong not in spite of having struggles, but because of them.

Self-improvement isn't easy, and it requires daily maintenance and ongoing effort. Just like losing weight, this work has no finish line, but self-reflection and inner work is one of the most important and overlooked steps for personal growth and healing. I realize firsthand that habits can be hard to break. I'm there in the trenches with you. Sometimes I find myself right back in a broken place, and I have to stop myself from being overly critical, take a big deep breath, and find my way back to operating from a place of positivity in which I remember to honor my worth.

I challenge you (as well as myself) to start today and every day with gratitude for your life, your imperfections, your health, your body, and the people you love. Know your worth as you are now and love yourself during each step of your journey. Set goals and take consistent action to accomplish them. Know that your worth is not dependent on a number on a scale or the size of your clothing. Invest deeply in becoming the best version of yourself, one step and one day at a time. After all, we can't heal by hating or being hypercritical of ourselves. I don't have to know your exact story to know that we are all exhausted by this relentless pressure to be, look, and act perfect. Enough is enough! We all have walked the path of "I'm not good enough," and we all know it's not working or making any of us feel good. It's way past time to shift to a more supportive approach. On the following pages, I want to share with you three focal points for putting this plan into action.

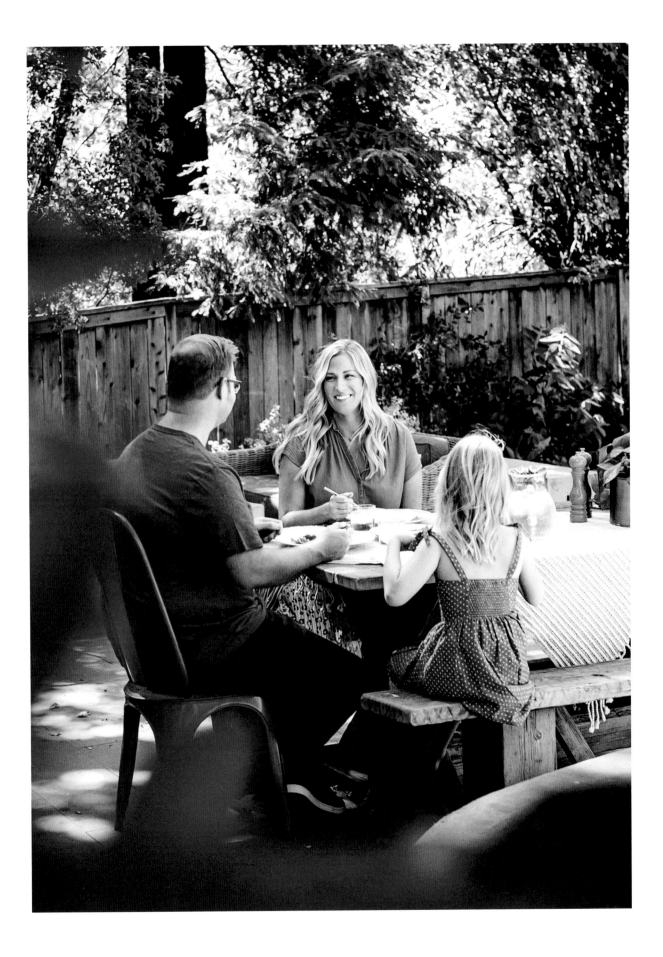

GOING BEYOND KETO: THREE FOCAL POINTS

Once I realized that I needed to work on more than just following keto and losing weight, I was able to determine three main areas that I feel are the keys to facilitating positive change and inner healing: inner voice, influence, and action. Each of these steps has made a big impact in my life as I grow and strive to live a healthy, positive, and fulfilling life. In this section, I'll share with you how and why each of these focal points is important and include a few examples of how to make them work in your life. Whether your goal is to get healthy, lose weight, start a business, or fulfill some other dream, these touchstones are sure to help you along the way.

> "Talk to yourself like you would to someone you love."
>
> —BRENÉ BROWN

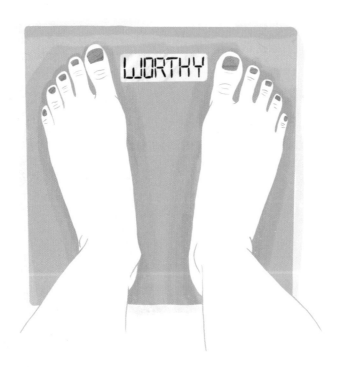

INNER VOICE

Face and overcome your biggest critic of all: yourself.
Get out of your own way and learn to tame your inner critic.

Many of us are way too hard on ourselves. I want you to think about the words you use to describe yourself both mentally and physically. These words guide your actions and beliefs, so bringing mindfulness to the things you say is a very important step to work on. If you find yourself saying something critical, try to stop yourself and swap your thoughts for more positive ones. Ask yourself, if I wouldn't say these words to my spouse or best friend, then why am I saying them to or about myself? Although none of us will fully master this 100 percent of the time, you will form new habits with practice and time. Remember, it's about progress, not perfection.

1. Be vulnerable.

As Brené Brown so beautifully says in her book *Daring Greatly,* "Vulnerability is the birthplace of love, belonging, joy, courage, empathy, accountability, and creativity." I suffered in silence behind a big smile for most of my life. When I finally had the courage to share my heart and hurt with others, I was able to genuinely be me and be seen instead of pretending that everything was fine. The goal here is to open your heart and to be seen for who you truly are. Vulnerability allows us the space to have the much-needed conversations that free us from the armor we put on to keep ourselves small and "safe."

2. Prioritize self-care.

As a busy working mom, wife, daughter, and friend, I have found prioritizing self-care to be a very important and necessary change in my life. If you are running on empty all the time, you can't be at your best for the people who mean the most to you. Self-care looks different for everyone, but some great examples are going for a walk, journaling, meditating, getting adequate sleep, doing deep-breathing exercises, practicing yoga, connecting with a loved one, learning a new hobby, eating healthy, learning to say no, learning to say yes, organizing the space around you, cleaning the house, and reading a book. Take some time to explore the possibilities and figure out what self-care looks like for you.

3. Don't believe everything you think.

Often we make assumptions based on fear—for example, when someone takes longer than normal to text or call you back, and you make up a story in your mind that involves the other person being mad at you. The issue with this way of thinking is that you have to experience and process every complex emotional possibility that you dream up, which is exhausting and anxiety-producing. When you find yourself headed down this path, try to relax, take a deep breath, and assume the best of people and situations until proven otherwise.

4. Seek help.

I feel it is really important that we, as a society, normalize the pursuit of mental health just as much as we have normalized the pursuit of physical health. I encourage you to reach out for support in whatever way feels appropriate to you. For me, therapy has been a really big help. I used to brush off ideas like "heal your inner child," but the truth is, we all carry things that have shaped us in some way. Call it what you like, but sometimes situations or emotions can take us right back to an age when we were hurt, felt abandoned, judged, neglected, or teased, or were made to feel that we weren't good enough. Acknowledging and working on the experiences that lie at the core of the many beliefs we have formed about ourselves and others can be really beneficial. So, whether you decide to see a therapist, call a supportive friend, go to group meetings, or join an online support group, know that seeking help is an important investment in your well-being.

5. Have a growth mindset.

I highly recommend *Mindset* by Carol Dweck. This book talks about our thoughts and why it's important to have a growth mindset instead of a fixed mindset. Let me briefly explain how similar thoughts can look completely different based on mindset. A person with a fixed mindset often sees challenges or setbacks as a stopping point, or the limit of their abilities. This mindset stops innovation, growth, and success in their tracks. A person with a growth mindset sees challenges or setbacks as opportunities to grow, adapt, and overcome. A growth mindset enforces the idea that we aren't born with inherent limitations, skills, or intelligence; instead, we have the ability to develop them with hard work. Therefore, having a growth mindset reinforces a healthier view of yourself and your ability to overcome obstacles, reach your goals, and grow as a person. We often stand in our own way, and this shift in mindset is a crucial part of healing your inner voice and developing self-confidence.

GROWTH MINDSET	vs.	FIXED MINDSET
Understands that failure is a part of success, which helps us learn, improve, and grow	« FAILURE »	Sees failure as proof that they aren't capable or good enough and shouldn't even try
Understands that skills, intelligence, and talents are developed through hard work, dedication, and persistence	« SKILLS »	Believes that skills, intelligence, and talents are innate and therefore cannot be changed or improved
Is open-minded and accountable to constructive feedback	« FEEDBACK »	Is closed-minded and avoids constructive feedback
Seeks out opportunities to learn new skills, methods, and advances	« LEARNING »	Prefers things to stay the same and resists change
Is persistent and eager to overcome challenges and setbacks	« CHALLENGES »	Gives up easily and often avoids challenges

INFLUENCE

You are the sum of the five people you spend the most time with. Who and what you spend your time and energy on matters.

In the past, I often overextended myself and found myself around others who were both draining and toxic. I realized that due to a lack of self-worth for most of my life, I became a people-pleaser, and often I wasn't selective enough about who I spent my time and energy on. When I realized the detrimental impact of negativity, I slowly made my inner circle of friends much smaller. This step wasn't easy, but the outcome of emphasizing quality over quantity is less stress and anxiety, and that is priceless. This focal point includes being aware of the effects that the people and things around you have on you and your energy. From family members to spouses to friends to what you watch and listen to—all of them have an impact. Sadly, there is no shortage of drama and negativity in this world, so be mindful of what you allow into your life. Long story short, you are in control of who and what you allow to influence you. Choose well.

1. Choose your circle wisely.

There's a saying that you are the sum of the five people you spend the most time with, and I have found it to ring true in my life. People can lift you up and root for your rise, or they can hold you back, leaving you feeling drained, stressed, or incapable. Surround yourself with people who support and encourage you while also challenging you to learn, improve, and grow. When I started working on my mental health and mindset, my outlook and perspective changed in certain ways. Along with that, some of my friendships and other relationships evolved. These shifts can be difficult at first, but they are sometimes a necessary part of becoming your best and happiest self. I'm truly happier and healthier having developed an inner circle of people who value gratitude, positivity, compassion, and empathy.

2. Don't compare yourself to others.

"Comparison is the thief of joy" is another saying I like to remember. In this world of social media highlight reels and aggressive lifestyle marketing, you don't have to look far to play the comparison game. I urge you not to go down that path. No one is perfect and happy all the time, no matter what they project to the world. The only person you should be comparing yourself to is who you once were in order to see how you've grown. If you find that social media exacerbates any feelings of unworthiness that you have, feel free to unfollow or hide certain people's profiles or accounts. I like to follow people who keep it real and share the kinds of ups and downs that we all experience as human beings.

3. Be mindful of how you spend your time and energy.

Everything we watch, read, and listen to has an effect on us. It is really important to be mindful of the things you allow into your life and to be aware of the kinds of things that drain you. Sometimes it's a little too easy to get caught up in spending hours on social media or watching Instagram or Facebook videos. It always breaks my heart when I see a family or group of friends out to dinner, and everyone's on their phones. I understand firsthand how addicting technology can be, but it's important to set boundaries. You can start small with approachable steps—for example, in my family, we make an effort to put our phones away during meals.

Another factor that often comes to mind with influence is the news. While it can be important to stay up-to-date with what's going on in the world around you, a lot of media is made for ratings and shock value, and this type of "news" can be exhausting rather than informative. For this reason, I rarely watch the news on TV; instead, I get my news from selective online sources.

4. Identify toxic relationships and deal with them appropriately.

If you have relationships that are toxic in nature, it is best to end those relationships or at least distance yourself from the negativity. I get that this is a difficult step, especially when it comes to toxic family members. However, you have many options aside from a black-and-white "don't ever talk to me again" approach. When I was dealing with the toxic people in my life, I generally either ended the relationship altogether, or if it was more complex or involved a family member, I chose to maintain the relationship but limit time spent with that person as well as what I shared with them.

5. Don't overextend yourself.

I am a recovering people-pleaser—someone who would never say no and would go out of my way to put the needs of others first, even before my own. Why did I do this? In part because I wanted people to like me, and in part because helping people has always been a passion of mine. I often felt that if people couldn't see the value in my physical self, then maybe they would be able to see my heart and how much I care, or how much I do. The bad news is that people-pleasers are often running on empty. I've learned that I truly can't take care of others without taking care of myself first.

> "You may not control all the events that happen to you, but you can decide not to be reduced by them."
>
> —MAYA ANGELOU

ACTION

Don't just dream it, do it! Invest deeply in the pursuit of your dreams, goals, and legacy.

Your inner voice and influences will have an effect on your willingness to take the third step: action. Your inner voice may tell you to play it safe or that you aren't capable of doing big things with your life. Your influences can either build you up and help you believe in yourself or keep you feeling small and incapable. If you've struggled to take action in your life, try working on the first two steps and then revisit this one when you realize what I already know about you (without even knowing you): that you are worthy and capable of accomplishing your goals, whatever they may be. When you have a dream, you must take steps to make it a reality; otherwise, it's a stagnant idea that will never go anywhere.

1. Journal.

Put pen to paper and organize your thoughts and ideas. Don't be afraid to dream really big or to pour your heart out onto each page. Along with your goals and dreams, it's important to plan a few new action items and assign deadlines for meeting them. If you have a tendency to procrastinate, like I do, then it's really helpful to keep things going by scheduling small tasks, and action steps to help you accomplish the larger goals that you set. For example, if you break larger goals down into smaller, and more approachable steps, it feels way less intimidating and approachable. When writing this book (and my last book), it felt very overwhelming at first, but then I set small goals with a schedule to do one topic, or a few recipes a day. Little by little it all adds up to one great outcome, so don't be afraid to break things up into bite-size pieces. You can buy a simple notebook, use a guided journal, or use the free printable worksheet pages that can be found on my blog (ketokarma.com/printables).

2. Redefine how you view success and failure.

Many people look at setbacks or failure as a sign that they aren't good enough or capable enough, and that couldn't be further from the truth. On the next page is an image of what hard work, failure, and success actually look like together. Many times people see someone who is successful and see only part of their story, only the upsides of success. What people often overlook or fail to realize is that every successful person isn't accomplishing great things because they never failed or experienced setbacks; instead, they are successful because they didn't let failures, setbacks, or people saying no deter them from pushing forward. This step has been an important focus for me because I learned to expect failures and learning curves without allowing them to diminish my sense of self-worth. When you expect bumps along the way, you are better prepared to know that although things won't always be easy, you are capable of accomplishing any goal that you set your mind and effort toward.

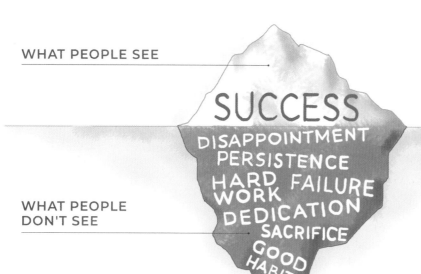

WHAT PEOPLE SEE

SUCCESS

WHAT PEOPLE DON'T SEE

DISAPPOINTMENT
PERSISTENCE
HARD FAILURE
WORK
DEDICATION
SACRIFICE
GOOD
HABITS

3. Overcome impostor syndrome.

I used to have this idea of what successful and happy people must be like. I assumed they had amazing and steadfast skills and confidence and never struggled with self-doubt. This is a perfect example of the stories we tell ourselves that keep us small. Many of us suffer from impostor syndrome. In our careers and in our personal lives, impostor syndrome can be debilitating. We tell ourselves that we are a fraud, that everyone around us knows more or is better than we are, and that it's only a matter of time before they realize we don't belong. When this feeling starts to kick in, it's important to stop and remind yourself that we are all equal, and no one is better or more capable than you. Almost every successful or admirable person I've met shares a similar message that they didn't reach a goal or achieve success because they are better than anyone else, but because they found a mission, goal, or passion and went all in, overcoming setbacks, self-doubt, and struggles along the way.

> "Everything around you that you call life was made up by people that were no smarter than you. And you can change it, you can influence it… Once you learn that, you'll never be the same again."
>
> —STEVE JOBS

4. Feedback—know when it counts and when it doesn't.

When it comes to taking action, often you will get solicited and unsolicited feedback or criticism regarding your choices. Some feedback can be really helpful, and it's important to be open to constructive criticism without letting it eat away at your self-worth or self-esteem. However, other feedback is better to block out or avoid altogether, so consider the source. "Keyboard warriors" online with no stake in the game, who aren't involved or invested in your life or mission, should be ignored. This is perfectly summed up by the "man in the arena" quote from Theodore Roosevelt, which is another gem that I learned from Brené Brown in her book *Daring Greatly*:

> *It is not the critic who counts; not the man who points out how the strong man stumbles, or where the doer of deeds could have done them better. The credit belongs to the man who is actually in the arena, whose face is marred by dust and sweat and blood; who strives valiantly; who errs, who comes short again and again, because there is no effort without error and shortcoming; but who does actually strive to do the deeds; who knows great enthusiasms, the great devotions; who spends himself in a worthy cause; who at the best knows in the end the triumph of high achievement, and who at the worst, if he fails, at least fails while daring greatly, so that his place shall never be with those cold and timid souls who neither know victory nor defeat.*

Therefore, make it a priority to seek out mentors whose feedback you value. This can be one or two people, like a therapist or someone in your life that you admire, or many people, like an encouraging support group. Either way, it is important to have a good outlet for positive and helpful feedback that will help you grow and reach your personal goals.

5. Make time for what matters, and drop the excuses.

Excuses are a dime a dozen, and trust me, I've used them all. My classics were always "I'll start after the weekend," "I don't have the time to do that," and "I don't know how to do that." The truth is, we all have the ability to make time for what matters. Let's say you work eight hours a day and sleep eight hours at night. That means you still have as much as eight hours of your day to take care of the kids, bills, and household responsibilities along with going for a walk, working on a side hustle, or learning a new skill. No one is going to be more committed to accomplishing your goals than you, so prioritize taking time for yourself and what is important to you!

I want to wrap up this chapter by reminding you that these are steps on a lifelong journey to be the best version of yourself. For a long time, I struggled with feeling like I had never quite mastered self-care, self-esteem, or personal goals—but then I realized that facilitating positive change is not a one-and-done thing; it is an ongoing practice to form new habits.

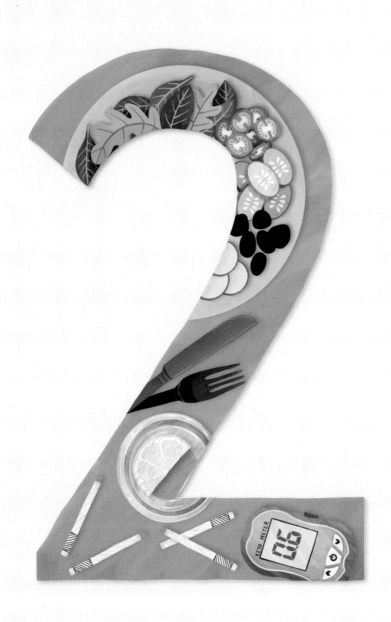

chapter 2:

WHAT IS KETO?

Throughout the majority of my life, as I struggled with my weight, I looked at healthy eating as a sacrifice or a punishment. But as I began working on my mental health and mindset, things started to change. Now, I view eating keto as a form of self-care and self-love. I know now more than ever that the food we consume has an effect on our bodies and our minds. While my path has involved some unexpected realizations with regard to weight loss, I am deeply thankful for and passionate about living a ketogenic lifestyle. I realized in going through all of these changes that weight loss wasn't the key to my happiness. However, it was a key to health in many other ways and completely transformed my addiction to food.

Before keto, food dominated my thoughts, and I was hungry all. the. time. On top of being an emotional eater, I was eating foods that made matters worse, like pouring gasoline onto a fire. The chips, pasta, bread, soda, and desserts were enjoyable for a brief moment, but they were very much my drug of choice that kept me craving more and more.

A few weeks after starting keto, I felt my first sense of food freedom. What a relief to finally feel like I was in control of what and why I was eating! It took consistency and hard work, but I knew it was time for real, lasting change. Eating a ketogenic diet is now my normal, my lifestyle. I don't have to obsess or really even think about it; it just works for me.

My biggest advice is to keep things simple. This lifestyle is really quite straightforward, and truthfully, sustainable change is about mind over matter. So don't overcomplicate things: stick to whole foods as much as possible, toss the bun, skip the fries, and eat foods that work with your body, not against it.

As you become keto-adapted, prepare for your tastes and preferences to change in unexpected ways. I used to swear that I couldn't live without certain foods, but now I no longer crave or miss them at all. Keep an open mind, stay focused, be consistent, and remember to love yourself through each and every step, setback, and in between of your journey.

You got this.

KETO 101

The ketogenic diet (or "keto" for short) is a high-fat, low-carbohydrate, moderate-protein way of eating. Essentially, eating a ketogenic diet will naturally change your body's primary energy source from glucose (carbs/sugar) to ketones (fat).

How does keto work in the body?

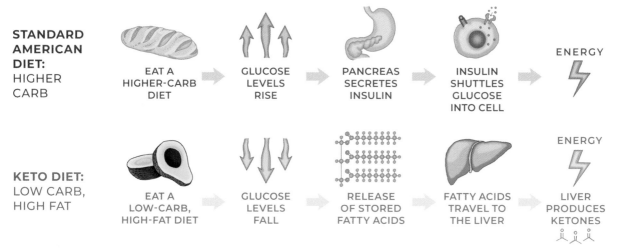

STANDARD AMERICAN DIET: HIGHER CARB	EAT A HIGHER-CARB DIET	GLUCOSE LEVELS RISE	PANCREAS SECRETES INSULIN	INSULIN SHUTTLES GLUCOSE INTO CELL	ENERGY
KETO DIET: LOW CARB, HIGH FAT	EAT A LOW-CARB, HIGH-FAT DIET	GLUCOSE LEVELS FALL	RELEASE OF STORED FATTY ACIDS	FATTY ACIDS TRAVEL TO THE LIVER	LIVER PRODUCES KETONES

What are ketones, and where are they produced?

Ketones (ketone bodies) are a natural lipid-based energy source used by the body and brain. Ketones are produced in the liver as a result of the body breaking down fat for energy—a process known as *fat oxidation*.

There are three types of ketone bodies:

- **Acetone** is measured in the breath using a breath meter.
- **Acetoacetate (AcAc)** is measured in the urine using urine test strips.
- **Beta-hydroxybutyrate (BHB)** is measured in the blood using blood test strips—the most accurate method for testing ketones.

note Acetone is technically a by-product produced during the breakdown of acetoacetate, but it is often referred to as a ketone body.

How long does it take to get into ketosis?

The timing varies from person to person, but it generally takes a few days to a week after dialing in your personal macros to get into ketosis. (More on macros below.)

What does it mean to be keto-adapted?

The term *keto-adapted* basically means that your body has been in ketosis for a consistent period to the point that it is fully adjusted and is using ketones as its primary energy source. The amount of time it takes to become keto-adapted varies from person to person, but it generally takes a few weeks to a month.

What are the health benefits of the ketogenic diet?

While the ketogenic diet has been proven to be a very effective way to lose weight, weight loss is just one positive outcome in a long line of potential health benefits. Research is being done all over the world regarding the use of ketogenic diets to treat many conditions, including heart disease, cancer, Alzheimer's disease, autism, epilepsy, Parkinson's disease, polycystic ovarian syndrome (PCOS), brain injuries, post-traumatic stress disorder, depression, acne, and so many more.

Will my cholesterol go up if I eat a lot of fat?

Cholesterol is a complex subject, and there are a lot of opinions and misinformation out there (even in the medical community). I recommend that you do some research beyond the "standard" cholesterol guidelines and think outside the box—as that box might just be a stage for profit and fearmongering. The book *Cholesterol Clarity* by Jimmy Moore with Eric C. Westman is a great place to start, as are David Diamond's lectures (specifically "Dietary Sense and Nonsense in the War on Saturated Fat," which you can watch for free on YouTube).

What are macros, and what macros should I aim for on the ketogenic diet?

Macros is short for *macronutrients*. The three primary macronutrients found in foods are fat, protein, and carbohydrate.

When people in the keto community talk about macros, they are referring to the breakdown of fat, protein, and carbohydrate in a meal or in a person's overall diet. Macros are often expressed as percentages, like this:

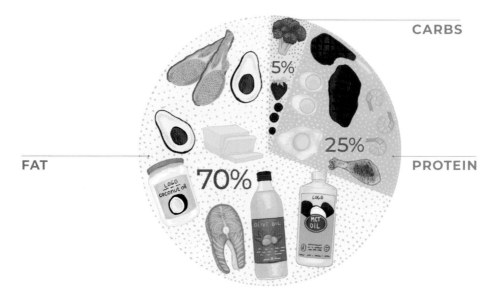

- **Carbs are kept to a minimum,** at around 5 percent of total caloric intake (which typically translates to 20 to 25 grams of net carbs a day; more on net carbs in a bit). Most often, the goal is to keep net or total carbs at or below 20 to 30 grams each day. (I personally count net carbs; find more on net versus total carbs on the next page.)

- **Protein is moderate,** at around 25 percent of total caloric intake. Protein is a very important macronutrient, so be sure to eat an adequate amount to keep your body functioning well and burning fat, not muscle tissue. When protein intake is lower than what your body requires, your body can start burning your lean body mass (muscle tissue) instead of fat, which should be avoided. While each person's protein intake will be different based personal stats and activity level, a great starting point can be found by using a keto calculator.

- **Fat is high,** at around 70 percent of total caloric intake. If you find yourself feeling full or satisfied, however, don't feel pressured to eat more fat just to "balance" your macros. Ultimately, don't fear fat, but don't force it, either.

These percentages are not set in stone; each person's ideal macros will be different. You can easily calculate your personalized macro targets by using a calculator like the one on my blog (ketokarma.com/macros), which takes into account your age, gender, activity level, and other factors. While macro calculators are a great place to start, you may need to make some adjustments to fine-tune your macros for optimal results, weight loss stalls, or if your weight or activity level changes.

tip Some people track everything they eat, especially at the beginning, but if that seems overwhelming to you, try focusing solely on keeping net carbs at or below 20 grams for the first week or two. Once you get used to this step, you can begin tracking your other macros (protein and fat) as well as your caloric intake, if you choose.

Do I need to track calories, too?

I believe that when it comes to weight loss, calories in versus calories out will always matter. There is no arguing that not all calories are created equal, but if you have struggled with overeating or emotionally eating, you may find it very helpful to learn portion control through tracking calories, even for a short time. In addition to tracking macros, I tracked calories during my first year on keto, and it gave me valuable insight into proper portion sizes for my body and lifestyle, as well as providing a great learning experience regarding the macros and ingredients in various foods.

Why is keto a moderate-protein diet?

When you eat more protein than your body requires, a natural process called gluconeogenesis leads to the conversion of a percentage of non-carbohydrate sources (in this case, protein) into glucose upon breakdown. If your glucose levels become too high, you may risk being kicked out of ketosis. Therefore, while it's not necessary to fear protein, and it's important to reach your protein goal to preserve your lean body mass, remember that consuming excessive amounts of protein could kick you out of ketosis.

What are total carbs and net carbs?

Among people who follow keto and other low-carb diets, you often hear the terms "total carbs" and "net carbs." Here's a quick breakdown of what those two terms mean.

Total carbs is exactly what it sounds like: a calculation of all the carbohydrate in a food, including dietary fiber, sugar, and sugar alcohols.

To arrive at the amount of *net carbs* in a food, you subtract dietary fiber (and sugar alcohols, if applicable) from the total amount of carbohydrate in that food, as shown in the example below. Dietary fiber and sugar alcohols generally have a minimal impact on blood sugar; therefore, some people choose not to count them as part of their target carbohydrate intake. Instead, they focus on net carbs.

TOTAL CARBS — DIETARY FIBER — SUGAR ALCOHOLS = **NET CARBS**

Here's an example of a food that contains both dietary fiber and sugar alcohols. As you can see from this nutrition label from Good Dee's Yellow Snack Cake low-carb baking mix, the total carbohydrate per serving is 13 grams. To calculate the net carbs, you subtract the 6 grams of dietary fiber and the 5 grams of sugar alcohol from the total carb count, which gives you only 2 grams of net carbs per serving.

NUTRITION FACTS	
Serving Size 1/12 pkg (22g mix)	
Servings Per Container 12	
Amount Per Serving	
Calories 70 Calories from Fat 50	
	% Daily Value*
Total Fat 6g	9%
Saturated Fat 0g	0%
Trans Fat 0g	
Cholesterol 0mg	0%
Sodium 100mg	4%
Total Carbohydrate 13g	4%
Dietary Fiber 6g	24%
Sugars 0g	
Sugar Alcohol 5g	
Protein 2g	

Here's another example. Three ounces of cauliflower has 4 grams of total carbs. When you subtract the 2 grams of dietary fiber, you get 2 grams of net carbs per serving.

Note: The nutrition information found on food labels may be calculated differently from country to country. In the United States, total carbs currently includes both fiber and sugar alcohols.

NUTRITION FACTS	
Serving Size 3oz (85g)	
Amount Per Serving	
Calories 20 Calories from Fat 0	
	% Daily Value*
Total Fat 0g	0%
Saturated Fat 0g	0%
Trans Fat 0g	
Cholesterol 0mg	0%
Sodium 25mg	1%
Total Carbohydrate 4g	1%
Dietary Fiber 2g	8%
Sugars 2g	
Protein 2g	

Lastly, here's an allulose example: The total carbohydrates are 24 grams. To calculate net carbs, you subtract 7 grams of fiber, 3 grams of sugar alcohol, and 13 grams of allulose, which equals 1 gram of net carbs, seen here as 1g total sugars. *Note:* Each brand that uses allulose should give you the exact amount of allulose to subtract from total carbs. If it doesn't, you can generally tell the difference by what is left in total sugars, which will be included in your net carb count.

NUTRITION FACTS	
Servings per container	
Serving Size (55g)	
Amount Per Serving	
Calories 200 Calories from Fat 135	
	% Daily Value*
Total Fat 15g	19%
Saturated Fat 3.5g	18%
Trans Fat 0g	
Cholesterol 0mg	0%
Sodium 150mg	7%
Total Carbohydrate 24g	9%
Dietary Fiber 7g	25%
Total Sugars 1g	
Includes 0g Added Sugars	0%
Sugar Alcohol 3g	
Protein 11g	

24g TOTAL CARBS — 7g FIBER — 3g ERYTHRITOL — 13g ALLULOSE = 1g NET CARB

note If a product is sweetened with allulose, which is a rare sugar, not a sugar alcohol, the allulose is included under either total carbs (as shown) or total sugars. When tallying net carbs, subtract allulose from the total carbs, along with fiber and sugar alcohols. Allulose has a glycemic index of zero and less than 0.4 calorie per gram.

AN APPROACHABLE STEP-BY-STEP GUIDE TO STARTING KETO

Starting a ketogenic diet is actually pretty simple. It's about mind over matter and allowing your body time to detox from sugar and the cravings that come along with eating sugar. Trust me, I know what it's like to feel controlled by food. With consistency, this will ease up over time, and you'll gain the upper hand.

Many of us have tried many diets, and sometimes the struggle to lose weight can wear on your view of your ability to switch to a healthier way of eating. For this reason, it's often beneficial to take things one step at a time instead of forcing yourself into an all-or-nothing approach. I used the following method to break up with sugar and ease my way into this healthy way of eating. Setting smaller, more approachable goals that didn't feel overwhelming helped build my confidence. So, if you're feeling overwhelmed or unsure of where to start, give this method a try!

STEP 1:
Remove one item from your "normal" diet that is high in carbs/sugar.
(Feel free to skip to Step 2 if you are ready to begin tracking carbs.)

Never underestimate the impact that small steps can make. I had spent so many years starting and stopping diets that I had lost confidence in my ability to stick to healthier eating habits. So, as a first step, I chose to give up regular soda. Soda was one thing that I consumed daily, but I knew it had no nutritional value and was loaded with sugar. Growing up, I drank soda with almost every meal, so leaving it behind was a bit of a challenge for me. I switched to sparkling water and focused on that one goal for a few weeks. Five years later, I still haven't gone back to regular soda, and I truly don't miss it. Once you build momentum from this initial success, go on to Step 2.

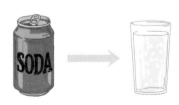

> "If you do what you've always done, you'll get what you've always gotten."
> —TONY ROBBINS

STEP 2:
Keep carbs under 20 to 30 grams.

Track only carbs, and keep them to under 20 to 30 grams. Don't worry about tracking anything else. You can choose to track net or total carbs; I count net carbs (for more information, see page 31). It's no surprise that changing your eating habits is an adjustment, but once you get the hang of it, it truly becomes your new normal and doesn't require a lot of thought. Simply keep a running tab on your carb intake for two to three weeks, and then move on to Step 3.

STEP 3:
Track your macros.

There are many free tools for tracking your macros, including apps like MyFitnessPal and Carb Manager. Use a keto calculator to find a good macro starting point. You can find these calculators in multiple places online, including my blog (ketokarma.com/macros). Once you have your personal macros, you can plug them into your tracking app. I recommend tracking your food for a minimum of two to three weeks, because during this time, you will get a grasp on how a normal day of eating looks within your macro and caloric goals. When I started tracking, I discovered that many foods that I thought were healthy or low in carbs are actually high in carbs or sugar. Think of tracking as an investment or learning opportunity, not something you have to do forever (unless you want to).

"It does not matter how slowly you go as long as you do not stop."

—CONFUCIUS

TESTING FOR KETONES

The presence of ketones in your urine, breath, and blood is an indicator that you are in ketosis. Here are the three options for checking your ketone levels:

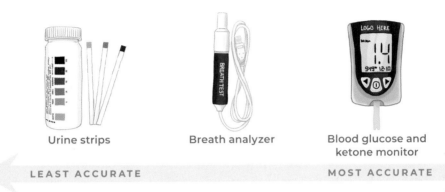

| Urine strips | Breath analyzer | Blood glucose and ketone monitor |

LEAST ACCURATE → MOST ACCURATE

- **Urine strips: Urine test strips turn purple in the presence of acetoacetate; the darker the color, the more ketones are present.** This method is the least accurate, especially after keto-adaptation. Due to the number of false negatives and positives I've seen, I don't recommend using urine strips for ketone testing.

- **Breath analyzer:** A breath analyzer gives you a good range to determine whether you are in ketosis but does not tell you your exact ketone level. This method is more reliable than urine testing, but still not the most accurate form of testing.

- **Blood glucose and ketone monitor (I use the Precision Xtra or Keto Coach meter):** Testing a tiny blood sample is the most accurate way to measure ketones. It's easy to do at home and requires only a simple prick of your finger. The ideal range is between 0.5 and 5 mM/L. Take it from me, I'm a complete wimp when it comes to anything involving pain or blood, and even I find it pretty painless. Here's a tip: when using the lancet, prick the side of your fingertip, which is a lot less sensitive than the pad of your finger. Be sure to wash your hands before testing, or use an alcohol wipe to cleanse your finger before using the lancet.

Unless you are doing keto for the treatment of a medical condition, you don't have to test right away. I recommend checking your blood ketones at some point, especially when dialing in your personal macros, as it will allow you to see if you are truly in a state of ketosis, but the timing is totally up to you. While your ketone level will vary quite a bit based on your eating window, the time of day, and your activity level, you can use your results to determine whether too much carbohydrate or protein is sneaking into your diet and possibly kicking you out of ketosis, or whether specific foods are having a negative effect. My main goal is to see my ketone level at or above 0.5 mM/L, which is the blood-level threshold of being in a state of nutritional ketosis.

Nutritional ketosis range: serum ketones range from 0.5 to 5 mM/L

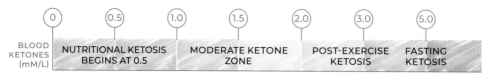

Having higher ketone levels doesn't necessarily equal better results or faster weight loss. Unless you are doing keto for therapeutic reasons, I wouldn't obsess over having higher levels. (Note, however, that dangerously high blood ketone levels of 15 to 25 mM/L, along with high blood sugar and a low blood pH, are characteristic of diabetic ketoacidosis, a life-threatening condition that can affect people with unmanaged diabetes.)

Ketone levels are often lowest in the morning and peak later in the day. Try to test at the same time each day for a more accurate day-to-day comparison. When testing to determine whether a specific food affects your ketone levels, it's smart to test your blood ketones one to two hours after consuming that food to check for changes. A significant drop in blood ketones or increase in blood sugar (if you check your blood sugar), may mean that it would be wise for you to stay away from specific food items that have been shown to negatively impact your ketone or glucose levels.

Considering Exogenous Ketones

Exogenous means "originating from an external source," and by now you know what ketones are. Exogenous ketones (sometimes abbreviated as EKs and also known as ketone supplements) are currently available in two main forms: ketone salts (also referred to as beta-hydroxybutyrate salts or BHB salts) and ketone esters. Both are lab created.

While exogenous ketones show great potential as a treatment for various medical conditions, including epilepsy, cancer, and Alzheimer's disease, I do not believe they should be marketed as weight-loss supplements. Sustainable weight loss will never come from a pill, wrap, or supplement; it comes from lifestyle change. If you are looking into these products for weight-loss purposes, I urge you to save your money. I've seen some pretty awful marketing and false information related to exogenous ketones, so please don't believe everything you read.

During my weight-loss journey, I never took ketone supplements, and I never obsessed over having high ketone levels. With the ketogenic diet increasing in popularity, there are a lot of companies out to make money, so do your research before making any purchases. One of my favorite features of the keto lifestyle is that the only thing you need to buy to be successful is the right food. After trying to buy my way out of my weight problem for years, I know the feeling of wanting a quick fix, but real and lasting change can't be bought; it comes from within.

KETO HEALTH

Let's go over some basic health topics that you should be aware of, as well as some tips for how to avoid unnecessary symptoms. Knowledge is power, and a well-formulated ketogenic diet should leave you feeling your best!

Keto flu

During the first few weeks of eating keto, it's common to develop an electrolyte imbalance. If not properly managed, this imbalance can lead to a temporary condition known as the "keto flu." It is associated with unpleasant symptoms such as headaches, dizziness, brain fog, lethargy, constipation, and leg cramps. These symptoms occur primarily in the early phases of keto, and things often balance out once a person becomes keto-adapted. Even after keto-adaptation, some people (especially those who are very active) may require electrolyte supplements if they do not consume enough foods that are rich in electrolytes (see below). (Remember that it's important to talk with your doctor before taking supplements, especially if you have health issues.) On a ketogenic diet, the main electrolytes to focus on are sodium, magnesium, potassium, and calcium.

Here are a few key ways to prevent or minimize the symptoms of keto flu:

- **General symptoms:** Add sodium (salt) to your diet. The general recommendation is to supplement with 2 to 9 grams of sodium per day: 2 to 4 grams for the average person or up to 7 to 9 grams for very active people or during intermittent fasting (see page 40 for more on fasting). Boosting your sodium intake is easy; simply drink 1 or 2 cups of bouillon or salted broth or add more quality salt to your food or beverages.

  tip Try to purchase quality real salt (from a mine), which contains trace minerals and no chemicals. Himalayan pink salt is another great option. Also, be sure to drink lots of water and other fluids! Dehydration can make you feel pretty awful, so be sure to stay hydrated.

- **Leg cramps:** Increase your intake of magnesium.

- **Constipation:** Drink more water and increase your fiber intake. Coffee sometimes does the trick, too!

Mg Magnesium-rich foods:

- Avocados
- Broccoli
- Dark chocolate
- Fish
- Kale
- Mushrooms, especially white button and portabella
- Nuts, especially almonds
- Seeds, especially pumpkin seeds
- Spinach

K Potassium-rich foods:

- Artichokes
- Asparagus
- Avocados
- Broccoli
- Brussels sprouts
- Fish, especially salmon
- Kale/leafy greens
- Mushrooms
- Tomatoes

Ca Calcium-rich foods:

- Almonds
- Bok choy
- Broccoli
- Celery
- Cheese
- Dark leafy greens (spinach, kale, collard greens, and so on)
- Sardines
- Seeds, like sesame and chia

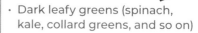

Hair loss

Hair loss is not a common side effect of a well-formulated ketogenic diet that provides you with adequate calories, macronutrients, hydration, and electrolytes. If you are experiencing hair loss, it could be due to the following insufficiencies:

- Not consuming enough calories.
- Not eating an adequate amount of protein.
- Zinc deficiency. To address this problem, add a zinc supplement and/or eat foods that are high in zinc, including cheese, dark chocolate, eggs, meat (especially red meat), mushrooms, nuts, seeds (flax, hemp, and pumpkin), shellfish (crab, lobster, and oysters), and spinach.

Keto rash

Keto rash is relatively rare, and the cause is currently unknown. The rash manifests in itchy, raised skin lesions that can be red, brown, or light pink. Although it's uncomfortable, it is not life-threatening; however, if you develop any form of rash, it's best to be evaluated by your doctor to understand the cause and your treatment options. This type of rash tends to occur early in the course of a ketogenic diet when weight loss is rapid. Treatment sometimes includes adding back enough carbs to suppress nutritional ketosis. According to a blog post by Dr. Stephen Phinney on Virta Health, some people reported that resuming nutritional ketosis caused the rash to recur, but in a milder form, and eventually they could sustain nutritional ketosis with higher ketone levels of 1 to 3 mM/L without a rash.

FASTING 101

Some people choose to incorporate fasting as a part of their ketogenic lifestyle. Before I started keto, fasting seemed impossible to me because I was always hungry. But after a few weeks, I found that my appetite had changed and my cravings had subsided. Intermittent fasting has been done safely for centuries and has some health benefits, so let's go over some general fasting guidelines and how to fast safely.

During a fast, you abstain from eating for a period of time, but you can consume any of the following beverages to stay hydrated:

- Water, with or without added salt to replenish electrolytes
- Black coffee (regular or decaf)
- Bone broth
- Unsweetened tea (regular or decaf)

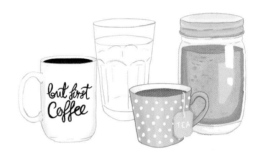

Supplement your electrolytes, as needed, with the following:

- $_{11}$ **Na** **Sodium** (buy a quality salt with trace minerals, like Redmond Real Salt)
- $_{19}$ **K** **Potassium** (powder or pill form)
- $_{12}$ **Mg** **Magnesium** (powder or pill form)

Because electrolyte supplementation is based on multiple factors, such as the type and longevity of each fast, the amount of each electrolyte that is needed can vary greatly. You can purchase a premixed electrolyte supplement, which will contain at least the three main electrolytes mentioned above, or purchase each type separately. Each product will list the recommended dosage on the packaging, but be sure to research the quality of each product before buying. Also, make sure your doctor is aware of what you want to take and gives you the green light.

note It is best to check with your doctor before fasting (especially if you plan to fast for more than 24 hours). Some people should not fast for specific health or medical reasons. Fasting is not a requirement, and it's important to be safe and do what works best for you!

Types of fasting

First, let's go over some of the most popular types of fasting:

TIME-RESTRICTED EATING/INTERMITTENT FASTING (IF): This type of fasting involves restricting your eating to a certain window of time. The most common fasting period is 16:8, so the goal is to eat all meals within an eight-hour period and then fast for the remaining 16 hours of the day. This type of fasting is often done three to seven days a week.

EXAMPLE: *Eat only between 11 a.m. and 7 p.m. Often, people doing this style of fasting skip one meal, usually either breakfast or dinner.*

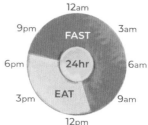

SPONTANEOUS FASTING: This is the type of fasting I often do. With spontaneous fasting, you randomly skip a meal or two on various days. Some mornings I wake up and don't feel hungry, or I have a really busy schedule, so I just make myself a cup of coffee and skip breakfast. This is an unstructured form of intermittent fasting, which is more in tune with mindful eating and listening to your body's hunger signals.

EXAMPLE:

Skip breakfast.

Eat lunch as normal.

Eat dinner as normal.

ALTERNATE-DAY FASTING: "Eat-stop-eat" involves a 24-hour fast followed by a 24-hour eating window. Another similar method is known as 5:2, in which you eat normally five days a week and then limit your calorie intake to 500 to 600 calories on the other two days (or fast completely).

EXAMPLE:

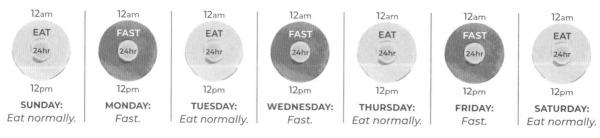

ONE MEAL A DAY (OMAD) FASTING: With this form of fasting, you skip two meals a day and eat just one larger-than-usual meal.

EXAMPLE: *Skip breakfast and lunch and eat a larger dinner.*

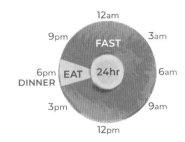

EXTENDED FASTING: This type of fasting involves abstaining from eating for a period of 24 hours or more. It may require doctor supervision as well as a multivitamin and electrolyte supplementation and hydration management. Women especially need to be cautious with fasting for longer than 48 hours due to the possibility of affecting hormones.

When it comes to fasting, it's a good idea to start with shorter fasts and build your way up. For example, try pushing breakfast from 7 a.m. to 10 a.m., or stop eating after 6 p.m. This way, you can take it one step at a time and get your body used to fasting before doing a full 24-hour or longer fast.

Benefits of fasting

Why fast on a ketogenic diet? Research has shown that fasting may deliver the following key health benefits:

- Lowers inflammation
- Improves brain function and cognitive focus
- Improves blood sugar and insulin levels
- Promotes weight loss/body fat loss
- Increased autophagy (cellular cleaning; see sidebar)

One of the biggest and often overlooked benefits of fasting is putting appetite back under your control. How often have you felt controlled by food? How often have you felt compelled to grab a chocolate bar or a bag of chips because you thought you were hungry when you were actually bored or stressed? Fasting, especially in conjunction with a ketogenic way of eating, allows you to understand that you are in control of the food you put into your body and that food no longer controls you.

What Is Autophagy?

Autophagy ("ah-TAH-fah-gee") is a form of cellular cleaning and repair. The word comes from the Greek words *auto* (self) and *phagein* (to eat). "Self-eating" describes an important cleansing/recycling process that enables the body to get rid of old cells and damaged proteins that it no longer needs and reuse anything that is still good; then new cells are created to replace the old ones.

While autophagy naturally occurs without fasting, fasting causes it to happen at an increased rate, as does eating a ketogenic diet and exercising.

EXERCISE ON KETO

Being active is beneficial for both your physical health and your mental health. The key is to find a form of exercise that is sustainable and enjoyable. Luckily, there are many types to choose from. I easily get burned out on going to a traditional gym, but I love taking walks with my best friend. We often walk around a half-mile circle, and by the time we've caught up on work, kids, and life, we have walked 3 to 4 miles, which is not only great exercise but also very cathartic! I encourage you to try a few things and see what feels right to you. Remember, it's okay to start small, such as by taking the stairs instead of the elevator, going for a short walk, or going for a swim.

> "Food is the most abused anti-anxiety drug, and exercise is the most underutilized antidepressant."
>
> —BILL PHILLIPS

MAINTENANCE MODE TIPS

"Maintenance mode" means that you've reached your goal weight and wish to maintain your current weight rather than continue to lose. Because keto is not a diet that you use just to shed pounds, but a lifestyle that keeps you feeling your best, I encourage you to stay in maintenance mode for the long term. Here are a few commonly asked questions and my recommendations for those who have reached this stage of their keto journey.

What do I do when I reach my goal weight?

In weight-loss culture, people tend to assume that they will eat healthy until they lose weight and then go back to the way they used to eat. I think we all know what generally follows. Keto isn't a temporary diet; it's a lifestyle change. Once you know what works for you, it's best to stay the course and continue your journey toward health and wellness.

Here are a couple of suggestions for maintenance mode:

- **If you are tracking calories and macros:** Once you have reached your goal weight, not much will change, except your caloric intake may increase if you have been maintaining a caloric deficit for weight loss. I recommend recalculating your macros with your updated weight and activity level and setting your deficit to zero. This will give you a new baseline for maintenance.

- **If you are not tracking macros:** Most people who choose not to track macros practice intuitive eating, which involves paying attention to your body's hunger and fullness signals. In this case, you can simply continue to listen to your body.

Can I have cheat meals?

Cheat meals are a personal choice. Some people allow them, and others feel that they lead to too much temptation or to falling off the wagon. I primarily (and happily!) eat keto but allow myself some "off-plan" meals on special occasions or while traveling. That said, there are some items that I have no desire to consume ever again, such as sugary soda. Once you are keto-adapted, your tastes are likely to change, and some foods that you once couldn't imagine life without will no longer have the same grip on you. Even more unexpected, you'll find that you don't miss them or even enjoy them anymore. I strive to be mindful and to be accountable to my health and goals while having a livable balance. Ultimately, you have to do what's best for you. There truly is no right or wrong approach!

How to restart after falling off track

I often get messages from people who say, "Help, I fell off the wagon! What do I do now?" My answer is almost always the same: just get back on track with your next meal. One bad habit that I had to break after many years of yoyo dieting was thinking that if I ate one thing that was "off-limits," I had blown it for the entire day, so I might as well eat whatever junk I wanted and start over tomorrow. This is a classic example of an excuse that kept me stuck and unaccountable for years. If you go off-plan, leave the guilt trips at the door and get right back to healthy eating with your very next meal.

"Success is not final, failure is not fatal; it is the courage to continue that counts."

—WINSTON CHURCHILL

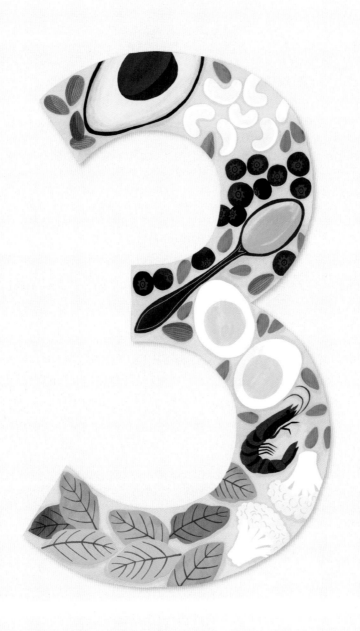

chapter 3:

SIMPLY KETO KITCHEN

It's time to stock up your kitchen and dig into all the delicious and wholesome foods that you can enjoy while living a ketogenic lifestyle!

My biggest advice here is to focus on the flavorful and nutrient-dense foods you get to enjoy and not on the things you "can't" have. After all, eating healthier isn't a punishment; it's an investment in you, your health, and your quality of life. So leave the food-shaming days behind you and choose to primarily eat foods that work *with* you, not against you. At the end of the day, we all know that sugar is very addicting, so avoiding it will enable you to take back control and end the days of insatiable hunger and food cravings.

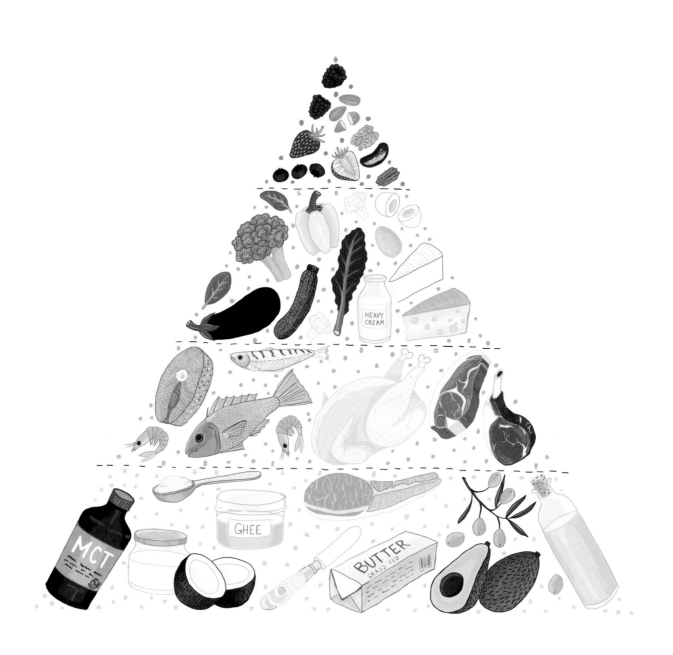

THE KETOGENIC FOOD PYRAMID

FATS AND OILS

While keto is a high-fat diet, it is important to educate yourself as to which types of fat are good to eat and which should be avoided:

ENJOY
saturated and monounsaturated fats such as

- Beef
- Pork
- Eggs
- Dairy (butter, cheese, heavy whipping cream, and so on)
- Tropical oils (avocado, coconut, olive)
- Avocados

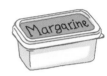

AVOID
trans and processed polyunsaturated fats such as

- Margarine
- Vegetable oils
- Vegetable shortening

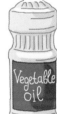

Like many of you, I was taught to stay away from saturated fat. But saturated fat has been made out to be the bad guy without proper cause for far too long. In fact, as Stephen Phinney and Jeff Volek point out in their excellent book *The Art and Science of Low Carbohydrate Living,* "Scientific evidence clearly shows that dietary intake of saturated fat compared to serum (blood) levels of saturated fat show little if any correlation." They go on to say that research has shown that an increase in dietary carbohydrate is linked to higher levels of saturated fat in the blood.

So enjoy those tasty saturated and monounsaturated fats, including the following:

- Avocado oil*
- Bacon fat*
- Beef tallow
- Butter (salted and unsalted)*
- Coconut oil*
- Ghee
- Lard
- Macadamia nut oil
- MCT oil*
- Olive oil*
- Palm oil

These fats and oils are used in the recipes in this book. Feel free to try the other keto fats and oils in this list to diversify your cooking. If you cannot tolerate dairy, ghee is an excellent substitute for butter.

tip Read ingredient labels and steer clear of products made with unhealthy oils. For example, you can now buy mayonnaise made with avocado or olive oil, and buy natural peanut butter without added oils or sugar. Small steps add up, so while you won't always be able to control ingredients when dining out, you *can* reduce your intake of unhealthy oils at home!

PROTEINS

Let's talk about the different types of protein that you can enjoy simply cooked as is or incorporated into a variety of flavorful dishes. Try to work within your budget to buy the best-quality proteins possible (organic, grass-fed, hormone-free, and so on), which truly is an investment in your health.

Red Meat

- Beef
- Bison
- Goat
- Lamb
- Pork

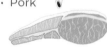

Game Meats

- Bear
- Boar
- Elk
- Rabbit
- Venison (deer meat)

Poultry

- Chicken
- Duck
- Game hen
- Pheasant
- Quail
- Turkey

Eggs

- Chicken eggs
- Duck eggs
- Goose eggs
- Ostrich eggs
- Quail eggs

Fish

- Anchovies
- Bass
- Burbot
- Carp
- Catfish
- Cod
- Flounder
- Haddock
- Halibut
- Herring
- Mackerel
- Salmon
- Sardines
- Snapper
- Sole
- Swordfish
- Tilapia
- Trout
- Tuna
- Walleye

Shellfish and Other Seafood

- Clams
- Crabmeat*
- Lobster
- Mussels
- Octopus
- Oysters
- Prawns
- Scallops
- Shrimp
- Snails

Avoid imitation crabmeat; it is not low-carb and has about 13 grams of carbs per 3 ounces.

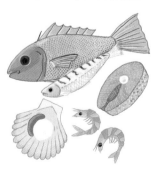

Dairy

- Butter (salted and unsalted)
- Cheeses
  Blue cheese
  Brie
  Camembert
  Cheddar
  Cottage cheese (watch the carb count)
  Cream cheese (full fat)
  Feta
  Goat cheese
  Gouda
  Gruyère
  Mascarpone
  Mozzarella (whole milk)
  Muenster
  Parmesan
  Pepper Jack
  Provolone
  Ricotta (whole milk; watch the carb count)
  Swiss
  Tilsit
  Various other specialty cheeses (watch the carb count)
- Greek yogurt (full fat—use sparingly)
- Half-and-half
- Heavy whipping cream
- Sour cream (full fat)

Safe Minimum Cooking Temperatures for Meat and Seafood

	FOOD	Temperature (°F)
GROUND MEATS	Beef, lamb, pork, veal	160°F
	Turkey, chicken	165°F
BEEF, LAMB, VEAL	Steaks, roasts, chops	145°F
PORK	Fresh pork	145°F
	Fresh ham (raw)	145°F
	Precooked ham (to reheat)	140°F
POULTRY	Chicken and turkey, whole	165°F
	Breasts, roasts	165°F
	Thighs, legs, wings	165°F
	Duck, goose	165°F
SEAFOOD	Finfish	145°F, or cook until flesh is opaque and separates easily with a fork.
	Shrimp, lobster, crabs	Cook until flesh is pearly and opaque.
	Clams, oysters, mussels	Cook until shells open.
	Scallops	Cook until flesh is milky white or opaque and firm.

Judgment-Free Keto

Are carrots keto? Is diet soda keto? Are low-carb wraps keto? Is low-carb fast food keto?

Just remember that keto is a metabolic state, not a food.

While certain foods—pasta, bread, sugar, and so on—are best avoided, there are a lot of gray areas when it comes to what people choose to eat while remaining keto. There is no one-size-fits-all approach; everyone has varying metabolic rates, food sensitivities, and health goals.

My hope is that we come together as a community in an effort to support and encourage one another instead of drawing lines in the sand. It's important to remember that we all come from different walks of life and are on our own individualized paths. Now that keto has achieved a degree of popularity, there are so many classifications of keto. And while I understand that people like to put things in boxes, I think we need to be mindful of how labels can affect people, especially ones like "dirty keto." Can we just not label things this way? After all, our words matter, and we all come together from a common space of wanting to improve our health and quality of life—*all* are equally welcome and worthy.

The last thing we need in this space is judgment or keto police. This community is full of people who come for support, advice, friendship, and kindness. It is up to each of us to foster a safe space where people can be vulnerable, ask questions, share struggles and triumphs, and be seen and heard. Although it may be tempting, try not to offer your opinion on what others choose to eat or do unless they specifically ask for advice. And when giving advice in response to a request for it, try to be warm, considerate, and judgment-free. The last thing you want to do is push people away, tear people down, or make people feel like they aren't doing enough. Many already struggle with insecurities, so let's not add to that pile. We rise by lifting others, and kindness *always* wins.

VEGETABLES

When it comes to vegetables, one rule that never fails is to stick to leafy green cruciferous veggies. Think mostly nonstarchy veggies that grow above ground. The following are some popular low-carb options:

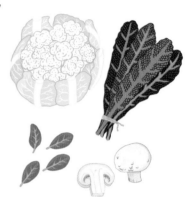

- Artichokes
- Arugula
- Asparagus
- Bok choy
- Broccoli
- Broccoli rabe
- Brussels sprouts
- Cabbage
- Cauliflower
- Celery
- Chard
- Chicory greens
- Endive
- Fennel bulb
- Garlic*
- Green beans
- Hot peppers (such as jalapeños)
- Kale
- Kohlrabi
- Lettuce (butter, romaine, radicchio, and so on)
- Mushrooms
- Onions*
- Radishes
- Seaweed
- Spinach
- Swiss chard
- Watercress

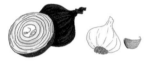

Onions (especially red onions and shallots) and garlic should be eaten in moderation because of their carb content.

FRUITS

Often referred to as "nature's candy," fruit contains a natural sugar called fructose. The following fruits are lower in carbs, but keep in mind that berries and tomatoes should be eaten in moderation. Besides, we all know that avocado is the real MVP in this category!

- Avocados
- Bell peppers (all colors)
- Blackberries
- Blueberries
- Cucumbers
- Lemons
- Limes
- Olives
- Pumpkin
- Raspberries
- Spaghetti squash
- Strawberries
- Tomatoes
- Zucchini

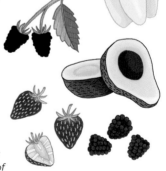

Berry Macros by Type,
per 100-gram serving of raw berries (about ⅔ cup)

TYPE	Total Carbs	Net Carbs
Blackberries	10g	5g
Raspberries	12g	5g
Strawberries	8g	6g
Blueberries*	21g	17g

Blueberries are on the higher end, at 17 grams of net carbs (21 grams of total carbs) per 100-gram serving, so it's best to limit them.

Whether or Not to Buy Organic Produce

The Environmental Working Group (www.ewg.org) maintains two lists to help you decide which fruits and vegetables you should buy organic versus conventionally grown. The Dirty Dozen is a list of the veggies that are best to purchase organic due to the use of pesticides and other chemicals, and the Clean Fifteen is a list of the veggies that are generally safe to buy non-organic. So, if you're on a budget and can buy only a few organic foods, here are the keto-friendly fruits and veggies that made the lists in 2019.

Low-carb items from the "Dirty Dozen" list— *recommended to buy organic*

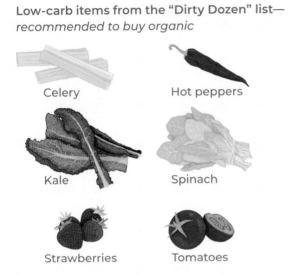

Celery   Hot peppers

Kale   Spinach

Strawberries   Tomatoes

Low-carb items from the "Clean Fifteen" list— *okay to buy conventionally grown*

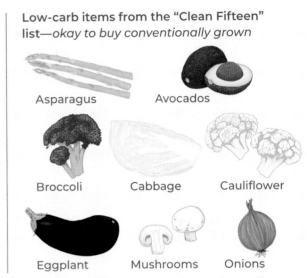

Asparagus   Avocados

Broccoli   Cabbage   Cauliflower

Eggplant   Mushrooms   Onions

NUTS, SEEDS, AND NUT BUTTERS

Feel free to enjoy nuts and seeds as a snack or in recipes like Crunchy Keto Granola (page 122) or Tina's Candied Pecans (page 280). For snacking, I recommend portioning out your desired amount rather than eating them straight from the bag or jar, as they are easy to overeat.

- Almonds
- Brazil nuts
- Cashews*
- Coconut (unsweetened shredded)
- Hazelnuts
- Macadamia nuts
- Peanuts
- Pecans
- Pili nuts

- Pine nuts
- Pistachios*
- Walnuts
- Chia seeds
- Flax seeds
- Hemp seeds
- Poppy seeds
- Pumpkin seeds
- Sesame seeds

- Sunflower seeds
- Almond butter (unsweetened)
- Peanut butter (no sugar added; made from only peanuts and salt)

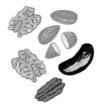

Pistachios and cashews are higher in carbs, so limit or avoid them.

HERBS AND SPICES

Fresh and dried herbs and spices can add a lot of flavor to your meals. These are the varieties that I like to have on hand:

- Allspice
- Basil
- Bay leaves
- Caraway seeds
- Chili powder
- Cilantro
- Cinnamon
- Cream of tartar
- Cumin
- Curry powder
- Everything bagel seasoning
- Garlic powder
- Ginger powder
- Italian seasoning
- Mint
- Old Bay seasoning
- Onion powder
- Oregano
- Paprika
- Parsley
- Peppercorns
- Red pepper flakes
- Rosemary
- Salt (Redmond Real Salt is my favorite)
- Steak seasoning (sugar-free)

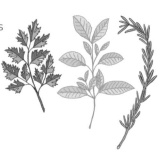

BAKING INGREDIENTS

Here are some of my favorite ingredients for keto baking:

- Almond flour (blanched)
- Almond meal
- Baking powder (aluminum-free)
- Baking soda
- Cocoa powder (unsweetened)
- Coconut flour
- Flaxseed meal
- MCT powder (vanilla-flavored or plain)
- Protein powder (sugar-free)
- Psyllium husk powder
- Stevia-sweetened dark chocolate chips (I use Lily's brand, which now offers stevia-sweetened semisweet chocolate chips as well)
- Unsweetened baking chocolate

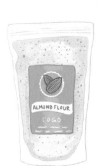

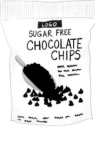

SWEETENERS

In the recipes in this book, I use Swerve brand sweeteners, which are erythritol-based blends. It comes in three forms:

- Brown sugar
- Confectioners' style
- Granular

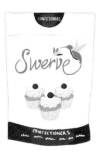

Here are a few additional sweeteners that I use and recommend:

- Allulose
- Erythritol, 100% (I like Whole Earth Erythritol)
- Monk fruit
- Stevia (I prefer the liquid form for cold drinks because it blends better, but I do use powdered stevia in one recipe in this book)
- Xylitol

note Animal lovers, take note: Although xylitol is safe for human consumption, it is toxic to some animals, especially dogs. Be sure to keep items containing xylitol out of the reach of your pets!

What Is the Glycemic Index?

The glycemic index (GI) is a scale that gives you an idea of how quickly a food will cause blood sugar to rise.

- Foods with a high GI should be avoided; they cause a rapid spike in blood glucose.
- Foods with a low GI are ideal; they have a slow and steady effect, or even no effect, on blood glucose. Selecting foods with a lower GI has been shown to aid in weight loss.

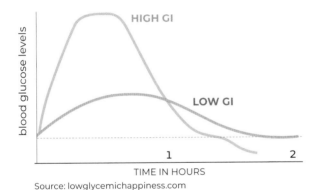

Source: lowglycemichappiness.com

High GI foods *cause blood sugar to rise rapidly. After about 30 minutes, blood sugar begins to plummet. Notice that it falls below its starting point. When blood glucose falls below normal levels, foggy thinking, tiredness, and depression can result.*

Low GI foods *cause blood sugar to rise gradually. After about 30 minutes, blood sugar begins to fall gently. Notice that it returns to the same level at which it started.*

The GI range is zero to 100, with 100 being pure glucose (sugar). On the other end of the scale is erythritol, which has a GI of zero.

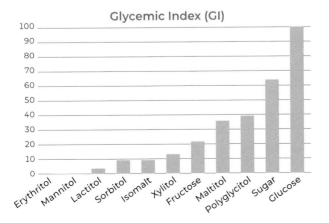

note Maltitol is a sugar alcohol that is used in some low-carb bars, ice cream, candy, and chocolate. As you can see in the chart, maltitol has a pretty high GI of 36. I highly recommend that you stay away from maltitol and pick a lower-GI sweetener.

DRESSINGS AND SAUCES

A lot of store-bought dressings and sauces contain added sugar and unhealthy oils, so be sure to read the labels. When dining out, I usually play it safe and ask for sauces on the side or substitute something that I know is low-carb, like ranch dressing or mayonnaise. Here are some keto-friendly sauces that you can add to your meals for more fat and flavor:

- Béarnaise
- Blue cheese dressing
- Buffalo sauce
- Chimichurri (page 88)
- Horseradish
- Hot sauce
- Italian dressing (check the labels, but most are low-carb)
- Keto Yum Yum Sauce (page 89)
- Marinara Sauce (page 82)
- Mayonnaise
- Mustard, yellow and Dijon

- Pesto
- Ranch Dip/Dressing (page 86)
- Simple Vinaigrette (page 84)
- Soy sauce (check for gluten-free options, if needed, or substitute coconut aminos)
- Sriracha
- Sugar-Free Ketchup (page 87)
- Sugar-Free Thousand Island Dressing (page 83)

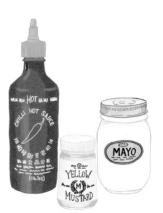

FLAVORING INGREDIENTS AND OTHER PANTRY ITEMS

When purchasing these items, always check the labels and choose the products that are the lowest in carbs, especially with tomato-based foods.

- Artichoke hearts
- Banana peppers
- Bouillon cubes (great for electrolytes!)
- Broth
- Canned tuna and other fish
- Capers
- Chocolate (sweetened with stevia or erythritol; stay away from maltitol)
- Coconut milk (full fat)

- Coconut oil or olive oil cooking spray
- Green chilis
- Keto bars (like those from Heka Foods)
- Olives
- Pickled jalapeños
- Pickles
- Pork rinds
- Red wine vinegar
- Roasted red pepper

- Sardines
- Sauerkraut
- Sun-dried tomatoes
- Tomato paste
- Vanilla extract

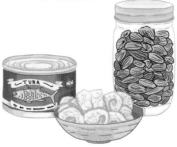

BEYOND SIMPLY KETO PANTRY ITEMS

The following list contains 15 pantry items that are used in the recipes in this book, with detailed explanations and tips. If you are new to keto, some of these foods may be new to you, but once you stock your keto kitchen, you'll be ready to make all kinds of delicious low-carb recipes!

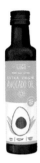

AVOCADO OIL. Avocado oil has a high smoke point—it can be used in high-heat cooking up to 520°F—and is known to have anti-inflammatory properties, lower cholesterol, and help with the absorption of other nutrients. It doesn't have a strong flavor, which makes it very versatile; it can be used for baking, grilling, and sautéing as well as in dressings. I used it for stir-frying in recipes like Beef and Broccoli (page 220) and Egg Roll in a Bowl (page 226).

BAKING POWDER. Baking powder is used to increase the volume and lighten the texture of baked goods. Since almond flour and coconut flour are more dense than regular flour, extra baking powder is needed in many keto baking recipes, including my Pumpkin Pecan Pancakes (page 100), Lemon Blueberry Scones (page 114), and Cheddar Chive Biscuits (page 268). For the best results, make sure your baking powder isn't expired!

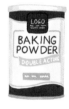

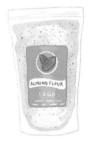

BLANCHED ALMOND FLOUR. Almond flour is made from ground blanched almonds and is used to replace traditional flour in many keto baked goods. It can also be used to replace breadcrumbs, like in the Meatloaf Muffins (page 206) and Baked Scotch Eggs (page 104).

COCONUT FLOUR. Coconut flour is also used as a low-carb flour substitute. It is often combined with almond flour in recipes. Coconut flour is very absorbent, so it cannot be used to replace an equal amount of regular flour or almond flour. For this reason, many recipes that call for coconut flour also have extra liquid. I use coconut flour in the 5-Minute Strawberry Shortcake Parfait for Two (page 284) and Olivia's Snickerdoodles (page 286).

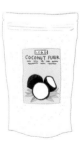

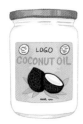

COCONUT OIL. Versatile coconut oil has a high smoke point and can be used as a dairy-free replacement for butter in almost any recipe. Coconut oil contains medium-chain triglycerides (MCTs), so it has similar benefits to MCT oil (see below). It does have a mild coconut taste, but I love to cook veggies with it, like Lemon Parmesan Asparagus (page 262), or to roast a nonstarchy veggie such as broccoli with it. I also like to combine it with sugar-free chocolate chips to make chocolate coatings for different desserts, like Boardwalk Chocolate-Covered Bacon (page 290).

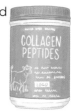

COLLAGEN PEPTIDES. Collagen peptides often come in powdered form, which easily mixes into hot or cold drinks and can even be used in baking. Collagen is virtually taste-free and is a great supplement for hair, skin, nail, and joint health. You can purchase collagen peptides online or in local grocery or convenience stores. I love to use collagen peptides when I make a Blueberry Collagen Smoothie (page 298), and I often stir it into my morning coffee.

CREAM OF TARTAR. Cream of tartar is found in the baking aisle and is often used to stabilize egg whites. I use it in my Three-Cheese Soufflés (page 102) to help them puff up. Cream of tartar is also used in keto frosting recipes and baked goods like meringues.

FLAXSEED MEAL. Flaxseed meal is high in omega-3 fatty acids and fiber, so it's great for heart health. You can use it as a breading or when making keto-friendly baked goods like Everything Bagels (page 106).

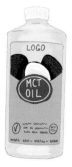

MCT OIL. MCT oil is derived from coconut oil but does not have a coconut taste. It has a low smoke point, so it's not recommended for use in high-heat cooking, but it can be used to make dressings or fat bombs or added to coffee. Medium-chain triglycerides are a type of healthy fat, so MCT oil is a great way to add healthy fat to your diet. It also acts as a natural energy source for your body and brain. If you find that MCT oil is hard to blend or upsets your stomach, MCT powder is a great alternative. My Blueberry Collagen Smoothie recipe (page 298) calls for MCT powder.

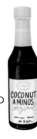

SOY SAUCE OR COCONUT AMINOS. Soy sauce is great for marinating meat, like the Maui Short Ribs (page 212), and can be used in moderation in various dishes. There are gluten-free soy sauce options, or, if you want to stay away from soy altogether, you can use coconut aminos instead. Coconut aminos is a liquid condiment similar to soy sauce but is made from the fermented sap of the coconut palm tree. Coconut aminos is slightly sweeter than soy sauce.

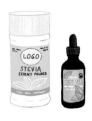

STEVIA. Stevia is a natural low-carb, zero-calorie sweetener that does not affect blood sugar or insulin levels. Because it can have a bitter aftertaste, stevia is often paired with other sweeteners, like erythritol, for a balanced sweetness. I like to use liquid stevia to sweeten coffee or tea and as an alternative to Swerve in the Chai Tea Latte (page 296) or Virgin Mojito (page 304). The conversion of replacing Swerve and stevia in drinks is two to four drops of liquid stevia per teaspoon of Swerve.

SUGAR-FREE CHOCOLATE CHIPS. When buying sugar-free chocolate bars or chips, look for products that are sweetened with stevia, allulose, or erythritol. Try to avoid maltitol, a sugar alcohol that can affect blood sugar and cause an upset tummy. You can try sugar-free chocolate chips in the Chocolate-Coated Cookie Dough Bites (page 274). Another great tip for a sweet tooth is to get a tablespoon of natural peanut butter and sprinkle it with a few sugar-free chocolate chips for a quick-and-easy dessert!

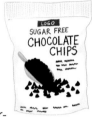

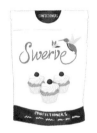

SWERVE (confectioners' style, granular, and brown sugar). Swerve is a sweetener blend that is mostly made from a natural sweetener called erythritol. It measures cup-for-cup as regular sugar, so it's great for converting traditional recipes into sugar-free keto versions. Unlike other low-carb sweeteners, Swerve does not raise blood sugar or insulin levels and has zero calories. It comes in three varieties: confectioners' style, granular, and brown sugar. I mostly use the confectioners' style, which blends well into hot and cold beverages, like a Café Mocha (page 294), and also bakes well. Swerve brown sugar is great for marinades, like the Maui Short Ribs (page 212), and makes Candied Bacon (page 276) extra delicious. The granular style is sometimes used in baking, like Jess's Keto Coffee Cake (page 120), and it dissolves well in hot beverages like coffee and tea.

TOASTED SESAME OIL. Due to the levels of polyunsaturated fat found in sesame oil, this oil should be used on an occasional basis and not in large amounts. The good news is that it has a strong and distinct flavor, so you need only a little bit in recipes. I use it in Asian-inspired dishes like Beef and Broccoli (page 220) and the peanut sauce that goes with my Chicken Satay Skewers (page 180).

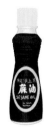

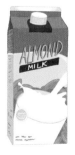

UNSWEETENED ALMOND MILK. Almond milk can be used as a low-calorie, low-carb, and dairy-free alternative to milk. It comes in plain and vanilla-flavored, but make sure you buy it unsweetened. I use it in a variety of recipes, including the Chai Tea Latte (page 296), Roasted Garlic Cauliflower Mash (page 266), and Blueberry Collagen Smoothie (page 298). I also like to pour it over Crunchy Keto Granola (page 122). Coffee shops may offer almond milk as an alternative to dairy milk, but check to be sure it isn't sweetened.

DRINKS

Drinking enough water has always been a struggle for me. If you aren't a huge fan of plain water, try sparkling water (LaCroix is my favorite, or you can purchase a SodaStream and make your own sparking water at home) or sugar-free flavored water. Here are some other options:

- Almond milk (unsweetened, plain or vanilla-flavored)
- Bone broth
- Cashew milk (unsweetened)
- Coconut milk (full fat, unsweetened)
- Coffee
- Macadamia nut milk
- Stevia- or erythritol-sweetened soda (Zevia is my favorite)
- Tea (unsweetened, iced or hot)

 note Although unsweetened coconut milk is keto-friendly, coconut water is not low in carbs and should be avoided. Coconut water averages 15 grams of sugar per 11.1-fluid-ounce serving.

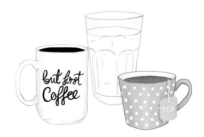

Low-Carb Alcohol

Whether or not to drink alcohol is a personal choice. If you do choose to imbibe, keep in mind that alcohol should be consumed responsibly and in limited quantities. I enjoy a drink on occasion (not daily), but I limit myself to one or two drinks. Keep in mind that keto is a lifestyle change, so find a livable balance that works for you. In my opinion, it's okay to enjoy an occasional drink that is low in carbs, but make sure you keep your health and goals in mind when deciding how much or how often. Moderation is key!

Wine
Wine is generally my go-to option when it comes to low-carb alcoholic beverages. Be sure to stay away from dessert wines, however, as they are loaded with sugar! The following are some of my favorite wine choices.

Serving size is 5 ounces.

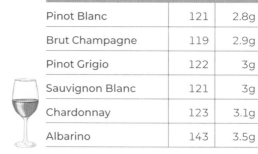

RED WINE	Calories	Carbs
Pinot Noir	122	3.4g
Merlot	123	3.7g
Cabernet Sauvignon	123	3.8g
Syrah	123	3.8g
Petite Syrah	126	3.9g
Zinfandel	131	4.2g

WHITE WINE	Calories	Carbs
Pinot Blanc	121	2.8g
Brut Champagne	119	2.9g
Pinot Grigio	122	3g
Sauvignon Blanc	121	3g
Chardonnay	123	3.1g
Albarino	143	3.5g

Liquor

The majority of liquors contain zero net carbs as long as they are unflavored and unsweetened. Check each brand to be sure. The following chart shows the averages across most brands per 1½-ounce serving.

Stay away from the majority of liqueurs and mixers, as most are not low-carb. Here are some low-carb mixer options:

- Flavored unsweetened sparkling water (such as LaCroix)
- Stevia- or erythritol-sweetened soda (such as Zevia)
- Sugar-free energy drinks (check the macros and look for brands sweetened with erythritol or stevia)
- Sugar-free water enhancers
- Lime juice (pair with tequila, crushed ice and the sweetener of your choice for a low-carb spin on a margarita)

LIQUOR	Calories	Carbs
Brandy	103–126	0–3g*
Gin	100	0
Rum	72–105	0
Tequila	96–104	0
Vodka	97–105	0
Whiskey/Scotch/Bourbon	96–105	0

*check labels for added carbs

Beer

In my opinion, beer should be your last choice as far as alcoholic beverages are concerned, especially if you are trying to lose weight. Most beer contains gluten, and beer is often referred to as "liquid bread." Again, keto is a lifestyle change; I don't expect that you will never drink a beer again if you enjoy beer. Keep in mind, though, that beer has the potential to affect ketosis more so than other alcoholic options. I personally enjoy a low-carb beer on occasion, but for the most part I stick to wine.

If you do choose to have a beer once in a while, here are some lower-carb options. The calorie and carb counts are based on a single-serving can or bottle.

BEER	Calories	Carbs
Budweiser Select 55	55	1.9g
Miller 64	64	2.4g
Rolling Rock Green Light	83	2.4g
Michelob Ultra	95	2.6g
Budweiser Select	99	3.1g
Miller Lite	96	3.2g
Busch Light	95	3.2g
Natural Light	95	3.2g
Michelob Ultra Amber	95	3.2g
Beck's Premier Light	64	3.9g
Miller Chill	100	4.1g
Coors Light	102	5g
Amstel Light	95	5g
Keystone Light	104	5g
Budweiser Light	110	6.6g
Heineken Light	99	6.8g

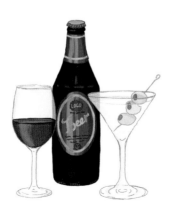

SIMPLY KETO ON A BUDGET

Now that we've gone through all the types of foods you can enjoy on keto, let's talk about budget, because keto gets an unfair reputation for being an expensive way of eating. You don't have to spend a lot of money to eat healthy! There are many tips and tricks for buying in bulk or cost-effective options. However, as consumers, we decide how and where we budget and spend our money, while considering that the food we eat greatly contributes to our overall health. My husband always jokes that you never want to cut back on toilet paper or food! The takeaway is to try to buy the best quality that you can afford knowing that you're investing in your health and quality of life.

One of my favorite strategies for saving money at the grocery store is to buy foods in bulk. Here are my top 15 items for buying in larger quantities, along with tips on how to store them:

ALMOND FLOUR. Buying in bulk greatly reduces the price per ounce of almond flour. My favorite is the blanched almond flour sold at Costco. Almond flour can be stored for up to a year when kept in an airtight container away from light and heat. After opening the bag, it's best to store your flour in the refrigerator.

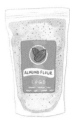

AVOCADOS. Avocados are tricky to buy in bulk because of the ripening time. You don't want to end up with ten avocados ripe all at once! If you place your ripe avocados in the fridge, however, the cold will stop them from ripening as fast, and you'll have an extra three to five days to enjoy them. If you don't have any ripe avocados, you can speed up the process by placing them in a brown paper bag on the counter for two to three days. Once they are ripe, store them in the refrigerator until ready to eat.

BACON. You can store vacuum-sealed bacon in the freezer for up to six months. Thaw it by placing it in the fridge for 24 hours in advance of using, or quickly defrost it by placing the entire unopened package in a bowl of cool water for about an hour, changing the water after 30 minutes.

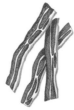

BUTTER. Good-quality grass-fed butter can be a little expensive, so buying this keto staple in bulk is a great option. Most unopened butter will last up to three months in the fridge or up to a year in the freezer.

CHEESE. Cheese is a staple in my house, and I eat it almost daily, so the more the merrier. Hard cheese, like Parmesan, has a pretty long shelf life when stored in the fridge. When it comes to preshredded cheese in a zip-top bag, remember that after you open the bag, it's best to remove as much air as possible before resealing it, which will keep the cheese fresher. When buying blocks of cheese, once opened, make sure to cover the cheese with plastic wrap or seal it in wax paper to keep air from getting to it.

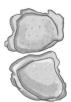

CHICKEN (thighs, breasts, and wings). Chicken is versatile and affordable, so I almost always have some on hand. Any cut of raw chicken can be kept in the freezer for six to nine months when vacuum-sealed. Another way you can freeze chicken is by removing the original packaging and separating into individual freezer bags, with a low-carb marinade if you like, according to serving size or the size of your family. Lay the bags flat and expel as much air as you can before sealing the bags. Also, you can cook chicken breasts in a slow cooker to make shredded chicken. Once cool, separate the shredded meat into 1- to 2-cup bags to freeze for up to six months, and then thaw to use for chicken salad, tacos, and other quick-and-easy meals.

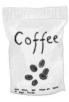

COFFEE. Whether you buy whole beans, ground beans, or K-cups, buying coffee in bulk greatly reduces the price per cup. Most wholesale clubs have a great selection. Store whole beans or grounds in an airtight container at room temperature.

EGGS. Eggs are a keto staple; you may be surprised how many eggs you eat in a week between breakfasts, snacks, and use in recipes. Buying in bulk will save you money and help you avoid extra trips to the grocery store to keep stocking up. Hard-boiled eggs make a great grab-and-go snack!

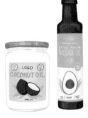

OLIVE OIL, AVOCADO OIL, AND COCONUT OIL. Virgin and extra-virgin oils have a longer shelf life than other types, but you can use whatever type of oil you would like. Store oils at room temperature, out of direct sunlight, for up to two years.

FROZEN SHRIMP. Not only is frozen shrimp the best bang for your buck, but you can buy it already peeled and deveined and either raw or cooked to save time! Frozen shrimp can last up to six months in your freezer. To thaw it, all you have to do is place the shrimp in a bowl of cool water for ten to twenty minutes, changing the water every five to ten minutes.

GROUND MEAT. Whether it is ground beef (I generally buy 80/20 lean to fat ratio), turkey (look for ground dark turkey meat), pork, bison, or chicken, ground meat can be stored in the freezer for up to four months in its original vacuum-sealed packaging. Place it in the refrigerator to thaw 24 hours before you want to use it.

NUTS. Nuts are a great keto-friendly snack. If you eat them often, buying nuts at a wholesale market can save you money. They can be stored at room temperature for up to three months or in the fridge for up to six months.

PEANUT BUTTER. Buying peanut butter in bulk usually means buying two large containers at the same time. Unopened peanut butter has a very long shelf life, so you can store it in your pantry. Once opened, it can be stored in the fridge for up to four months. When selecting peanut butter, look for one that contains only peanuts and salt to avoid unhealthy oils.

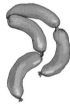

SAUSAGES/HOT DOGS. Depending on how large your family is and how big the package of hot dogs or sausages is, open all of the packages and lay each one on a cookie sheet to freeze. Once frozen, separate into freezer bags according to family and serving sizes, or put them all in one large bag and take out one or two as needed. To thaw them, take them out of the freezer and place in the refrigerator 24 hours in advance. Store in the freezer for up to two months.

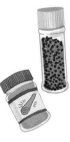

SPICES. When you buy spices in bulk, you may or may not have to transfer them to your own containers for storage. I store bulk spices in mason jars to ensure an airtight seal, which helps keep spices fresher longer. Examples of spices you may want to buy in bulk are whole peppercorns (for your pepper grinder), salt, garlic powder, and ground cinnamon.

Helpful Tips for Selecting Quality Foods

Here's a message from my good friend Dr. Ryan Lowery, CEO of Ketogenic.com and coauthor of *The Ketogenic Bible*, to help you be an informed consumer when selecting foods made from healthy ingredients that won't spike your blood sugar or leave you with an upset tummy! Remember, as consumers we get to "vote" with the money we spend, and together we are changing and demanding more from the food industry.

With the enormous number of keto products hitting the market, it is difficult to differentiate a legitimate product from one that might knock you out of ketosis. Unfortunately, some companies sell products that not only contain ingredients that can spike blood glucose or mess up your stomach, but also carry deceptive nutrition labels. Fortunately, the team at Ketogenic.com has created a Ketogenic Certified program (ketogenic.com/certified) for companies to submit their products for testing. Rather than just reading the labels, they use an advanced laboratory to look at glucose and ketone levels to make sure that the products they test fit the criteria of being "keto." Those products that pass muster can feature this label on the package:

In addition to looking for the Ketogenic Certified label on products, here are some of their top tips for avoiding "fake" keto products:

- Avoid products containing sugar alcohols (maltitol, sorbitol, and so on), with the exception of erythritol and xylitol.

- Watch out for sneaky names for sugar, like maltodextrin, dextrose, fructose, and sucrose.

- Be cautious about consuming products made with vegetable oils (i.e., canola or soybean). You commonly find these oils in foods like dressings and mayonnaise. Fortunately, there are plenty of healthy alternatives available, such as mayonnaise made with avocado oil.

- The fewer ingredients in a product, the better. Try to avoid products with a laundry list of ingredients that you can't pronounce or identify.

- Not all types of fiber are the same. For example, some products contain isomalto-oligosaccharides (IMO), which are listed as fiber. This ingredient is not a true fiber and can cause glucose and insulin response. Additionally, be cautious with chicory root or inulin. While it is commonly labeled as fiber and has prebiotic activity, it can lead to gastrointestinal distress and bloating.

If you have little storage space (hello, city living), or if you're cooking for one or for a smaller family, here are some great budget-friendly items that you can buy in small quantities:

- Bagged spinach
- Bone-in chicken thighs
- Broccoli
- Cabbage
- Canned tomato products
- Canned tuna, chicken, or salmon
- Celery
- Chuck roast
- Eggs
- Frozen nonstarchy vegetables
- Ground beef
- Ground turkey
- Hot dogs/sausages (check the carb counts)
- Kale and other leafy greens
- Pork chops

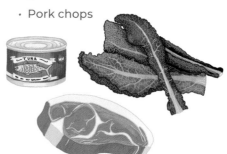

GROCERY SHOPPING IN STORES AND ONLINE

These are just a few of my favorite items from several common grocery stores in my area, along with Amazon, which is a great online source for shelf-stable keto ingredients. I also have several grocery haul videos on my YouTube channel (youtube.com/ketokarma2015) for even more shopping ideas and recommendations.

Costco

- Almond flour, blanched
- Almonds
- Avocado oil
- Avocados
- Bacon
- Berries
- Bone broth
- Carnitas
- Cheeses
- Cheese crisps
- Cheese wraps
- Chicken salad
- Coconut oil
- Coffee
- Cream cheese
- Deli meat
- Dips and spreads (check the carb counts)
- Eggs
- Egg wraps (crepini)
- Grilled chicken skewers
- Guacamole cups
- Hard-boiled eggs, individually wrapped
- Heavy whipping cream
- Kerrygold butter
- Macadamia nuts
- Meats, fresh or frozen
- Nonstarchy veggies, fresh or frozen
- Pesto
- Pork belly
- Rao's Marinara Sauce
- Riced cauliflower
- Rotisserie chicken
- Sausages
- Seafood, fresh or frozen
- Sparkling water
- Spinach
- Three Bridges Egg Bites
- Wild Planet canned tuna

Safeway

- Aidell's Italian meatballs
- Aidell's sausages (check the carb count on each flavor)
- Almond flour, blanched
- Avocados
- Bacon
- Butter
- Cheeses
- Coconut cream, unsweetened
- Coconut oil
- Cream cheese
- Deli meat
- Halloumi
- Keto-friendly ice cream (check the ingredients)
- Low-carb condiments (ranch dressing, mayonnaise, hot sauce, and so on)
- Meats, fresh or frozen
- Nonstarchy veggies, fresh
- Pork rinds
- Quest bars
- Rao's Marinara Sauce
- Rotisserie chicken
- Seafood, fresh or frozen
- Sour cream
- Sparkling water
- Spices
- Stevia

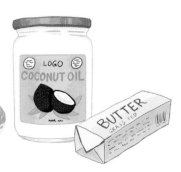

Trader Joe's

- Almond flour, blanched
- Almond meal
- Avocados
- Bacon (the thick applewood-smoked bacon is my favorite)
- Cauliflower (whole heads, fresh riced, and frozen riced)
- Cheese bites
- Cheeses
- Chicken fajitas, refrigerated
- Chili lime chicken burgers, frozen
- Coconut cream, unsweetened
- Coconut flour
- Coconut oil
- Coconut oil spray
- Cream cheese
- Eggs
- Everything but the Bagel Sesame Seasoning Blend
- Grass-fed burgers, frozen
- Half-and-half
- Hard-boiled eggs
- Heavy whipping cream
- Hollandaise
- Kerrygold butter
- Marinated goat cheese
- Meats, fresh or frozen
- Mini Brie Bites
- Nonstarchy veggies, fresh or frozen
- Pork belly
- Prosciutto
- Quest bars
- Salad greens
- Seafood, frozen
- Seaweed snacks
- Zucchini spirals, fresh or frozen

Whole Foods

- Avocado oil
- Bacon pieces, precooked
- Butter
- Coconut flour
- Cream cheese
- Epic Bacon Bars
- Epic Pork Rinds
- Flaxseed meal
- Guacamole (found in the produce section)
- Half-and-half
- Hard-boiled eggs
- Heavy cream
- Hot bar meals
- Keto-friendly ice cream (check the ingredients)
- Lily's stevia-sweetened dark chocolate
- Meats, fresh and frozen
- Natural Calm
- Natural peanut butter, freshly ground
- Nonstarchy veggies, fresh or frozen
- Quest bars
- Seafood, fresh or frozen
- Sour cream
- Sparkling water
- Spices and specialty ingredients from the bulk bins
- Swerve sweeteners

Amazon

- Almond flour, blanched
- AlternaSweets Sweet & Smokey BBQ Sauce
- Avocado oil
- Cheese crisps
- Coconut flour
- Coconut oil
- Coffee
- Collagen peptides
- Golden flaxseed meal
- Good Dee's baking mixes and syrup
- Keto-friendly cookies (check the ingredients)
- Lily's stevia-sweetened dark chocolate
- Liquid stevia
- MCT powder/oil
- Moon Cheese
- Nut butters
- Nuts
- Pork rinds
- Primal Kitchen dressings
- Quest bars
- Quest chips
- Spices
- Swerve sweeteners
- Whole Earth erythritol

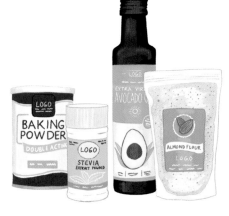

GRAB-AND-GO SNACK/MEAL OPTIONS

Although I hope that you'll take time to explore all the great new recipes in this book, I live in the real world, too. Life can be really busy, but we have to make time for the things that are important to us—and healthy eating should definitely be on that list! Luckily, there are a lot of items you can prepare ahead and grab and go with little to no effort:

- Ants on a log (celery and peanut butter with sugar-free chocolate chips, or spreadable cheese with chopped pecans)
- Avocado
- Beef jerky or meat sticks (check the carbs)
- Bell peppers, sliced
- Berries (blackberries, blueberries, raspberries, or strawberries, in moderation)
- Celery (on its own or paired with peanut butter, cream cheese, or dressing of choice)
- Cheese crisps
- Cheese slices or cubes
- Cherry tomatoes
- Chicken salad (or plain chicken in a can or packet)
- Chocolate-Coated Cookie Dough Bites (page 274)
- Crunchy Keto Granola (page 122)
- Cucumber spear or slices
- Deli meat (chicken, ham, roast beef, or turkey)
- Deviled eggs
- Egg bites (these can be purchased premade in many stores now, but check the ingredients; or they can be premade at home for a quick grab-and-go)

- Egg salad
- Guacamole
- Hard-boiled eggs
- Jicama slices
- Keto-friendly bars
- Lettuce-wrapped sandwiches/ burgers
- Little smokies or grilled sausages, cut up
- Low-carb dips (such as Buffalo chicken and spinach artichoke; check the carbs)
- Low-carb yogurt (check the carb counts/ingredients)
- Marinated artichoke hearts
- Meat and cheese tray
- Meat sticks (check the carb counts)
- Nonstarchy veggies (see the list on page 50), with or without dip (such as ranch or blue cheese dressing)
- Nuts (almonds, macadamia nuts, pecans, or walnuts) or seeds
- Nut butter
- Olives
- Pepperoncini or hot peppers
- Pickled asparagus
- Pickles
- Pork rinds

- Precooked sausages or hot dogs
- Raw broccoli or cauliflower
- Rotisserie chicken
- Salad
- Sauerkraut
- Seaweed snacks
- Sugar-free dark chocolate (avoid maltitol sweetened)
- Tomato slices
- Tuna salad (or plain tuna in a can or packet)
- Unsweetened coconut flakes

tip Everything bagel seasoning is great on hard-boiled eggs, avocados, and meat such as chicken, turkey, and ham.

With a few simple ingredients, you can make a delicious keto-friendly meal in a hurry without a recipe. Here are a few of my favorite quick-and-easy keto meal ideas:

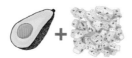 Avocado halves filled with premade chicken, egg, or tuna salad

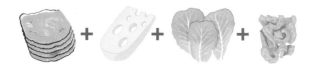 Deli meat and cheese lettuce wraps with pork rinds

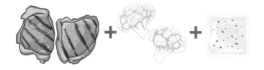 Grilled fish, chicken, pork, or beef with any side from the list below, paired with a keto-friendly sauce like ranch, blue cheese, or flavored butter to add fat and flavor

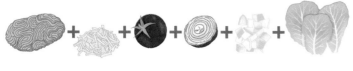 Low-carb taco salad (ground taco beef, shredded cheese, diced tomatoes, onions, and avocado or guacamole over chopped or shredded lettuce)

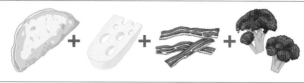 Omelets with a variety of fillings (cheese; sausage, bacon, or chicken; nonstarchy veggies; and so on)

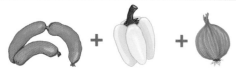 Pan-fried sausages with peppers and onions

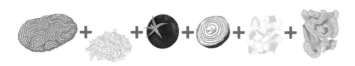 Pork rind nachos (ground taco beef, shredded cheese, diced tomatoes, onions, and avocado or guacamole over pork rinds)

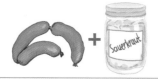 Sausage with sauerkraut

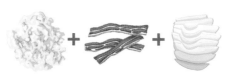 Scrambled eggs with bacon or sausage and sliced or diced avocado

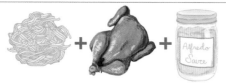 Zucchini noodles with rotisserie chicken or precooked sausage or meatballs (check the carbs) and Alfredo sauce or sugar-free marinara sauce (page 82)

I wrote the recipes in this book with "simple" in mind. Here are the some of the meals that can be prepared in 30 minutes or less:

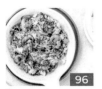 **96**
Jessica's Special

 100
Pumpkin Pecan Pancakes

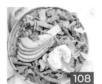 **106**
Everything Bagels

 108
Arugula, Avocado, and Asparagus Salad with Poached Eggs

 118
Pesto Chicken Egg Cups

 126
Smoked Salmon Salad with Creamy Dill Dressing

 128
Prosciutto Arugula Pizza

 130
Cheeseburger Salad

 134
Cilantro Lime Tuna Salad

 136
Spicy Italian Lettuce Wrap

 186
Zesty Ranch Turkey Burgers

 192
Caprese Chicken with Pesto for Two

 194
Crispy Baked Chicken Thighs

 196
Creamy Sun-Dried Tomato and Basil Chicken

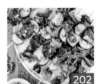 **202**
Skirt Steak Kabobs with Chimichurri

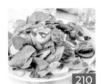 **210**
Mike's Spinach Salad with Warm Bacon Dressing

 226
Egg Roll in a Bowl

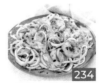 **234**
Shrimp Scampi with Zucchini Noodles

 238
Cod Veracruz

 240
Sriracha Lime Salmon

Finally, here are some quick and easy-to-prepare sides to pair with the meals listed above:

- Baked Spinach Chips (page 246)
- Cauliflower rice
- Grilled or baked asparagus
- Roasted Garlic Cauliflower Mash (page 266)
- Roasted or pan-fried Brussels sprouts
- Roasted or steamed broccoli
- Roasted or steamed cauliflower
- Sautéed zucchini slices
- Side salad
- Zucchini noodles

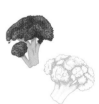

KETO BENTO BOXES

Bento boxes are a great option for kids' school lunches, as well as adult lunches! These make-ahead meals are customizable, quick, colorful, and healthy:

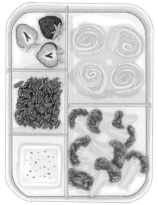

OPTION 1 (nut-free):
Turkey and cheddar cheese roll-ups, broccoli florets with ranch dressing, strawberries, sunflower seeds

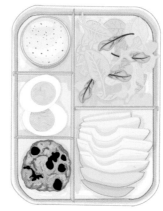

OPTION 4 (breakfast):
Lemon Blueberry Scone (page 114), hard-boiled egg, avocado slices, mixed greens with your favorite low-carb dressing

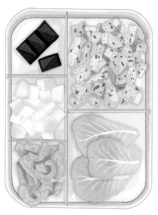

OPTION 2 (nut-free):
Chicken salad, butter lettuce, avocado slices, pork rinds, a few squares of sugar-free chocolate

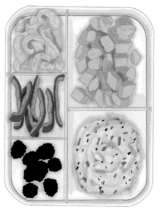

OPTION 5 (dairy-free and nut-free):
Diced cooked chicken, dairy-free guacamole, pork rinds, sliced bell peppers, blackberries

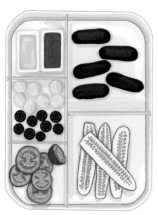

OPTION 3 (dairy-free):
Pre-grilled Little Smokies with mustard or sugar-free ketchup, pickle spears, cherry tomatoes, blueberries, macadamia nuts

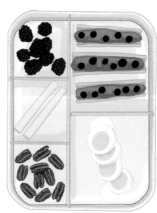

OPTION 6 (vegetarian):
Ants on a log (celery with peanut butter and sugar-free chocolate chips), cheese stick, hard-boiled egg, raspberries, pecans

DINING OUT

Now more than ever, there are low-carb and keto-friendly options everywhere. There's no need to always stay home to cook every meal—go out and enjoy some of the dining options below! Keto is so popular now that you don't even get weird looks anymore when you ask for no bun.

Restaurant options

Whether you're craving a juicy burger or Maine lobster with butter for dipping, you can eat keto at almost any restaurant. Here's a breakdown by type of restaurant/cuisine:

 BBQ: Pulled pork, brisket, sausage, ribs, smoked chicken, collard greens or other nonstarchy veggies, salads. The trick is to ask for no barbecue sauce on the meat. If you want to be extra careful, you can even ask if the seasonings or rubs are sugar-free.

 BREAKFAST/BRUNCH: Omelet, eggs Benedict (substitute avocado slices for the English muffin), eggs with bacon or sausage and avocado, steak and eggs.

 BURGER JOINTS: The majority will allow you to pass on the bun and give you a lettuce wrap if you ask. Be sure to have them leave off the ketchup, and add mayo if you like. Some burger places offer grilled chicken as an alternative, which you can eat with ranch dressing or on a salad (no croutons, and choose either ranch or Caesar dressing).

 PIZZA JOINTS: Just eat the pizza toppings, also known as a "meatza," a salad without croutons, or wings (not breaded).

 POKE: Poke bowl, start with a base of zucchini noodles or mixed greens, then choose your protein. Most places will have shrimp, ahi tuna, salmon, hamachi,

and so on; all of these choices are great. They will usually dress the fish with the sauce of your choice, spicy mayo, or soy sauce. For sides, green or white onion, pickled ginger, cilantro, sesame seeds, avocado, masago, jalapeño, and cucumber are good options. Stay away from crab salad containing imitation crabmeat (which has about 13 grams of carbs per 3 ounces) and seaweed salad (often contains sugar).

 SEAFOOD: Shrimp (not breaded), scallops, fish (not breaded), oysters, crab (but not imitation crabmeat; it is not low-carb), lobster, ask for calamari to be grilled instead of breaded, salads, nonstarchy veggies. Butter is a great no-carb accompaniment to seafood, but stay away from cocktail sauce as it usually contains sugar.

 SUB/SANDWICH SHOPS: Many offer lettuce-wrapped subs, sometimes called an unwich, or they will make any of your favorite subs into a salad.

 SUSHI: Sashimi, rolls with cucumber wraps (no rice, and sugar-free sauces only), miso soup, salad. Skip the imitation crabmeat, which is not low-carb.

VEGAN/VEGETARIAN: Salads, bunless Impossible or Beyond burgers or sausages, nonstarchy veggie stir fry, cauliflower rice with nonstarchy veggies topped with vegan pesto.

WING RESTAURANTS: Chicken wings (not breaded; sometimes called "naked" wings) are a good choice. Stay away from sweet sauces; stick to Buffalo sauce, Parmesan garlic sauce, salt, and pepper or dry rubs without sugar. Dip the wings in ranch or blue cheese dressing and enjoy them with a side of celery.

AMERICAN: Bunless burgers, sandwiches, or cheesesteaks, salads, side of avocado, side of pickles, sautéed veggies. If the restaurant serves breakfast, you can order eggs, bacon or sausage, and cheese; just ask for no bread, biscuit, or muffin.

CHINESE: Egg drop soup, chicken with mushrooms, beef or chicken and broccoli, garlic prawns. Watch for sugar in sauces; feel free to ask about ingredients before ordering.

GERMAN: Sausage, bunless burgers, sauerkraut, salads.

GREEK: Kabobs and Greek salads are great choices. Also, most tzatziki sauce is pretty low in carbs.

INDIAN: Tandoori chicken, kabobs, roasted eggplant (without breading), grilled halloumi cheese.

ITALIAN: Chicken Alfredo (substitute broccoli or asparagus for the pasta), steak and veggies, antipasto salad. (Remember that a lot of Italian dishes, such as meatballs, contain breadcrumbs, so watch out for hidden carbs.)

JAPANESE STEAKHOUSE: One of my favorites! Chicken, steak, shrimp, scallops, or lobster; skip the rice and ask for extra veggies (often mushrooms, zucchini, and onion; I ask for light onion). Skip the orange ("yum yum") sauce, as it's not low-carb. Brown ginger sauce is usually low in carbs—feel free to ask, or simply use a little soy sauce. Also, meals generally come with a clear broth soup and a salad with ginger dressing. (The ginger dressing at my local place has 2 grams of carbs per tablespoon, so use it sparingly or skip it altogether.)

MEXICAN (sit-down): Fajitas (skip the tortillas), taco salad with no beans and no tortilla bowl or tortilla pieces, carnitas with a side of guacamole; avocado stuffed with chicken, beef, or shrimp.

MEXICAN (fast-casual): Burrito bowl without dressing. Pick a protein and then add toppings—I like fajita veggies, pico de gallo, cheese, sour cream, and guacamole. Another option is to order several tacos or one large burrito with no beans or rice and ask for no shells/tortillas; they will serve it in a bowl or on a plate.

THAI: Garlic prawns (not breaded) with veggies instead of rice, Tom Kha Gai (coconut milk soup with chicken), red curry (ask if it contains added sugar), chicken satay (either skip the peanut sauce or ask if it contains sugar).

VIETNAMESE: Pho; select a protein (I get rare beef) and ask for no noodles. The server will bring you sprouts, jalapeño, and fresh basil to add. Some restaurants will even give you veggies (broccoli, cabbage, and so on) instead of noodles.

tip I find it really helpful to let the server know upfront that I would prefer not to be served a bread basket, chips and salsa, or pitas and hummus. It's better not to have the temptation, especially when you're hungry! If you're out with friends who aren't low-carb, then obviously this won't work. In that case, if you're feeling tempted, I recommend ordering a side salad (skip the croutons) with ranch or blue cheese dressing, or ordering a keto-friendly appetizer that you can enjoy before your meal.

Coffee shop options

Here are some safe drink options to order from your favorite coffee shop:

- Coffee (hot or iced) with or without half-and-half or heavy whipping cream
- Americano with or without half-and-half or heavy whipping cream
- Espresso
- Iced tea, unsweetened
- Hot tea
- Sparkling water

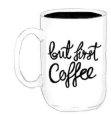

All of the above can be paired with your preferred low-carb sweetener. Some coffee shops, including Starbucks, offer sugar-free syrups that are sweetened with sucralose (Splenda). I don't add syrups to my coffee, but if you enjoy them, just be sure to use them in moderation. Also, Starbucks now carries a Whole Earth stevia and monk fruit blend (in a green packet), which is a great option!

If you get hungry at the coffee shop, here are some common keto-friendly food offerings:

- Avocado spread (eat with a spoon or use as a dip with meat, cheese, or veggies)
- Bunless breakfast sandwiches (for example, bacon, egg, and cheese with the bread removed)
- Egg bites (check the macros; some are higher in carbs, but I eat them on occasion)
- Hard-boiled eggs
- Meat and cheese trays
- Moon Cheese
- Salads (remove any croutons and stick to low-carb dressings)
- Salted almonds
- String cheese

tip When ordering a drink with heavy cream or half-and-half, ask for it on the side or specify an amount, like 2 tablespoons. If you don't give a specific amount, they often pour a lot in, and the calories or carbs can add up.

HEALTHY EATING FOR KIDS

As you may know, I am a mom to a sweet little girl named Olivia. People often ask me about the way she eats, and about how to navigate various dietary preferences under the same roof. While there is no one-size-fits-all approach, I'll share my outlook and routine with you. This is a judgment-free zone, and each family is different, so do what works for your schedule, budget, and lifestyle. Being a parent is amazing, stressful, joyful, anxiety-producing, fulfilling, and challenging all at the same time. Before having a child, I had many preconceived ideas about what I would and wouldn't do as a parent, many of which are laughable now that the real world of parenting has arrived. Like all things in life, parenting is a balancing act of compromising and holding your ground, laughing and crying, and having good days and bad.

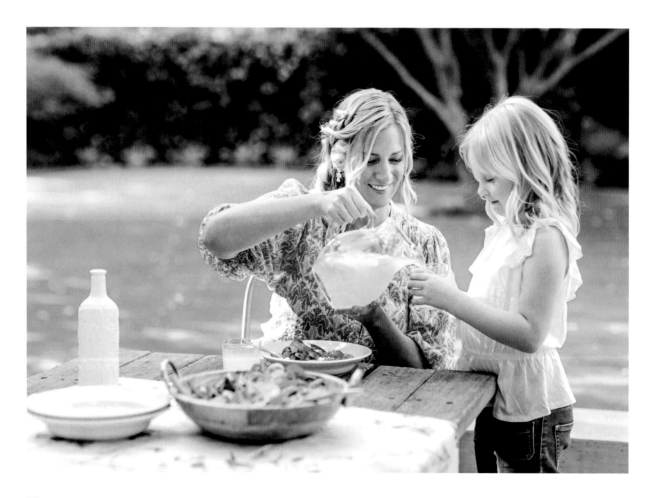

When I was growing up, there wasn't much focus on nutrition or healthy eating habits. My parents rarely cooked; we mostly ate processed foods, fast food, pizza, sandwiches, takeout, and microwaved items. Looking back, I truly don't think healthy eating was on my parents' radar. My dad often says that at the time, he was just trying to make us happy. Of course, at that age, I never complained about having pizza two or three times a week!

I think that with each generation, the hope is to learn and grow, to look back, not to play a blame game, but to see areas that need attention or adjustment. And trust me, as much as I love Olivia and try my best, I don't have everything dialed in or figured out. I hope that she will add new skills and improvements when it's time for her to raise her own kids. The bottom line is that none of us is perfect, so give yourself some grace. As Olivia's mom, my main goals are to make her feel loved and valued and to show and teach her the importance of empathy, positivity, growth mindset, and kindness.

Below, I'll share some of the adjustments and goals that I've made now that I'm a parent. While I find each of these points to be helpful and important, I think it's necessary to have realistic expectations and allow yourself some wiggle room because life just isn't perfect, nor should it be. Plus, kids are forever changing; one moment they love something, and the next they'll say it's yucky or gross. They sure do love to keep us on our toes!

- **Involve your kids in the kitchen.**
  Kids love to help in the kitchen, so let them be your assistants and find age-appropriate jobs that keep them involved and teach them how to prepare food. Olivia often helps me by cracking eggs, adding or mixing ingredients, or washing fruit. While we are cooking, I often tell her about different food items and which have a lot of sugar and need to be eaten in moderation and which are really healthy and help her body grow strong.

- **Give your kids a choice.**
  This doesn't happen every night, but I often ask Olivia to choose between two or three veggie side options for dinner. I find that she really loves being included in the decision-making. Another benefit is that when it comes time to eat, she generally eats her veggies without a fuss because it was her choice!

- **Encourage kids to try new things.**
  As parents, we play a big role in the development of our kids' food preferences and tastes, so it's helpful to expose them to new foods and encourage them to try new things. Olivia can be a picky eater, so I know firsthand that following this advice isn't always as easy as it sounds. I encourage her to take at least one bite of each new food, and she knows she can spit it out if she doesn't like it. This approach doesn't always work, though; sometimes she just says no, and that's okay.

- **Turn off phones and the TV during meals.**

  This is a big one, but it's one that I struggle with myself sometimes. When you are watching TV or distracted by your phone, you aren't paying as much attention to your hunger signals. Distracted eating has been shown to increase overeating, so as often as possible, I try to make dinnertime family time, with phones and the TV off. Sometimes, after a busy day, we find ourselves eating dinner in front of the TV in the living room, which is okay on occasion. But my goal is to have an uninterrupted dinner together at the table.

- **Pack your kids' lunches (or have them pack their own, if they're old enough).**

  Unfortunately, in most schools, lunch options for kids are very high in carbs and lacking in fresh ingredients. On occasion, I order Olivia school lunch, but for the most part I pack bento-style lunches for her containing a variety of items for snack time and lunch. (You can find a few examples on page 68.) Growing up, I almost always ate school lunch, which often had choices of mac 'n' cheese, nachos, corndogs, pizza, or chicken nuggets and potatoes or fries. While Olivia does eat a ketogenic diet, we try to focus on healthy eating habits and whole organic/pastured foods as much as possible, while also allowing her to eat a cupcake at a birthday party or share pizza with friends. Mick and I want her to be informed to make good choices, but not obsessive about or fearful of food.

- **Try to minimize using food as a reward or a comfort tool.**

  Like all things in life, this is a balancing act. Most kids have cake at birthday parties and pizza parties at school—food has deep roots in culture and celebration, after all. But keep in mind how easy it can be to use food to combat sadness, stress, and anxiety. Bad day at school or work? Let's grab a pizza or some chocolate and take our mind off things! Unfortunately, this coping mechanism often leads to emotional eating, which many people (myself included) struggle with. My advice is to find other ways to help your kids share and manage their emotions. When Olivia is either sad or celebrating something, I try to find non-food-related acknowledgments, like a new book, an art class, or a scooter ride to the park. You don't want to overcorrect and have your child learn to fear food, but be mindful about trying to reward happy moments or process complex emotions without food.

Ultimately, you should do what works for you and your family. Don't compare yourself, or your kids, to other people. These tips are only recommendations, and even I struggle to follow them on occasion. Progress, not perfection. Take small, sustainable steps to give your kids a healthy and happy foundation. Above all, don't be so hard on yourself. Mom guilt and Dad guilt are tough. There never seems to be enough time in the day, and although we all try our best, some days we have to give ourselves a little grace and know that we love our kids more than anything in the world, and that's enough.

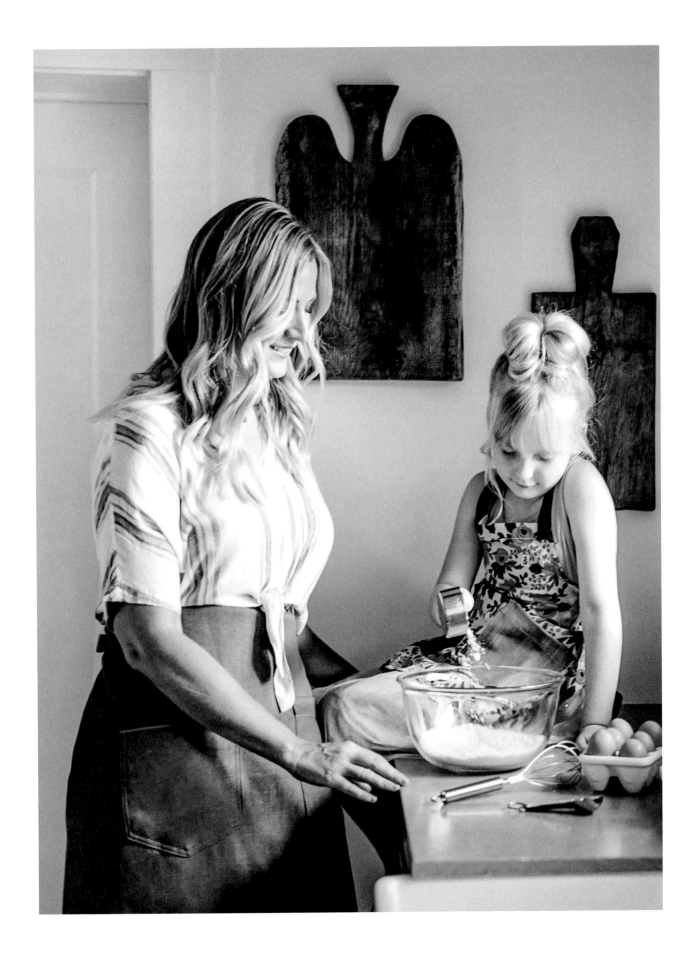

TEN HELPFUL AND TIME-SAVING KITCHEN TOOLS

Now that you know which kinds of foods you should be stocking in your kitchen, let's talk about some of the tools that can make keto cooking faster and easier. Aside from the basics, like a couple of sharp knives, a few pots and pans, and a mixing bowl or two, these are ten of my favorite kitchen tools.

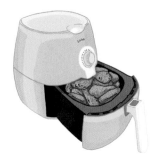

AIR FRYER. I absolutely love my air fryer. It saves so much time because you don't need to preheat it or deal with a lot of oil. Food always turns out perfectly cooked, crispy, and delicious. You can bake just about anything you would in a regular oven (as long as it fits); all you have to do is reduce the temperature by 25 degrees and the time by 20 percent. One of my favorite easy meals is boneless chicken thighs with the skin on. The skin turns out golden brown, crispy, and delicious. Naked chicken wings is also another great meal to make in an air fryer.

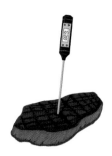

DIGITAL THERMOMETER. I almost always rely on a digital thermometer for grilling and roasting. It takes the guesswork out of getting poultry, meat, and fish to the perfect internal temperature. Most digital thermometers can be set to a specific temperature, and an alarm will let you know when the meat reaches that temperature. All of my recipes suggest cooking times; however, the actual times may vary depending on the thickness of the meat or the temperature accuracy of your oven or grill, so a thermometer is a good tool to have.

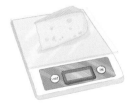

FOOD SCALE. A food scale is great to have on hand in order to follow recipes and to help understand portion sizes. If you are tracking your macros, knowing how much specific items weigh can be really helpful for more accurate macro tracking.

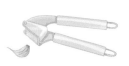

GARLIC PRESS. Using a garlic press is a quick and easy way to get very finely minced garlic in just a few seconds without getting your hands or a knife dirty. Plus, many presses are easy to clean, dishwasher-safe, and affordable. Garlic sent through a press has an almost pastelike texture that's smoother than you can get by mincing it with a knife. In some recipes in this book, where a superfine texture is best, I specify "pressed" garlic. If you don't have a garlic press, simply mince the garlic as finely as you can by hand.

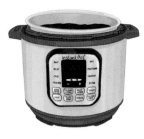

INSTANT POT OR SLOW COOKER. Almost anything you make in an Instant Pot, you can also make in a slow cooker and vice versa. Both are the kind of appliances that you cover with the lid, set a timer, and forget about until the timer goes off; and then you magically have a perfect, warm meal waiting. If you want to prepare in advance for a busy day ahead, you can make ingredient bags beforehand to just dump into the slow cooker or Instant Pot to make meals even easier. One special feature of the Instant Pot is that it has a sauté feature, so you can brown or sear the meat in the pot before using the pressure-cooking settings.

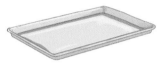

MEAT MALLET. When you pound chicken or beef to an equal thickness, the cooked meat will have a more even temperature throughout without running the risk of overcooking due to sections being thicker or uneven. You can also pound meat thin so that you can stuff it with sun-dried tomatoes, cheeses, herbs, spinach, and so on for a delicious meal.

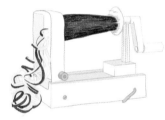

SILICONE BAKING MAT OR PARCHMENT PAPER. This is a must-have, especially if you want to dabble in keto baking. A silicone baking mat or simple parchment paper keeps foods from sticking to baking sheets and makes cleanup a breeze.

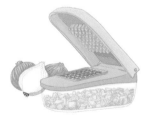

SPIRALIZER. It's no secret that zucchini noodles, or "zoodles," are a staple in the keto community. They bulk up your meals with vegetables and give you the feeling of eating pasta; it's such a fun way to eat your veggies. Before I owned a spiralizer, I used a vegetable peeler to peel thinly sliced "noodles" off of zucchini. Not only did that take a long time, but the noodles were flat and not uniform. You can find handheld spiralizers at most cooking stores for around $10 to $15, or you can order one from Amazon.

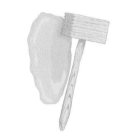

VEGGIE CHOPPER OR MANDOLINE. Most home cooks don't possess the knife skills to create perfectly even or very thinly sliced veggies like chefs can. I like to save time by using a veggie chopper or mandoline to quickly slice zucchini, eggplant, Brussels sprouts, asparagus, and other keto-friendly vegetables to sauté as a side dish, toss into salads, or layer into a casserole. You can also use this tool to grate cheese and shred cabbage or other vegetables. Just watch your fingers—these bad boys are sharp!

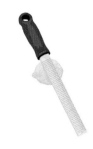

ZESTER OR MICROPLANE. Citrus zest gives a little zing to marinades, vegetables, and desserts. You can also use a zester or Microplane to grate hard cheeses, ginger, hazelnuts (great over a cup of keto coffee), whole nutmeg, and sugar-free chocolate.

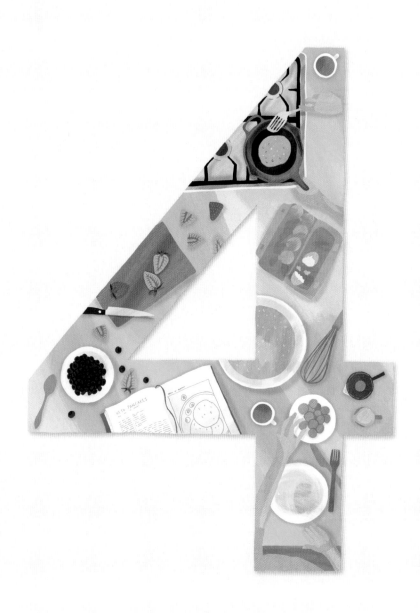

chapter 4:

RECIPES

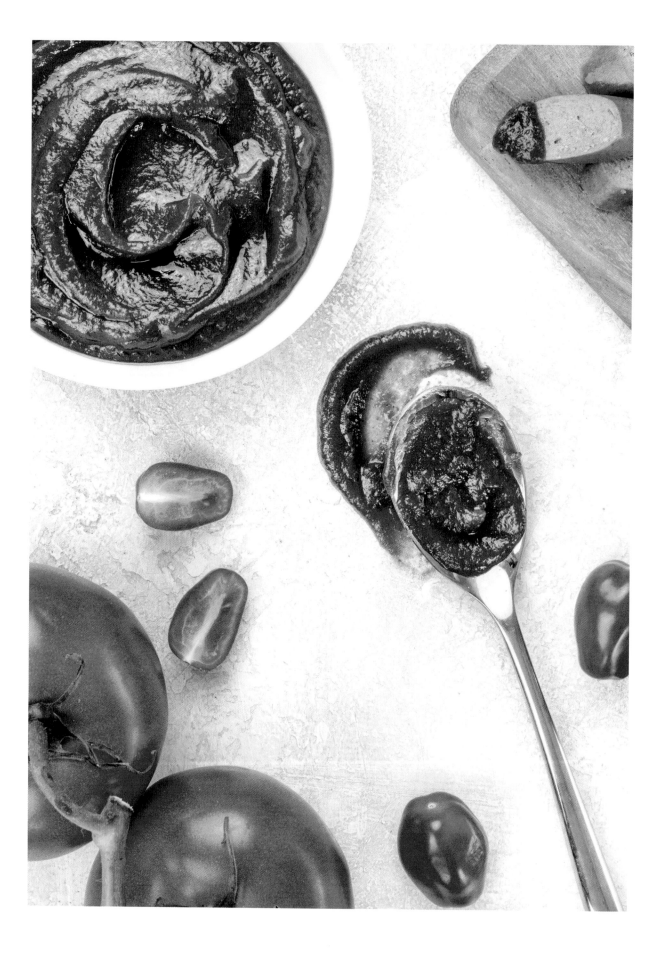

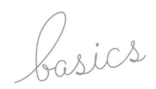

basics

MARINARA SAUCE

Yield: 2½ cups (¼ cup per serving)

Prep Time: 5 minutes

Cook Time: 35 minutes

¼ cup olive oil

4 cloves garlic, minced

1 teaspoon dried minced onions

1 (28-ounce) can crushed tomatoes

½ cup water

1 teaspoon salt

½ teaspoon dried oregano leaves

½ teaspoon dried basil

¼ teaspoon red pepper flakes (optional)

This simple and delicious marinara stores really well in the fridge or freezer and can be served over zoodles, spread lightly as a pizza sauce, or easily turned into a meat sauce.

1. In a medium saucepan, heat the olive oil over medium heat. Add the garlic and dried minced onions and cook for 1 minute.

2. Add the remaining ingredients and bring to a simmer. Continue to simmer for 30 minutes, until the sauce has thickened and darkened in color. Store leftovers in an airtight container in the refrigerator for up to 4 days, or 4 to 6 months in the freezer.

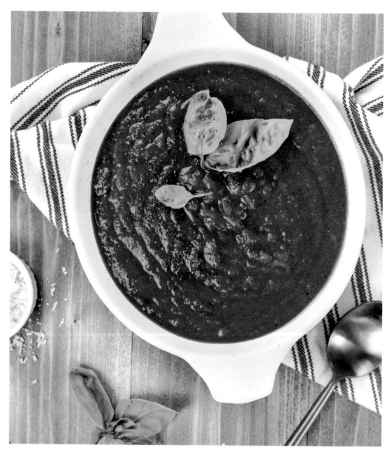

PER SERVING:

CALORIES **69** · FAT **5g** · PROTEIN **1g** · CARBS **4g** · FIBER **1g** · NET CARBS **3g**

SUGAR-FREE THOUSAND ISLAND DRESSING

Yield: 1½ cups (2 tablespoons per serving)

Prep Time: 5 minutes (not including time to make ketchup)

1 cup mayonnaise

1 tablespoon minced onions

¼ cup sugar-free ketchup, homemade (page 87) or store-bought

1 medium dill pickle, diced

1 tablespoon dill pickle juice (from a jar of pickles)

1 to 2 tablespoons prepared horseradish (optional)

After a lot of online research, I still don't understand the difference between Russian dressing and Thousand Island dressing. Can you believe that there are actually hundreds of articles on this topic? Whatever you want to call it, this salad dressing recipe is amazing and is delicious on sandwich "wraps," side salads, or, my favorite, the Reuben Casserole (page 228).

Mix together all the ingredients until well incorporated. Keep refrigerated until ready to use. Store in an airtight container for up to 1 week.

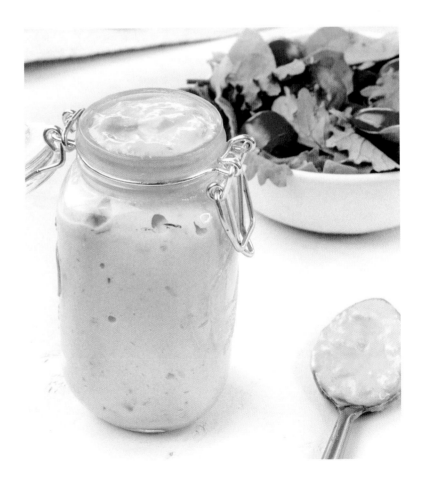

PER SERVING:
CALORIES **124** · FAT **13g** · PROTEIN **0g** · CARBS **4g** · FIBER **1.5g** · ERYTHRITOL **0.5g** · NET CARBS **2g**

SIMPLE VINAIGRETTE

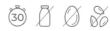

Yield: ½ cup (2 tablespoons per serving)

Prep Time: 5 minutes

⅓ cup olive oil

2½ tablespoons red wine vinegar

½ teaspoon Dijon mustard

½ to 1 tablespoon Swerve confectioners'-style sweetener

Salt and pepper, to taste

If you ever find yourself out of salad dressing and short on time, this vinaigrette is the recipe for you. It is so easy to whip up, and you likely already have all of the ingredients in your pantry! Sometimes I like it a little bit sweeter, sometimes a little more vinegary, and sometimes I like to add herbs and spices. Feel free to add various seasonings and play around with the amount of sweetener you use.

Place all the ingredients in a bowl and whisk with a fork until blended. You can also make this in a jar with a lid, close, and shake to blend. Store the extras in the refrigerator in an airtight container for up to 2 weeks.

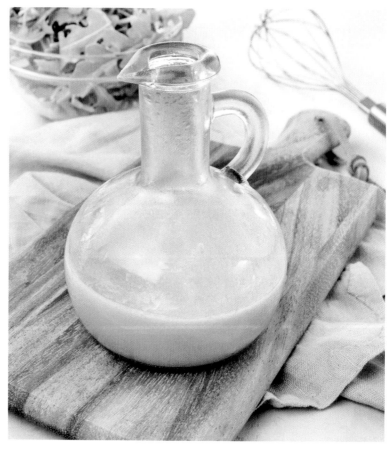

basics

PER SERVING (WITH 1 T. SWEETENER):
CALORIES **217** · FAT **24g** · PROTEIN **0g** · CARBS **3g** · FIBER **0g** · ERYTHRITOL **3g** · NET CARBS **0g**

RANCH HERB MIX

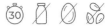

Yield: 14 tablespoons
(1 tablespoon per serving)

Prep Time: 5 minutes

6 tablespoons dried parsley

2 tablespoons dried dill weed

2 tablespoons dried chives

2 tablespoons onion powder

1 tablespoon garlic powder

1½ teaspoons salt

1 teaspoon ground black pepper

This mix of dried herbs adds a great herby zest to any recipe. I love to mix it into ground beef, sprinkle it over chicken before I roast it, or, of course, use it make a dip or dressing for veggies and salads.

Mix all the ingredients together in a small bowl or, for a powdery herb blend (my preference), pulse the ingredients in a blender cup or small food processor for 5 to 10 seconds. Store in an airtight container, and shake well before using. Will keep for up to 1 year.

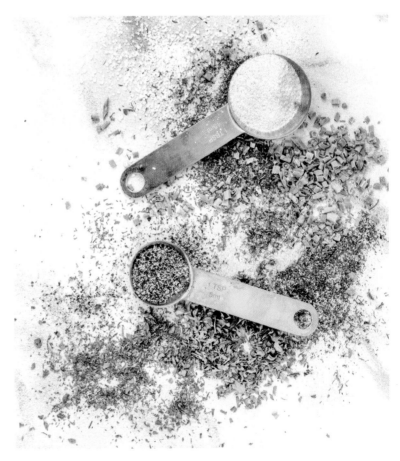

PER SERVING:

CALORIES **10** · FAT **0g** · PROTEIN **1g** · CARBS **3g** · FIBER **1g** · NET CARBS **2g**

RANCH DIP/DRESSING

Yield: 2¼ cups (2 tablespoons per serving)

Prep Time: 5 minutes, plus 1 hour to chill (not including time to make seasoning mix)

1 cup mayonnaise

1 cup sour cream

1 tablespoon fresh lemon juice

¼ cup ranch herb mix, homemade (page 85) or store-bought

You're going to love this delicious ranch dip, which is also easily converted into ranch dressing with the help of a little pickle juice (see below)! Both the dip and the dressing are great with nonstarchy veggies (see page 86), chicken, and salads!

Mix all the ingredients together, cover, and refrigerate for 1 to 2 hours before using. Store in the refrigerator in an airtight container for up to 1 week.

Variation: Pickle Juice Ranch Dressing. To use as a dressing, thin the dip mixture with ¼ cup of dill pickle juice.

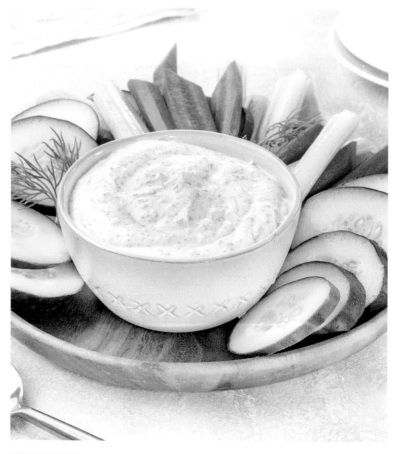

PER SERVING:

CALORIES **135** · FAT **13g** · PROTEIN **1g** · CARBS **1g** · FIBER **0g** · NET CARBS **1g**

SUGAR-FREE KETCHUP

Yield: 1½ cups (2 tablespoons per serving)

Prep Time: 5 minutes

Cook Time: 25 minutes

1 (6-ounce) can tomato paste

⅓ cup Swerve confectioners'-style sweetener

½ cup apple cider vinegar

¼ cup water

¼ teaspoon onion powder

¼ teaspoon garlic powder

⅛ teaspoon ground allspice (optional)

Store-bought sugar-free ketchup is expensive and sometimes you'll find questionable ingredients or sweeteners in it. Making ketchup at home is so easy, and it is used in many other dressings and sauces, like Sugar-Free Thousand Island Dressing (page 83) and Cocktail Sauce (page 162).

Place all the ingredients in a saucepan. Bring to a boil over medium heat, then reduce the heat to a simmer and cook for 20 minutes, stirring occasionally, until thick and deep red in color. Remove from the heat and let cool completely before refrigerating. Store in the refrigerator in an airtight container for up to 3 weeks.

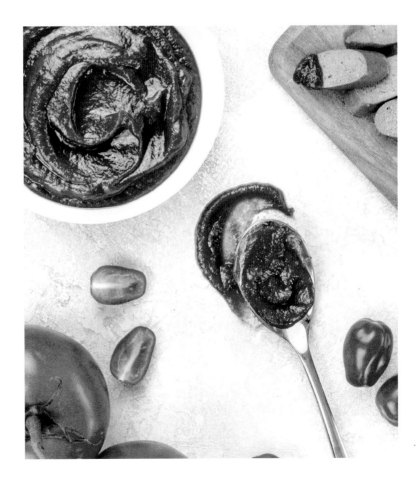

PER SERVING:
CALORIES **13** · FAT **0g** · PROTEIN **0g** · CARBS **8g** · FIBER **1g** · ERYTHRITOL **5g** · NET CARBS **2g**

CHIMICHURRI

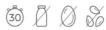

Yield: 1½ cups (2 tablespoons per serving)

Prep Time: 15 minutes

½ cup olive oil

2 tablespoons red wine vinegar or white vinegar

⅔ cup chopped fresh parsley

4 cloves garlic, minced

1 red chili pepper

1 teaspoon red pepper flakes

1 teaspoon dried oregano leaves

1 teaspoon coarse salt

½ teaspoon ground black pepper

This sauce is the king of sauces. It is so versatile, customizable, and flavorful! Chimichurri pairs well with a variety of foods, including steak, chicken, seafood, and grilled or baked non-starchy veggies.

Place all the ingredients in a bowl and stir well to combine. Store in an airtight container in the refrigerator for up to 1 week.

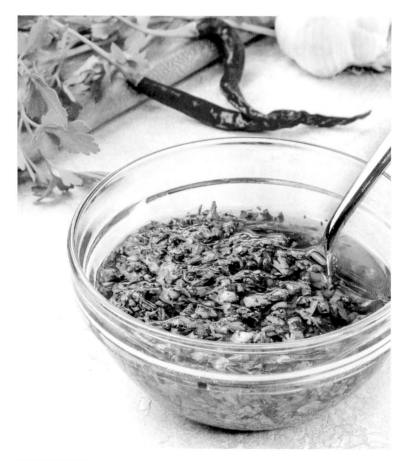

PER SERVING:

CALORIES **85** · FAT **9g** · PROTEIN **0g** · CARBS **1g** · FIBER **0g** · NET CARBS **1g**

KETO YUM YUM SAUCE

Yield: 1 cup plus 2 tablespoons
(2 tablespoons per serving)

Prep Time: 5 minutes, plus 1 hour
to chill

1 cup mayonnaise

1 tablespoon unsalted butter, melted

1½ teaspoons tomato paste, or 1 tablespoon sugar-free ketchup, store-bought or homemade (page 87)

1 tablespoon water

1½ teaspoons Swerve confectioners'-style sweetener

½ teaspoon garlic powder

½ teaspoon smoked paprika

Small pinch of salt

Yum yum sauce is often found in Japanese steakhouses as a dipping sauce for grilled shrimp, chicken, steak, or vegetables. Traditional recipes usually contain sugar and quite a few specialty ingredients. This recipe is quick, easy, and totally keto-friendly.

Put all the ingredients in a small bowl and mix until well blended. Taste and if desired add an additional ½ teaspoon of sweetener for a sweeter sauce. Cover and place in the refrigerator for at least 1 hour. Keep chilled until ready to use. Store leftovers in the refrigerator in an airtight container for up to 1 week.

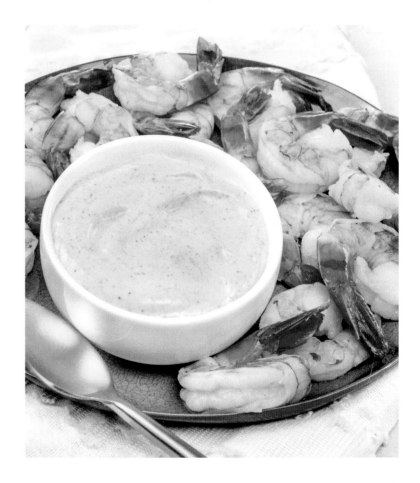

PER SERVING:

CALORIES **173** · FAT **19g** · PROTEIN **0g** · CARBS **1g** · FIBER **0g** · ERYTHRITOL **0.5g** · NET CARBS **0.5g**

ROSEMARY LEMON MARINADE

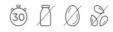

Yield: ½ cup (2 tablespoons per serving)

Prep Time: 5 minutes

¼ cup olive oil

1 teaspoon grated lemon zest

¼ cup fresh lemon juice (about 2 lemons)

2 cloves garlic, minced

2 tablespoons fresh rosemary leaves, finely chopped, or 2 teaspoons dried rosemary leaves

½ teaspoon salt

¼ teaspoon ground black pepper

A perfect all-purpose marinade, great for lamb, pork, chicken, steak, fish, and vegetables. Use ½ cup of marinade per 1 pound of meat or vegetables. Adjust recipe size accordingly.

Put all the ingredients in a gallon-size zip-top bag, seal, and shake. To use, place 1 pound of raw meat or vegetables in the bag with the marinade, then seal and lightly shake to coat the ingredients with the marinade. Place in the refrigerator to marinate for at least an hour.

note While the marinated meat or vegetables are cooking, use the excess marinade to make a sauce. Pour the leftover marinade into a small saucepan and bring to a boil. Boil for at least 5 minutes, stirring periodically, until the marinade thickens into a sauce.

PER SERVING:

CALORIES **126** · FAT **14g** · PROTEIN **0g** · CARBS **2g** · FIBER **0g** · NET CARBS **2g**

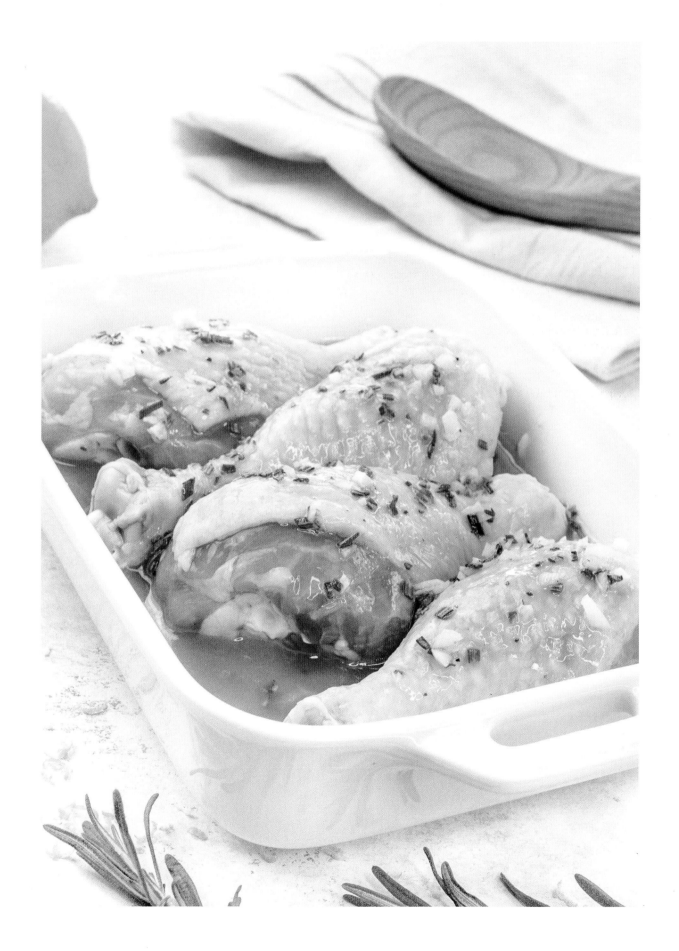

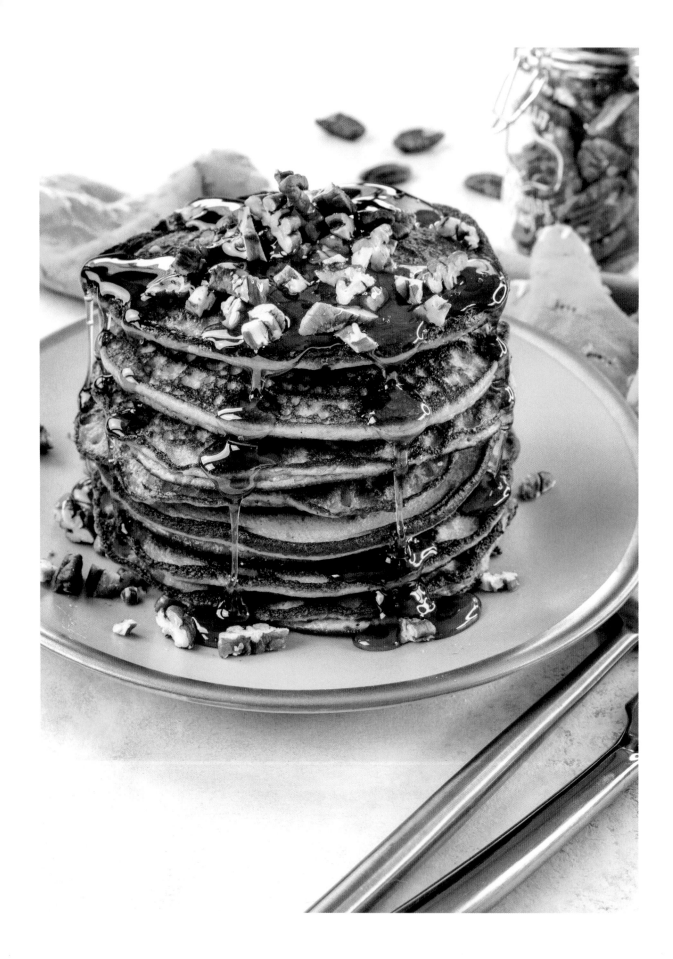

breakfast

SHAKSHUKA

Yield: 6 servings

Prep Time: 10 minutes

Cook Time: 27 minutes

2 tablespoons olive oil

½ cup diced yellow onions

½ red bell pepper, diced

3 cloves garlic, minced

½ teaspoon ground cumin

1 teaspoon paprika

¼ teaspoon red pepper flakes (optional)

1 (14½-ounce) can diced tomatoes

½ teaspoon salt

¼ teaspoon ground pepper

6 large eggs

½ cup crumbled feta cheese

2 tablespoons chopped fresh cilantro

I love one-skillet recipes, and shakshuka is a favorite among my family members. It looks fancy, but it's really simple and absolutely delicious!

1. Preheat the oven to 375°F.

2. Heat the oil in a large cast-iron or other oven-safe skillet over medium-low heat. Add the onions and bell pepper. Cook gently until softened, about 5 minutes. Add the garlic, cumin, paprika, and red pepper flakes, if using; toss together. Pour in the tomatoes and season with the salt and pepper. Simmer until the tomatoes have thickened, about 10 more minutes.

3. Make 6 shallow wells in the sauce and gently crack an egg into each well. Season with additional salt and pepper. Transfer the skillet to the oven and bake until the eggs are set, 8 to 12 minutes, depending on how you like your eggs (8 minutes will give you set whites with runny yolks; 12 minutes will give you set whites and yolks).

4. Sprinkle with the crumbled feta and cilantro before serving.

PER SERVING:

CALORIES **167** · FAT **12g** · PROTEIN **9g** · TOTAL CARBS **7g** · FIBER **2g** · NET CARBS **5g**

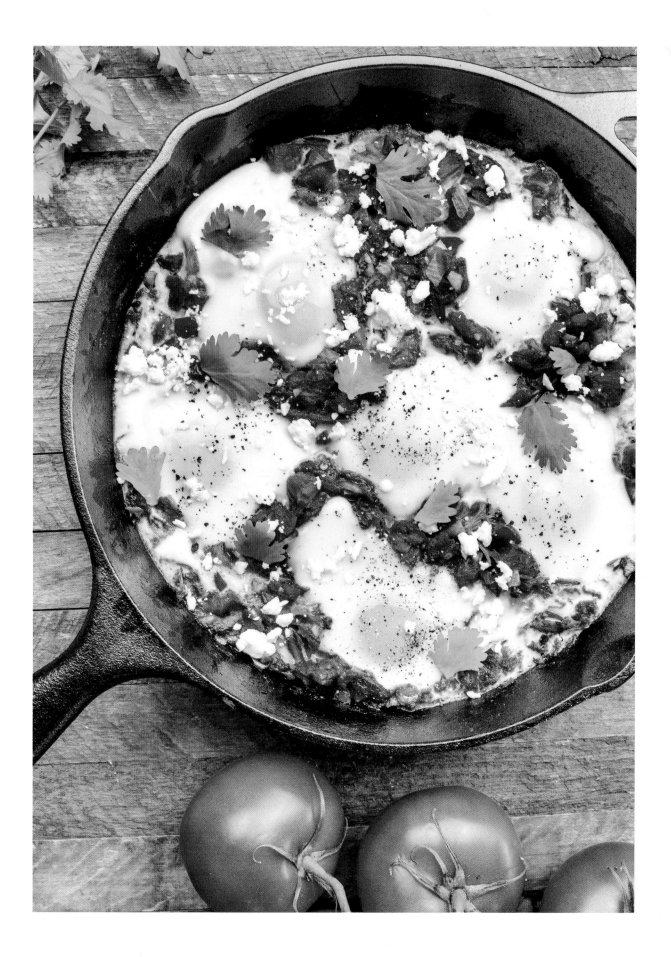

JESSICA'S SPECIAL

Yield: 6 servings (1 cup per serving)

Prep Time: 10 minutes

Cook Time: 20 minutes

3 tablespoons unsalted butter

8 ounces cremini mushrooms, sliced

3 cloves garlic, minced

1 pound ground turkey

¼ teaspoon salt

¼ teaspoon ground black pepper

Pinch of cayenne pepper (optional)

5 ounces baby spinach

6 large eggs, beaten

1 cup freshly grated Parmesan cheese

3 green onions, chopped

Thinly sliced chili pepper or red pepper flakes, for garnish (optional)

My amazing and talented assistant, Jessica, shared this delicious recipe, which has been passed down for generations in her family. It is a perfect example of how simple ingredients can come together to make something really special. This recipe is easy to make and reheats really well for leftovers or meal prepping!

1. Melt the butter in a large skillet over medium heat. Add the mushrooms to the pan and sauté until slightly soft, about 4 minutes.

2. Add the garlic, ground turkey, salt, pepper, and cayenne, if using, to the pan. Cook the turkey until no longer pink, about 5 minutes, using a wooden spoon to break up the pieces into crumbles. Toss the spinach in the hot pan just until wilted.

3. Create a well in the center of the meat/veggie mixture and pour the beaten eggs into the well. Stir the eggs in the center of the pan until curds begin to form, then start stirring the eggs and the meat together. Once the eggs are scrambled and everything is mixed together, stir in the Parmesan cheese and green onions. Serve garnished with sliced chili pepper, if desired.

PER SERVING:

CALORIES **338** · FAT **25g** · PROTEIN **26g** · TOTAL CARBS **3g** · FIBER **1g** · NET CARBS **2g**

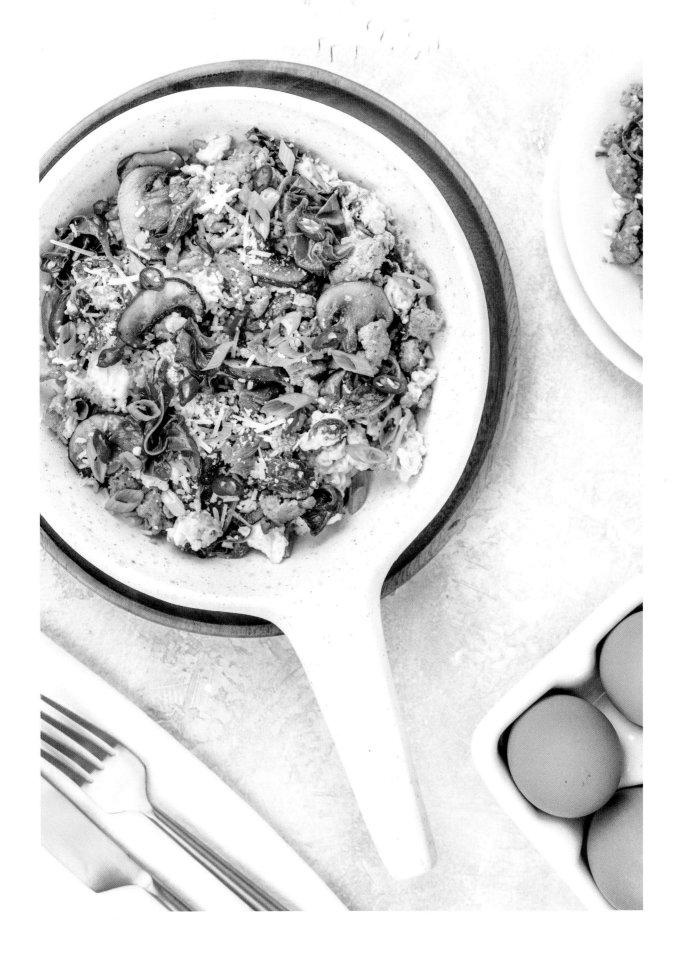

CHILE RELLENOS CASSEROLE

Yield: 6 servings

Prep Time: 10 minutes

Cook Time: 35 minutes

1 (27-ounce) can whole green chilies, drained

2 cups shredded cheddar cheese

4 large eggs

1 cup half-and-half

1 teaspoon hot sauce (optional)

½ teaspoon dried oregano leaves

½ teaspoon salt

SUGGESTED TOPPINGS

Sour cream

Chopped fresh cilantro

Sliced avocado

Sliced green onions

All the flavor of traditional chile rellenos, but without the carbs or the long preparation time! This casserole reheats really well for quick-and-easy breakfasts during a busy week. I like to top mine with sour cream, avocado, and green onion.

1. Preheat the oven to 350°F. Grease a 9 by 13-inch baking pan.

2. Open each chile lengthwise so that it lies flat. Arrange half of the chilies in the bottom of the baking pan in a single layer. Top with half of the shredded cheese. Arrange the remaining chilies over the cheese.

3. Beat the eggs, half-and-half, hot sauce (if using), oregano, and salt. Pour evenly over the chilies.

4. Top with the remaining cheese and bake for 35 minutes, until golden brown. Let stand for 10 minutes before cutting. Serve with the toppings of your choice.

PER SERVING (WITHOUT TOPPINGS):
CALORIES **277** · FAT **20g** · PROTEIN **15g** · TOTAL CARBS **6g** · FIBER **5g** · NET CARBS **1g**

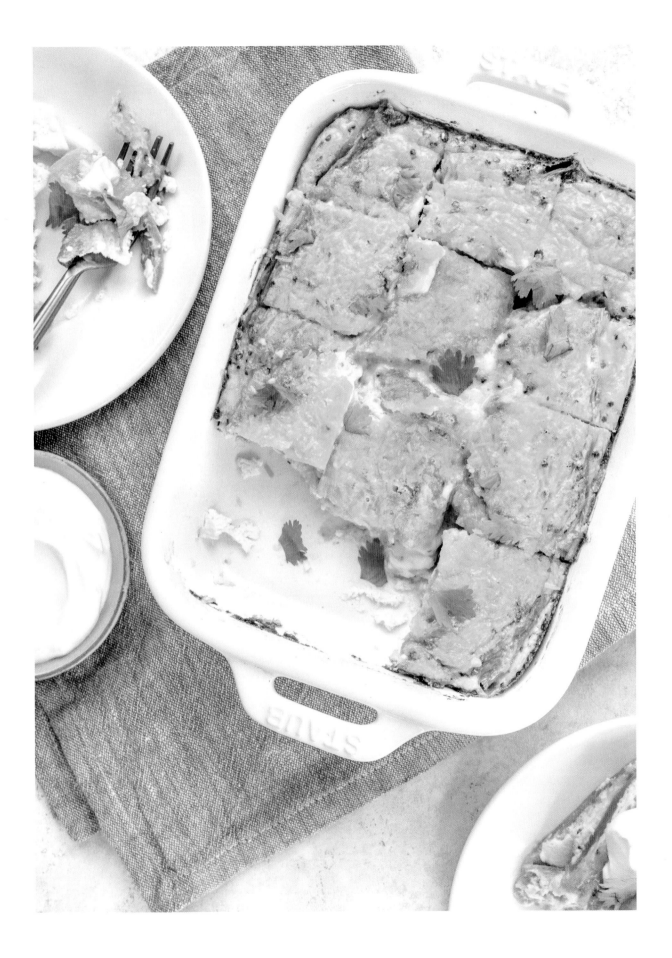

PUMPKIN PECAN PANCAKES

Yield: 6 pancakes (3 per serving)

Prep Time: 5 minutes

Cook Time: 14 minutes

¼ cup canned pumpkin puree

2 ounces cream cheese (¼ cup)

2 large eggs

½ teaspoon vanilla extract

2 tablespoons Swerve confectioners'-style sweetener

1 teaspoon pumpkin pie spice

½ cup blanched almond flour

½ teaspoon baking powder

3 tablespoons chopped raw pecans

FOR SERVING (OPTIONAL)

Butter

Sugar-free maple syrup

I took my original cream cheese pancake recipe and revamped it to incorporate the warm spices and flavors of fall, but these pancakes can be enjoyed all year long!

1. Place all the ingredients, except the pecans, in a blender and blend until smooth.

2. Heat a large skillet over medium-high heat and coat with cooking spray.

3. Pour ¼- to ⅓-cup portions of batter into the pan, two or three at a time, and top each pancake with ½ tablespoon of chopped pecans.

4. Cook until the sides are firm and bubbles appear evenly throughout the top, 3 to 4 minutes. Flip and cook for 2 to 3 minutes on the second side. Repeat with the remaining batter.

5. Serve with butter and sugar-free maple syrup, if desired.

note Double check to make sure you are buying 100 percent pumpkin puree and not "pumpkin pie filling"; the cans look very similar. Also, when you are selecting a sugar-free syrup, try to find one that is sweetened with allulose, stevia, or erythritol.

PER SERVING (WITHOUT BUTTER OR SYRUP):
CALORIES **239** · FAT **19g** · PROTEIN **9g** · TOTAL CARBS **14g** · FIBER **3g** · ERYTHRITOL **6g** · NET CARBS **5g**

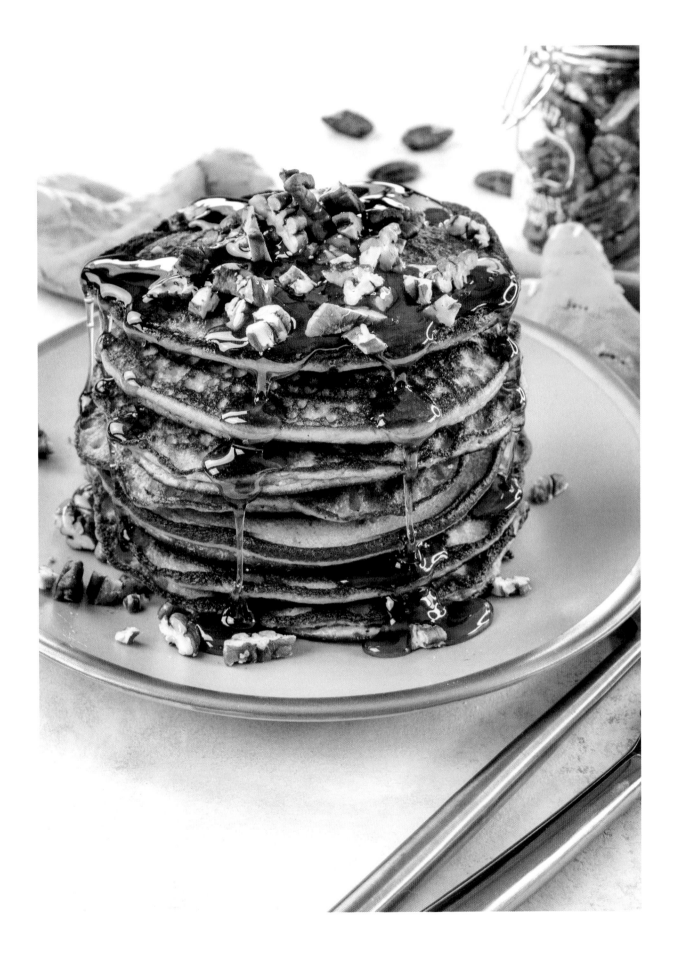

THREE-CHEESE SOUFFLÉS

Yield: 4 soufflés (1 per serving)

Prep Time: 15 minutes

Cook Time: 30 minutes

4 teaspoons unsalted butter, for greasing the ramekins

¼ cup freshly grated Parmesan cheese

½ cup crumbled goat cheese or diced cream cheese

¼ cup shredded Gruyère cheese

7 large eggs

½ cup sour cream

5 tablespoons half-and-half

1 tablespoon water

1 teaspoon Dijon mustard

½ teaspoon cream of tartar

¼ teaspoon salt

¼ teaspoon ground black pepper

Finely chopped fresh chives, for garnish

Special Equipment:
4 (8-ounce) ramekins

Don't worry, making a cheese soufflé is not as daunting as it sounds! Many traditional soufflé recipes have a long list of ingredients and an even longer list of instructions, so I tried to simplify the process. This recipe still achieves a beautiful golden-brown, light and puffy soufflé that's perfect for Sunday brunch. Feel free to experiment using your favorite types of cheeses in place of the Gruyère.

1. Preheat the oven to 350°F. Grease four 8-ounce ramekins with the butter.

2. Pour 1 tablespoon of Parmesan cheese into each ramekin and roll it around so that it coats the bottom and sides. Then sprinkle the other two cheeses evenly into the ramekins and set aside.

3. Using an electric mixer or a blender, beat the eggs, sour cream, half-and-half, water, mustard, cream of tartar, salt, and pepper until bubbles form and the ingredients are well incorporated, about 1 minute.

4. Slowly pour the egg mixture into the ramekins, filling each almost to the top. Bake for 30 minutes, or until the soufflés are puffed up and golden brown. Garnish with chopped fresh chives and serve immediately.

PER SERVING:
CALORIES **242** · FAT **28g** · PROTEIN **19g** · TOTAL CARBS **4g** · FIBER **1g** · NET CARBS **3g**

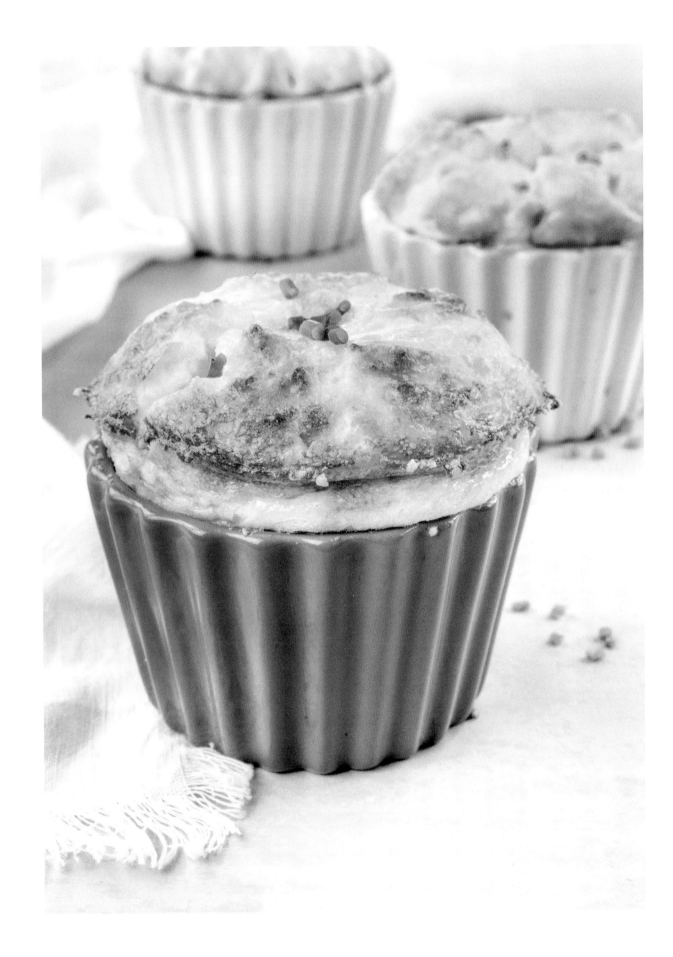

BAKED SCOTCH EGGS

Yield: 6 Scotch eggs (1 per serving)

Prep Time: 15 minutes (not including time to cook eggs)

Cook Time: 25 minutes

¼ cup blanched almond flour

1 large egg

¾ cup freshly grated Parmesan cheese

1 pound bulk pork sausage

6 hard-boiled eggs, peeled

Finely chopped fresh parsley, for garnish (optional)

These Scotch eggs are great served warm, cold, or at room temperature, which makes them the perfect grab-and-go breakfast or snack. They can be eaten as is or dipped in your favorite mustard.

1. Preheat the oven to 400°F. Line a rimmed baking sheet with parchment paper.

2. Place the almond flour in a shallow bowl. Set aside. Crack the raw egg into a second shallow bowl. Beat it slightly and set aside. Place the Parmesan in a third bowl.

3. Divide the sausage into 6 equal portions, then form each into a 3- to 4-inch diameter patty. Mold each sausage patty around a hard-boiled egg, until the sausage fully covers each egg. Pinch the edges together to seal.

4. Roll each sausage-wrapped egg in the almond flour, then dip it into the beaten egg on all sides. Finally, roll to fully coat in the Parmesan cheese. Set the coated eggs on the prepared baking sheet.

5. Spray each egg generously with cooking spray and place them into the oven. Bake for 25 minutes, until they are golden and the sausage is cooked through. Serve warm, cold, or at room temperature. Garnish with parsley, if desired.

note You can also soft-boil your eggs for about 5 minutes if you prefer a softer yolk.

PER SERVING:

CALORIES **367** · FAT **30g** · PROTEIN **24g** · TOTAL CARBS **2g** · FIBER **0g** · NET CARBS **2g**

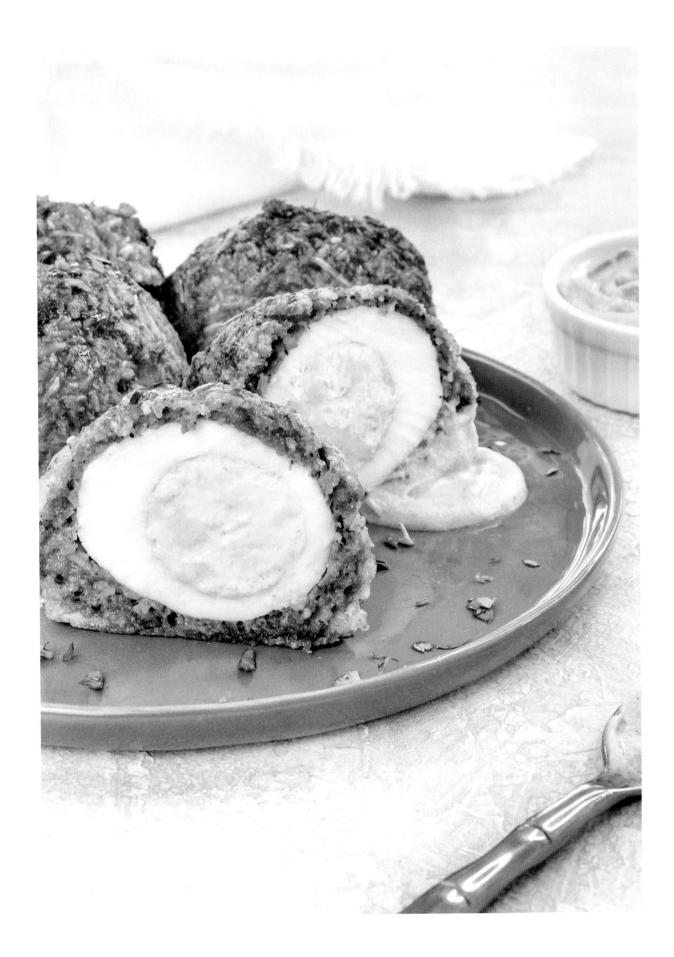

EVERYTHING BAGELS

Yield: 6 bagels (1 per serving)

Prep Time: 10 minutes

Cook Time: 15 minutes

3 cups shredded low-moisture mozzarella cheese

2 ounces cream cheese (¼ cup), cubed

1½ cups blanched almond flour

¼ cup flaxseed meal

1 tablespoon baking powder

Pinch of salt

2 large eggs

FOR THE BAGEL TOPS

1 large egg, for the egg wash

2 tablespoons everything bagel seasoning mix

Variation: Everything Bagel Personal Pizzas. Slice a bagel in half and top with no-sugar marinara sauce (page 82) and your favorite low-carb toppings. Put under the broiler until the cheese is melted.

There are a million keto bagel recipes out there, but I found that using flaxseed meal really makes this recipe special. Not only is flaxseed full of omega-3 fatty acids and fiber, but it also really changes the texture of these bagels to become more "breadlike" than most other keto bagels I've tried. These bagels are great to make the night before because they are even better once they are sliced and toasted!

1. Preheat the oven to 400°F. Line a baking sheet with parchment paper or a silicone baking mat.

2. Microwave the mozzarella and cream cheese for 2 minutes. Take out, stir, and microwave the cheeses for an additional minute. Take out and stir until the cheeses are combined and smooth.

3. In a large bowl, whisk together the almond flour, flaxseed meal, baking powder, and salt. Add the mozzarella mixture and eggs to the dry ingredients and start kneading with your hands. You can also do this in a stand mixer with a paddle attachment. Make sure everything is well mixed together.

4. Divide the dough into 6 equal portions, then form each into a round disk, about ½ inch thick. Using your finger, poke a hole into the center of each disk and mold to form a bagel shape.

5. Whisk the remaining egg in a small bowl. Brush the egg wash on the top of each bagel, then carefully sprinkle the bagel seasoning evenly onto the tops of the bagels.

6. Bake for 12 minutes, until lightly golden brown. Serve as is or slice in half and toast before serving. Store in the refrigerator in an airtight container or zip-top bag for 2 to 3 days or freeze for up to 6 months.

PER SERVING:

CALORIES **302** · FAT **23g** · PROTEIN **20g** · TOTAL CARBS **6g** · FIBER **4g** · NET CARBS **2g**

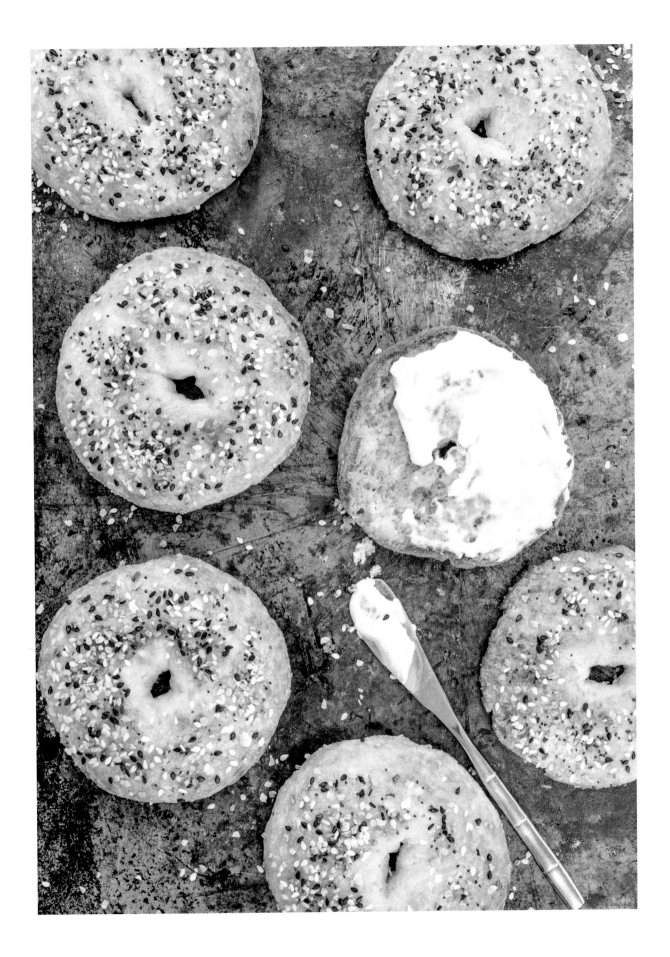

ARUGULA, AVOCADO, AND ASPARAGUS SALAD WITH POACHED EGGS

Yield: 2 servings

Prep Time: 10 minutes

Cook Time: 11 minutes

DRESSING

2 tablespoons olive oil

1 tablespoon fresh lemon juice

½ teaspoon Dijon mustard

Salt and pepper, to taste

SALAD

1 tablespoon olive oil

16 spears asparagus

Salt and pepper

1 teaspoon white or apple cider vinegar

2 large eggs

3 cups arugula

½ avocado, sliced

¼ cup shaved Parmesan cheese

Arugula is one of my favorite greens, and this fresh and delicious breakfast salad is my go to when I need a break from my standard scrambled eggs and bacon.

1. Make the dressing: Place all the ingredients in a bowl and whisk with a fork until blended. You can also make this in a jar with a lid, close, and shake to blend.

2. Fill a medium saucepan with about 2 inches of water and bring to a boil over high heat for poaching the eggs. While the water is coming to a boil, prepare the asparagus.

3. In a medium skillet, heat the tablespoon of oil over medium heat. While it's heating, prepare the asparagus by snapping off the thick ends and discarding. Cut the spears into 2-inch pieces, then add them to the hot oil and sauté for about 5 minutes, until fork tender. Season with salt and pepper to taste and slide the pan off the heat.

4. Once the poaching water is boiling, turn down the heat to maintain a low rolling boil and pour in the vinegar. Carefully crack the eggs into the water and cook for 3 to 6 minutes, depending on how done you like your eggs (3 minutes will give you runny yolks; 6 minutes will give you firm yolks). Remove the eggs with a slotted spoon, place them on a paper towel, and carefully pat them dry.

5. To assemble the salad, toss the arugula and the cooked asparagus with half of the prepared dressing. Divide the salad between 2 plates. Top each with half of the sliced avocado, half of the shaved Parmesan, and a poached egg. Drizzle with the remaining dressing and season with salt and pepper to taste.

PER SERVING:

CALORIES **361** · FAT **33g** · PROTEIN **12g** · TOTAL CARBS **6g** · FIBER **4g** · NET CARBS **2g**

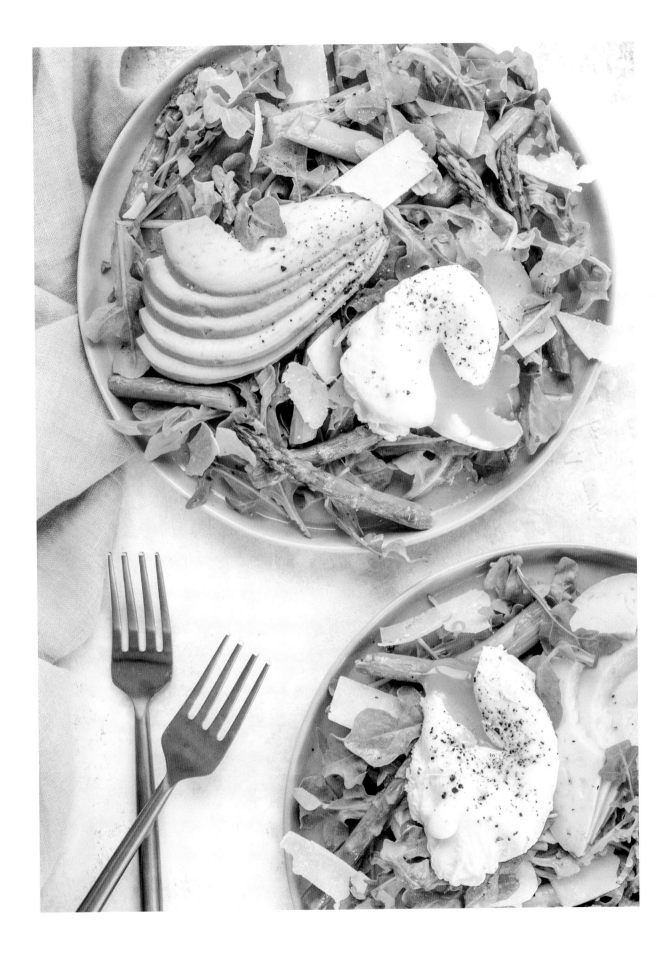

CORNED BEEF HASH WITH RADISHES

Yield: 4 servings (⅔ cup hash and 1 egg per serving)

Prep Time: 10 minutes

Cook Time: 26 minutes

3 tablespoons unsalted butter

12 radishes, quartered

1 small yellow onion, diced

½ green bell pepper, diced

Salt and pepper

1 pound precooked corned beef, diced

2 cloves garlic, minced

1 teaspoon white or apple cider vinegar

4 large eggs

Believe it or not, radishes have a very similar texture and appearance to red potatoes after they are sautéed. This dish pairs well with Sugar-Free Ketchup (page 87) or Sugar-Free Thousand Island Dressing (page 83).

1. Heat the butter in a large skillet over medium-high heat. Add the radishes to the pan and sauté for about 10 minutes, until fork-tender. Add the onion and bell pepper to the pan and continue to cook until they are soft, about 5 more minutes. Season with salt and pepper.

2. Add the corned beef and garlic to the skillet and sauté, stirring often, until the corned beef is crispy on the edges, about 5 minutes. Turn the heat to low to keep the hash warm while you poach the eggs.

3. Fill a large saucepan with 3 to 4 inches of water. Bring to a boil over high heat, then pour in the vinegar. Turn down the heat to maintain a low rolling boil. Gently crack the eggs into the water and cook for 3 to 6 minutes, depending on how done you like your eggs (3 minutes will give you runny yolks; 6 minutes will give you firm yolks). Use a slotted spoon to remove the eggs from the water and gently place them on a paper towel and carefully pat dry.

4. Spoon one-quarter of the hash onto a plate and top with a poached egg. Repeat with the rest of the hash and poached eggs.

PER SERVING:

CALORIES **364** · FAT **29g** · PROTEIN **22g** · TOTAL CARBS **4g** · FIBER **1g** · NET CARBS **3g**

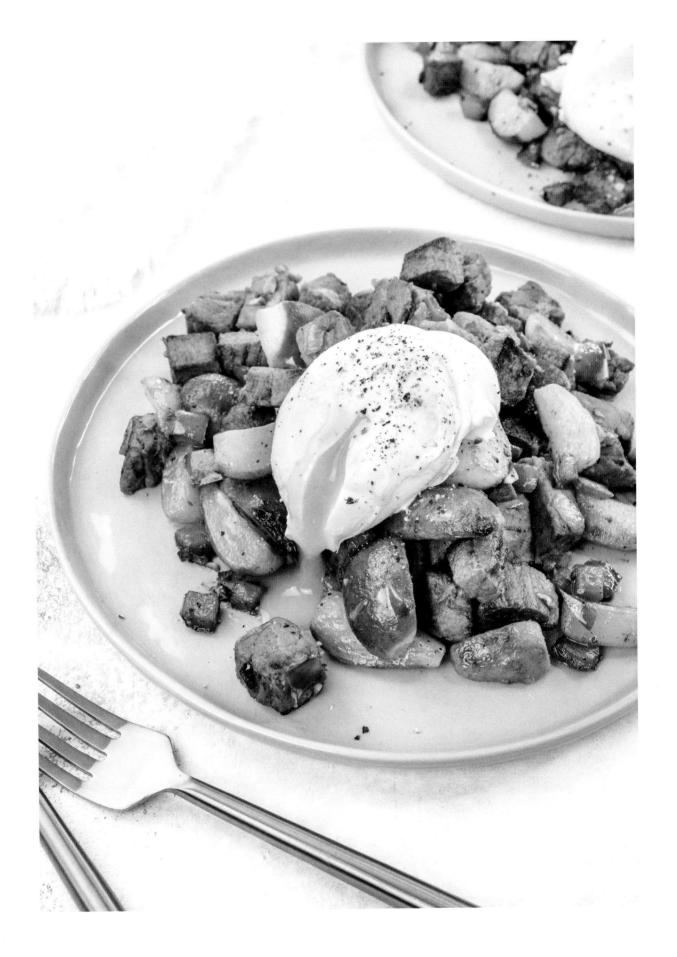

CAULI HASH BROWNS

Yield: 12 hash browns (2 per serving)

Prep Time: 15 minutes

Cook Time: 20 minutes

½ medium head cauliflower, cored and separated into florets

1 cup shredded cheddar cheese

1 large egg

¼ teaspoon onion powder

¼ teaspoon salt

⅛ teaspoon ground black pepper

These cauli hash browns are golden and crispy just like potato hash browns. Even people who claim not to like cauliflower are likely to love these, as they don't have a strong cauliflower taste. They pair perfectly with keto breakfast staples like bacon and eggs, or you can dip them in Sugar-Free Ketchup (page 87).

1. Preheat the oven to 400°F. Coat a standard-sized muffin pan with cooking spray.

2. Use a food processor or cheese grater to rice the cauliflower florets. You should get about 2 cups. Mix the riced cauliflower with the rest of the ingredients in a bowl until well combined.

3. Evenly distribute the hash-brown mixture among the prepared muffin wells, putting about 2 heaping tablespoons in each one. Press down to smooth the tops.

4. Bake for 12 minutes, then use a fork to flip each hash brown over and continue baking for 8 minutes more or until golden brown. Place on a cooling rack or paper towels and allow to set for 3 to 5 minutes. Hash browns will firm up as they cool. Serve immediately, while still warm.

note Use 2 cups of packaged riced cauliflower to save time!

PER SERVING:

CALORIES **99** · FAT **8g** · PROTEIN **6g** · TOTAL CARBS **2g** · FIBER **1g** · NET CARBS **1g**

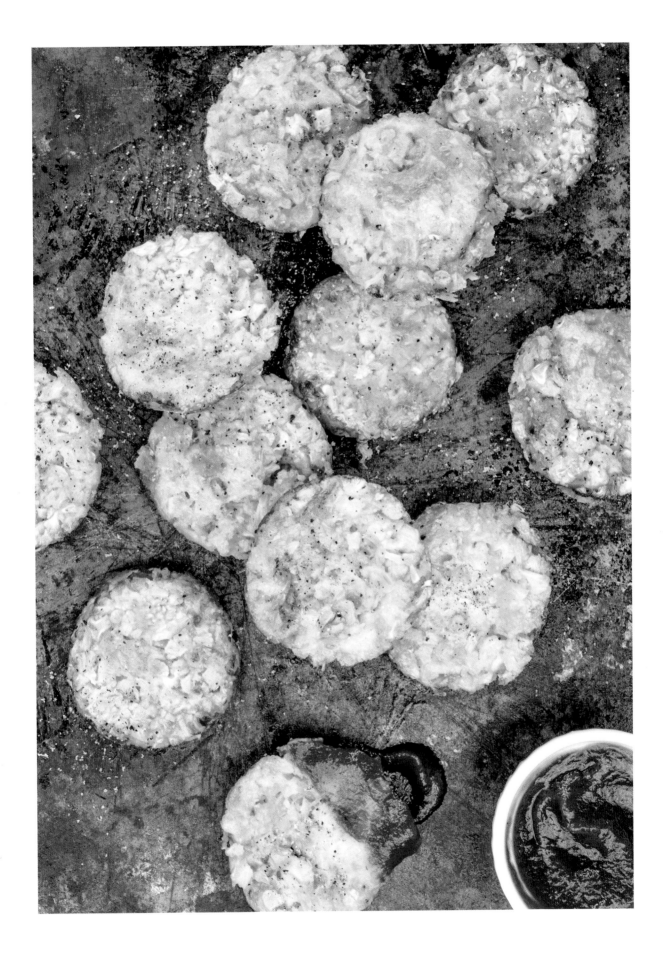

LEMON BLUEBERRY SCONES

Yield: 6 scones (1 per serving)

Prep Time: 15 minutes

Cook Time: 23 minutes

1¼ cups blanched almond flour

3 tablespoons Swerve granular sweetener

1½ teaspoons baking powder

⅛ teaspoon salt

Grated zest of 1 lemon

¼ cup whole-milk ricotta

1 large egg

1 teaspoon fresh lemon juice

2 ounces fresh blueberries (about ⅓ cup)

notes If you want to bake one or two scones at a time, after you slice the dough into 6 wedges, bake only the amount you would like. Wrap the leftover dough wedges in plastic wrap and then aluminum foil and freeze for up to 2 months. You can bake the frozen scone dough wedges straight from the freezer, per the original recipe, but add 3 to 5 minutes to the baking time.

Be sure to purchase a lower-carb ricotta. It should have no more than 1 gram of carbs per 2 tablespoons.

These scones are hands down my favorite recipe to make on a Saturday morning with Olivia. They are flaky and buttery and have the most amazing flavor, with just the right amount of sweetness. If you don't have lemons or you prefer a classic blueberry scone, I've included a simple blueberry variation below.

1. Preheat the oven to 325°F. Line a baking sheet with parchment paper.

2. Mix all the dry ingredients, including the lemon zest, in a medium mixing bowl.

3. Place the ricotta in the center of 2 layers of cheesecloth or a clean, thin kitchen towel. Gather up the sides and wring out excess liquid.

4. Add the strained ricotta, egg, and lemon juice to the dry ingredients, then mix until fully incorporated. Using a spatula, gently fold in the blueberries until combined.

5. Form the dough into a large ball, then place it on the prepared baking sheet. Flatten it to a 6-inch round disk.

6. Slice into 6 wedges as if slicing a pizza, then separate the scones and spread them evenly across the baking sheet.

7. Bake for 20 to 23 minutes, or until lightly golden brown on top. Allow the scones to cool on a cooling rack; they will firm as they cool. Once the scones are completely cooled, store the extras in an airtight container on the counter for up to 48 hours or in the fridge for up to 1 week.

Variation: Simple Blueberry Scones. Omit the lemon zest and lemon juice and add ½ teaspoon vanilla extract.

PER SERVING:

CALORIES **72** · FAT **5g** · PROTEIN **4g** · TOTAL CARBS **6g** · FIBER **1g** · ERYTHRITOL **2g** · NET CARBS **3g**

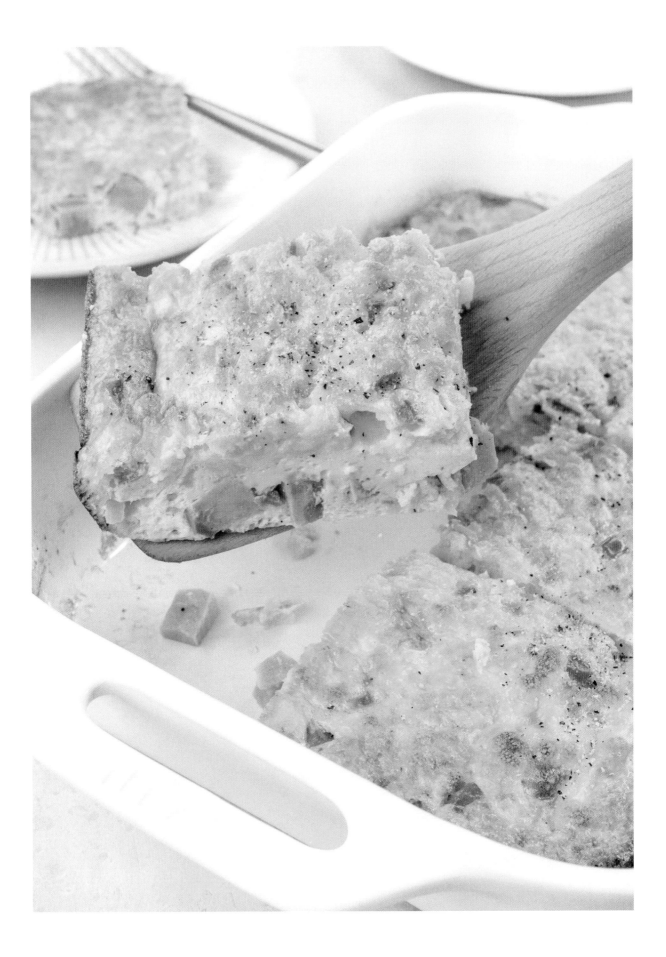

PESTO CHICKEN EGG CUPS

Yield: 4 egg cups (1 per serving)

Prep Time: 5 minutes

Cook Time: 15 minutes

4 slices deli chicken breast

4 tablespoons crumbled feta cheese

4 large eggs

4 teaspoons pesto

Made with only four simple ingredients, these egg cups are great for busy mornings. Feel free to scale the recipe up or down for your needs; for example, sometimes I bake just one or two if I'm running low on eggs.

1. Preheat the oven to 400°F. Coat 4 wells of a standard-size muffin pan with cooking spray.

2. Lay a slice of chicken breast in each prepared well, pressing it against the bottom and sides of the well to make a cup.

3. Put 1 tablespoon of feta into each cup. Crack an egg into each cup, being careful not to break the yolk. Top the egg whites in each cup with 1 teaspoon of pesto, avoiding the yolks.

4. Bake for 12 to 15 minutes, until the yolks are just set and the whites are firm.

PER SERVING:

CALORIES **225** · FAT **15g** · PROTEIN **19g** · TOTAL CARBS **2g** · FIBER **0g** · NET CARBS **2g**

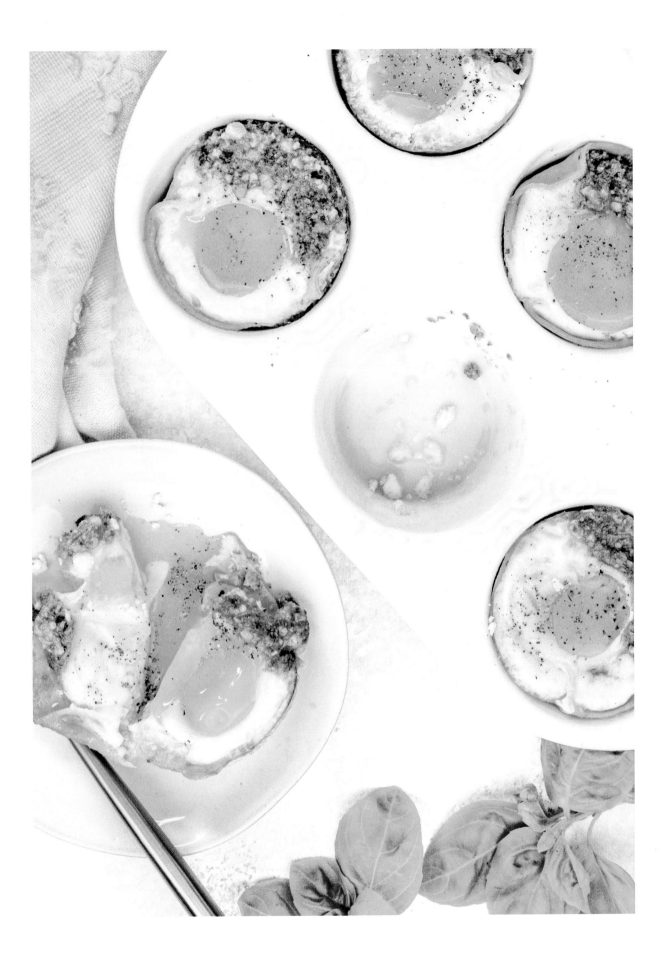

JESS'S KETO COFFEE CAKE

Yield: 9 servings

Prep Time: 20 minutes

Cook Time: 30 minutes

2½ cups blanched almond flour

⅓ cup Swerve granular sweetener

1 tablespoon baking powder

½ teaspoon salt

6 tablespoons (¾ stick) cold unsalted butter, finely diced

2 large eggs

⅓ cup whole-milk ricotta

¼ cup half-and-half

1 teaspoon vanilla extract

CINNAMON SWIRL

⅓ cup unsalted butter, softened

⅓ cup Swerve brown sugar

1 teaspoon ground cinnamon

Who says you can't have your cake and eat it, too? This delicious recipe was created by one of my best friends, Jessica. We had such a great time testing (and tasting) during the development of this recipe, which has turned out to be one of my favorites. Enjoy a slice of this cake with a cup of coffee and some good friends.

1. Preheat the oven to 325°F. Grease a 9-inch square nonstick baking pan with cooking spray.

2. In a large bowl, whisk together the almond flour, sweetener, baking powder, and salt, then work in the cold butter cubes with your hands until combined.

3. In a separate bowl, whisk together the eggs, ricotta, half-and-half, and vanilla until combined, then add to the flour and butter mixture and mix until smooth. Spread the batter evenly into the prepared pan.

4. Combine the ingredients for the cinnamon swirl, then sprinkle the mixture on top of the batter. Using a spoon, work the cinnamon swirl into the top ½-inch layer of the batter. The top layer should be a darker cinnamon swirl color.

5. Bake until the top is golden brown and a toothpick or knife inserted in the center comes out clean, 28 to 30 minutes. Allow to rest for 10 to 15 minutes before serving. Store leftovers in aluminum foil or plastic wrap on the counter for 1 to 2 days, or up to 7 days in the refrigerator.

PER SERVING:
CALORIES **216** · FAT **21g** · PROTEIN **4g** · TOTAL CARBS **17g** · FIBER **1g** · ERYTHRITOL **14g** · NET CARBS **2g**

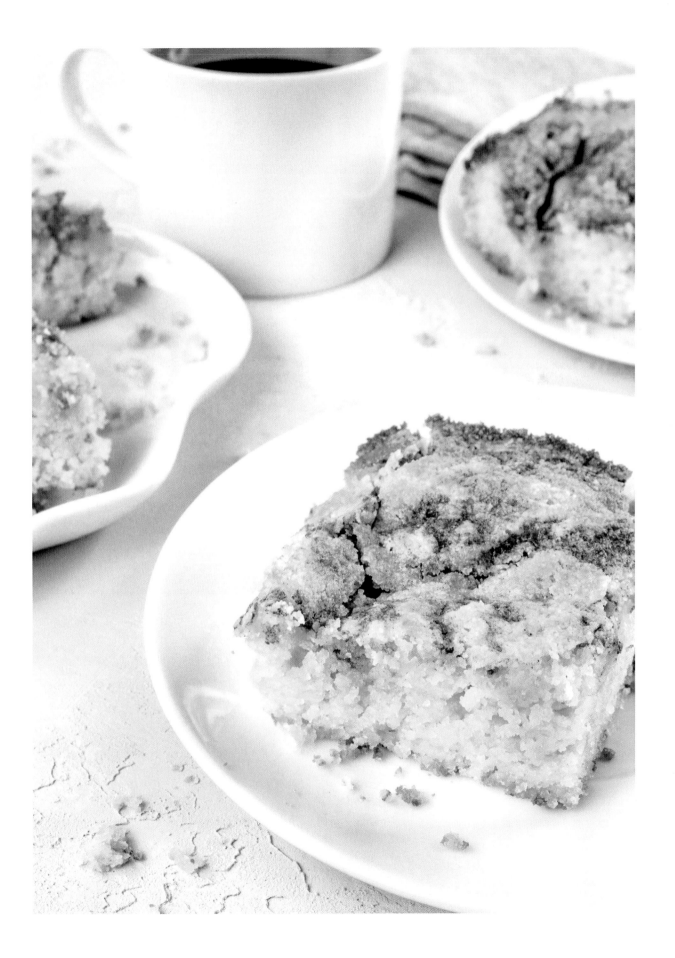

CRUNCHY KETO GRANOLA

Yield: About 8 cups (about ⅔ cup per serving)

Prep Time: 10 minutes

Cook Time: 19 minutes

1 cup slivered raw almonds

1 cup roasted salted peanuts

1 cup raw pecans

1 cup raw pumpkin seeds

½ cup unsweetened shredded coconut

½ cup flaxseed meal

¼ cup chia seeds

1 tablespoon ground cinnamon

¼ cup coconut oil

½ cup Swerve brown sugar or confectioners'-style sweetener

1 teaspoon vanilla extract

1 large egg white

Packed with nuts and seeds, these sweet and salty granola clusters are great for breakfast topped with your favorite nut milk or sprinkled over low-carb yogurt, or enjoyed as is for a quick snack during the day.

1. Preheat the oven to 325°F. Line a rimmed baking sheet with parchment paper or a silicone baking mat.

2. Coarsely chop the almonds, peanuts, pecans, and pumpkin seeds and place in a large bowl. Add the coconut, flaxseed meal, chia seeds, and cinnamon to the bowl with the nuts and mix together using a rubber spatula.

3. Heat the coconut oil in the microwave in a microwave-safe mug or small bowl until completely melted but not hot, 30 to 60 seconds. Whisk in the sweetener, vanilla, and egg white until it is well mixed and has a pastelike texture. It may separate a little bit, but that is normal.

4. Pour the wet ingredients over the nuts and seeds and mix with a rubber spatula until everything is coated.

5. Dump out the granola onto the prepared baking sheet and firmly press down with the back of the spatula until there is an even layer covering the entire baking sheet, about ½ inch thick.

6. Bake for 18 minutes, until golden brown. Take out of oven and let cool completely in the pan. Gently break into small pieces. Store in an airtight container at room temperature and enjoy within 2 weeks.

note You can also use a large food processor to make quick work of chopping the nuts and pumpkin seeds. Just place them in a food processor and pulse 5 or 6 times for a coarse chop.

PER SERVING:

CALORIES **285** · FAT **32g** · PROTEIN **17g** · TOTAL CARBS **17g** · FIBER **8g** · ERYTHRITOL **6g** · NET CARBS **3g**

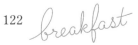

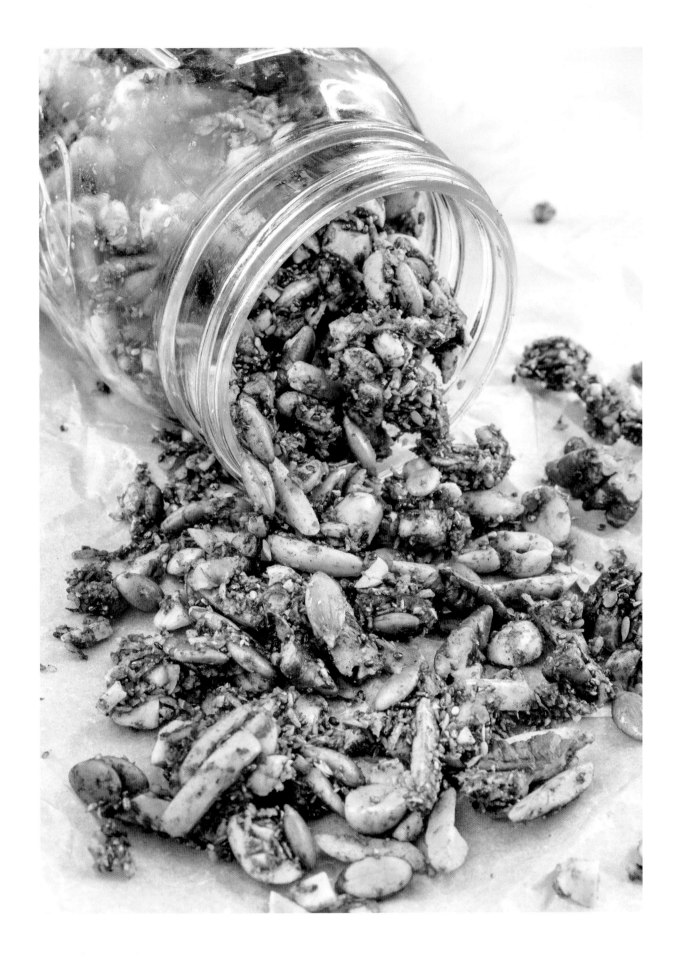

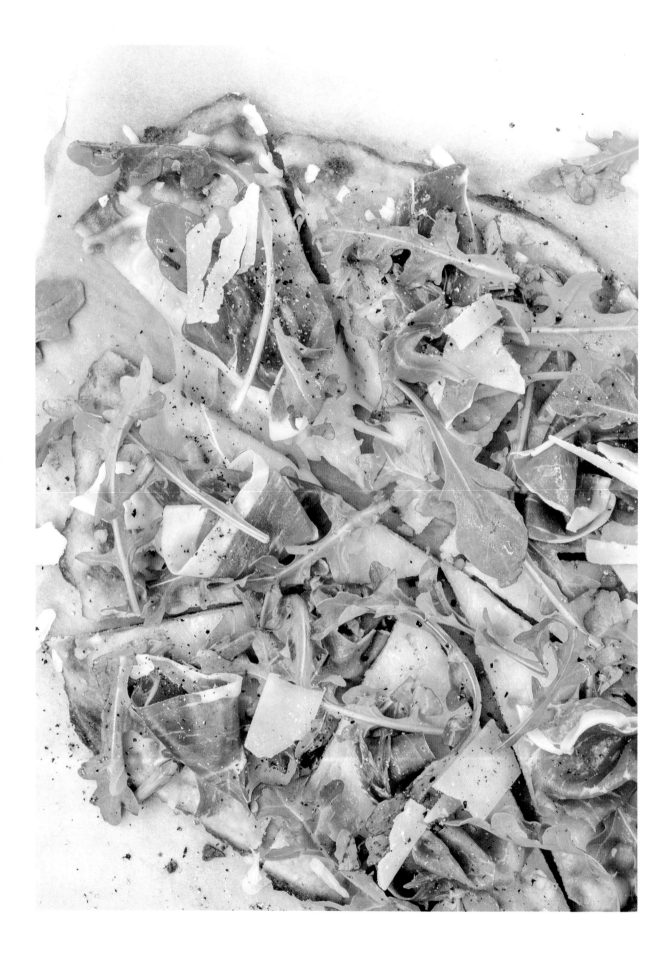

lunch & light meals

SMOKED SALMON SALAD WITH CREAMY DILL DRESSING

Yield: 4 servings

Prep Time: 15 minutes

DRESSING

½ cup crème fraîche or sour cream (see note)

Juice of 1 lemon

1 tablespoon chopped fresh dill, or 1 teaspoon dried dill

1 tablespoon chopped fresh chives, or 1 teaspoon dried chives

¼ teaspoon salt

⅛ teaspoon ground black pepper

SALAD

4 cups mixed greens

¼ red onion, very thinly sliced

8 cherry tomatoes, halved

⅓ English cucumber, peeled and diced

1 tablespoon capers, drained

6 ounces smoked salmon, torn into bite-sized pieces

It doesn't get much better than a nice salad for lunch, with no cook time and minimal cleanup. I love the combination of the crisp veggies with the creamy herbed dressing. If you have never heard of crème fraîche, it is basically sour cream's fancy cousin from France. It has a higher fat content than sour cream, making it an even better keto option.

1. Place all the dressing ingredients in a small bowl and whisk to combine. Set aside.

2. For the salad, toss together all the veggies and capers and divide among 4 plates. Top each salad with an equal amount of the smoked salmon.

3. Drizzle each salad with 2 tablespoons of the dressing.

note Add 1.25 to the total and net carbs if using sour cream instead of crème fraîche. As always, be sure to use full-fat sour cream.

PER SERVING:
CALORIES **167** · FAT **13g** · PROTEIN **9g** · TOTAL CARBS **7g** · FIBER **1g** · NET CARBS **6g**

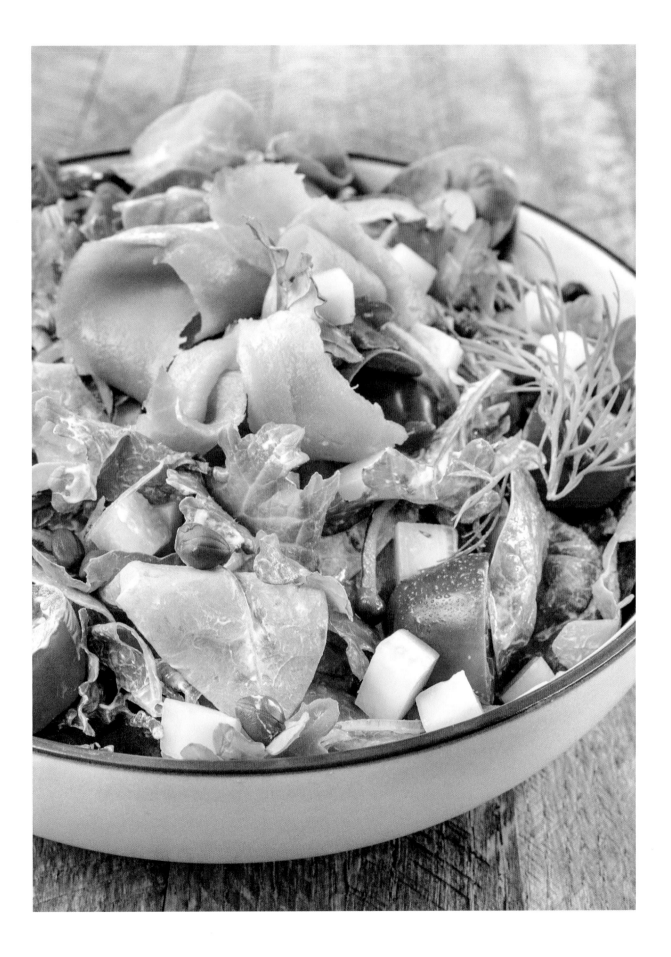

PROSCIUTTO ARUGULA PIZZA

Yield: 2 servings

Prep Time: 15 minutes

Cook Time: 15 minutes

CRUST

⅔ cup shredded low-moisture mozzarella cheese

½ cup blanched almond flour

¼ teaspoon garlic powder

Pinch of salt

2 large egg yolks

TOPPINGS

1 tablespoon plus 1 teaspoon olive oil, divided

1 clove garlic, pressed

1 cup baby arugula

1 teaspoon fresh lemon juice

Salt and pepper

½ cup shredded mozzarella cheese

2 ounces thinly sliced prosciutto

3 tablespoons shaved Parmesan cheese

This makes the perfect quick-and-easy meal for two, or for one with leftovers! (Because everyone loves leftover pizza for breakfast the next day, right?) At first, I was a little skeptical about putting a salad on top of pizza, but, I'm telling you, everything pairs together perfectly to create one of my all-time favorite pizzas. Feel free to swap the toppings to make your favorite pizza.

1. Place an oven rack in the top position. Preheat the oven to 425°F. Line a baking sheet with parchment paper.

2. Make the crust: In a microwave-safe bowl, mix together the mozzarella, almond flour, garlic powder, and salt. Microwave for 30 to 45 seconds, or until the cheese is soft. Knead with your hands until well mixed. Add the egg yolks to the still-warm mixture and continue kneading until incorporated and you can form the dough into a ball.

3. Place the dough on the prepared baking sheet and evenly roll it out to a ¼-inch-thick circle. Poke the crust with a fork a few times to prevent air bubbles from forming.

4. Par-bake the crust on the top rack for 10 minutes.

5. While the crust is baking, prepare the toppings: Mix together 1 tablespoon of the oil and the pressed garlic and set aside. In a separate bowl, toss the arugula with the remaining 1 teaspoon of oil and the lemon juice. Season with salt and pepper to taste. Set aside.

6. When the crust is done, take it out of the oven and flip it over. Brush the oil and garlic mixture on the flat side of the crust. Top the pizza with the mozzarella cheese and place back in the oven for another 4 to 5 minutes, until the cheese is melted.

7. Take the pizza out of the oven and top with thinly sliced prosciutto, then the prepared arugula, and finally the shaved Parmesan. Cut into slices with a sharp knife and enjoy! Store leftovers covered in the refrigerator for up to 4 days.

PER SERVING:
CALORIES **542** · FAT **46g** · PROTEIN **27g** · TOTAL CARBS **6g** · FIBER **3g** · NET CARBS **3g**

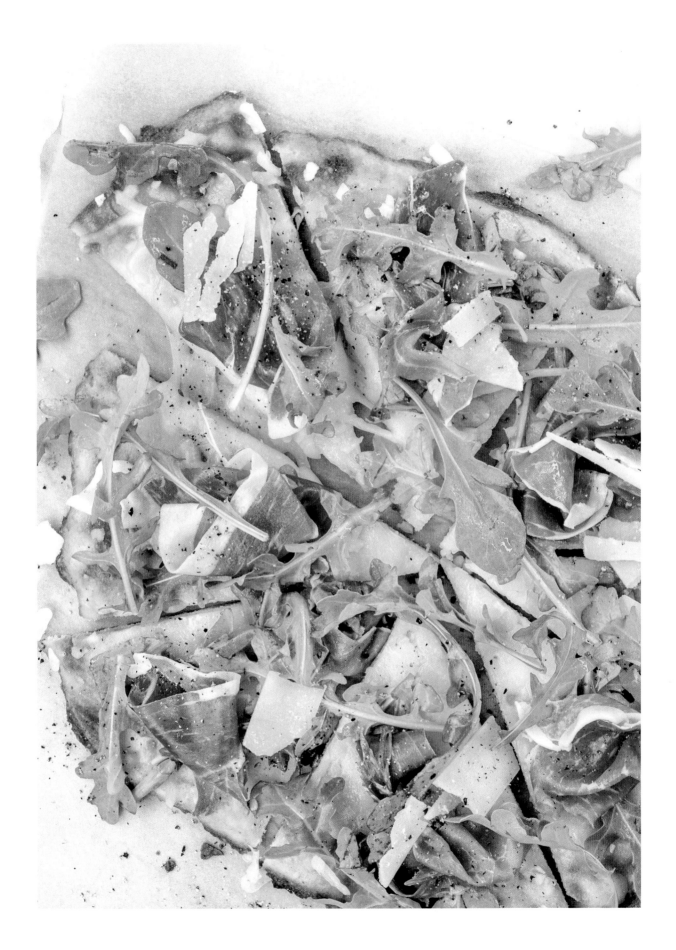

CHEESEBURGER SALAD

Yield: 4 servings

Prep Time: 5 minutes (not including time to make dressing)

Cook Time: 7 minutes

1 pound ground beef

Salt and pepper

6 cups chopped romaine lettuce

1 Roma tomato, diced

1 dill pickle, sliced into rounds

¼ cup very thinly sliced red onions

1 cup shredded cheddar cheese

Bunless burgers are a staple in the keto community. Why not bulk it up and add some extra greens and your favorite creamy salad dressing? I like to pair this salad with Sugar-Free Thousand Island Dressing (page 83) or ranch dressing.

1. Heat a large skillet over medium-high heat and spray with cooking spray. Add the ground beef and brown for 5 to 7 minutes, using a wooden spoon to break up the beef into crumbles. Drain the fat, season with to taste with salt and pepper, and set aside.

2. Divide the lettuce, tomato, pickle, and red onions evenly among 4 serving plates.

3. Top each salad with one-quarter of the ground beef and ¼ cup of the cheddar cheese.

PER SERVING (WITHOUT DRESSING):
CALORIES **345** · FAT **24g** · PROTEIN **30g** · TOTAL CARBS **3g** · FIBER **2g** · NET CARBS **1g**

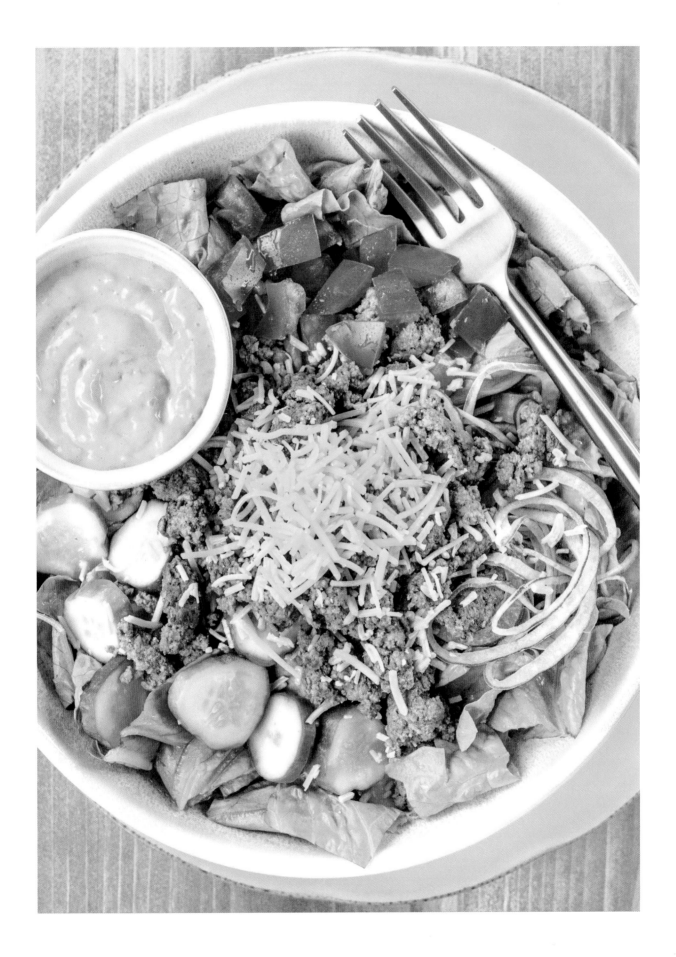

CURRY CHICKEN SALAD

Yield: 6 servings

Prep Time: 10 minutes, plus 1 hour to chill (not including time to cook chicken)

¾ cup mayonnaise

1 tablespoon fresh lemon juice

1 tablespoon curry powder

1 teaspoon turmeric powder

½ teaspoon garlic powder

3 cups cubed cooked chicken breast

2 green onions, chopped

1 stalk celery, chopped

1 tablespoon chopped fresh cilantro and/or parsley

½ cup slivered almonds, toasted

Salt and pepper

This flavorful and colorful chicken salad is perfect for lunch or dinner and is a great choice for meal prepping. This recipe is quick and easy to prepare, and you can save even more time by using rotisserie chicken.

1. In a large bowl, whisk together the mayonnaise, lemon juice, curry powder, turmeric, and garlic powder.

2. To the bowl, add the chicken, green onions, celery, cilantro, and toasted almonds. Stir to combine, then season with salt and pepper to taste. Refrigerate the salad for at least 1 hour to let the flavors meld. Store leftovers in an airtight container in the refrigerator for up to 4 days.

Serving tip:
Serve in butter lettuce wraps and top with additional fresh cilantro and/or parsley or toasted almond slices.

PER SERVING:
CALORIES **278** · FAT **15g** · PROTEIN **29g** · TOTAL CARBS **5g** · FIBER **2g** · NET CARBS **3g**

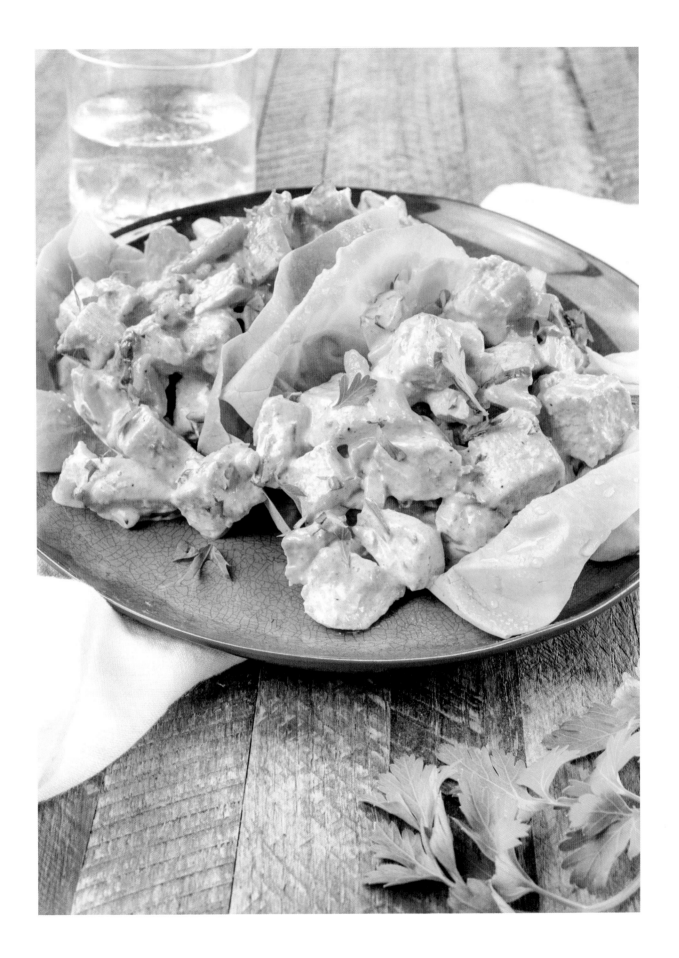

CILANTRO LIME TUNA SALAD

Yield: 2 servings

Prep Time: 10 minutes

1 (5-ounce) can tuna packed in water

3 tablespoons mayonnaise

3 tablespoons chopped red onions

2 tablespoons chopped fresh cilantro

1 avocado, diced

1 stalk celery, chopped (about ¼ cup)

1 teaspoon fresh lime juice

Salt and pepper, to taste

Tuna salad is a nice and simple option for a quick meal, and with a few fresh ingredients, like cilantro and avocado, it's really filling and flavorful! I like to serve it over fresh spinach leaves.

Drain the tuna and break it apart with a fork. Add the remaining ingredients and gently toss until incorporated.

PER SERVING:
CALORIES **313** · FAT **27g** · PROTEIN **12g** · TOTAL CARBS **8g** · FIBER **6g** · NET CARBS **2g**

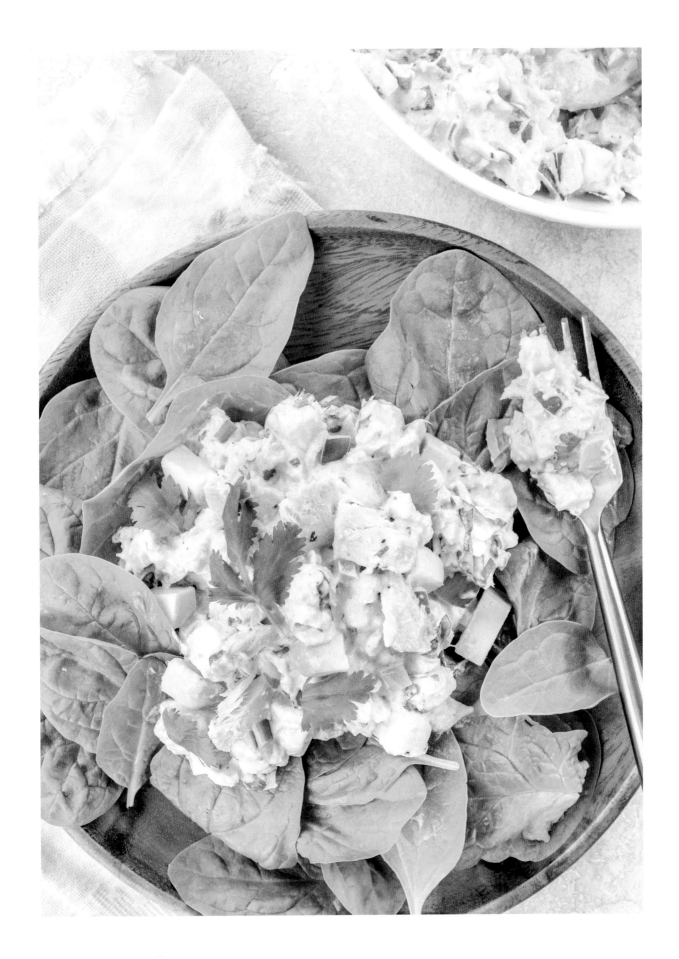

SPICY ITALIAN LETTUCE WRAP

Yield: 1 serving

Prep Time: 10 minutes

4 to 6 large leaves iceberg lettuce

6 slices salami

2 slices Black Forest ham

2 slices prosciutto

1 slice provolone cheese, cut in half

1 tablespoon mayonnaise

1 slice tomato, cut in half

6 slices pepperoncini or pickled banana peppers

Salt and pepper

Everything you love about a classic Italian sub, except wrapped tight in lettuce with a spicy kick.

1. Lay a large square piece of parchment paper (about 14 inches long) on a work surface and arrange the lettuce leaves to make a large rectangle on the parchment. Overlap the edges of the lettuce leaves so that you cannot see any parchment paper underneath.

2. Top the lettuce with the meats, cheese, mayonnaise, tomato, and pepperoncini, then season to taste with salt and pepper.

3. Using the parchment paper, lift up one long side of the lettuce leaf rectangle and begin to roll the lettuce over the fillings. When the fillings are halfway covered, use the parchment to fold in the sides, then finish rolling the wrap forward, as if rolling a burrito. Keep the wrap in the parchment paper and slice in half on the diagonal.

PER SERVING:
CALORIES **415** · FAT **32g** · PROTEIN **28g** · TOTAL CARBS **7g** · FIBER **3g** · NET CARBS **4g**

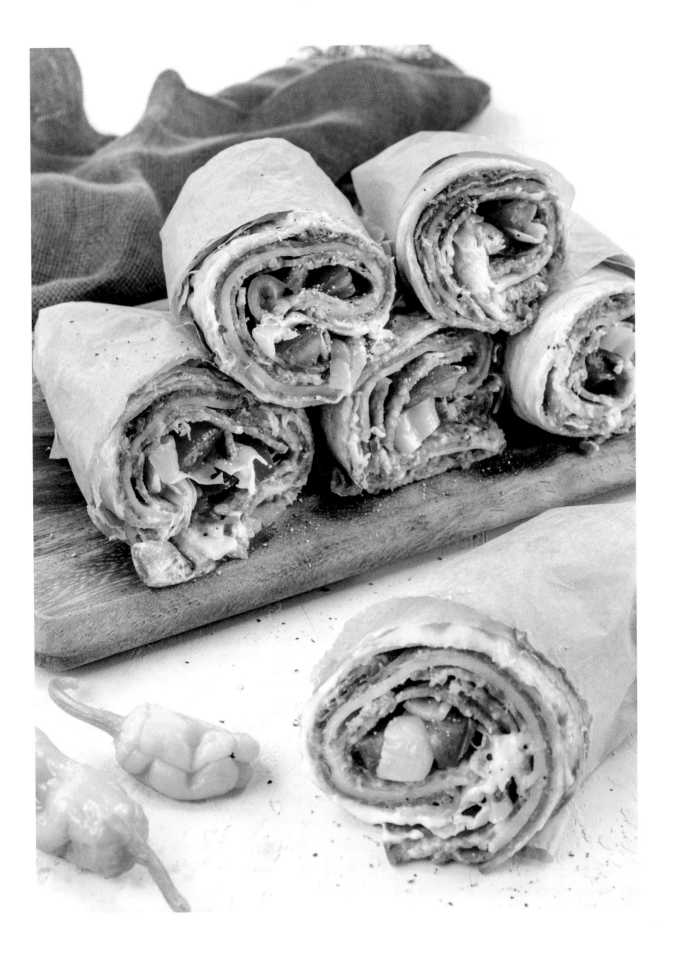

ON-THE-GO COBB SALADS

Yield: 5 servings

Prep Time: 15 minutes (not including time to make dressing or cook eggs or bacon)

10 tablespoons ranch dressing, homemade (page 86) or store-bought

15 cherry tomatoes, halved

2 mini cucumbers, sliced

½ cup sliced red onions

5 hard-boiled eggs, sliced

1¼ cups shredded cheddar cheese

5 slices bacon, cooked crispy and crumbled

10 slices deli turkey, cut into pieces

6 cups chopped romaine lettuce

Not only are these salads delicious, but they are fun to assemble and so convenient to make in advance for a busy week ahead. This recipe makes five salads—one for each day of the work week. I like to chop all the ingredients and then ask Olivia to help pour in each layer.

1. Divide the ingredients evenly among 5 quart-sized wide-mouth mason jars, placing the ingredients in the jars in the order listed. Store the jars in the refrigerator for up to 5 days.

2. When ready to eat, pour the salad from the jar into a serving bowl. Toss to combine the ingredients and enjoy!

Special Equipment:
5 quart-sized wide-mouth mason jars

note Remember that the salad dressing always goes in first to prevent the other ingredients from getting soggy.

PER SERVING:
CALORIES **218** · FAT **16g** · PROTEIN **14g** · TOTAL CARBS **5g** · FIBER **1g** · NET CARBS **4g**

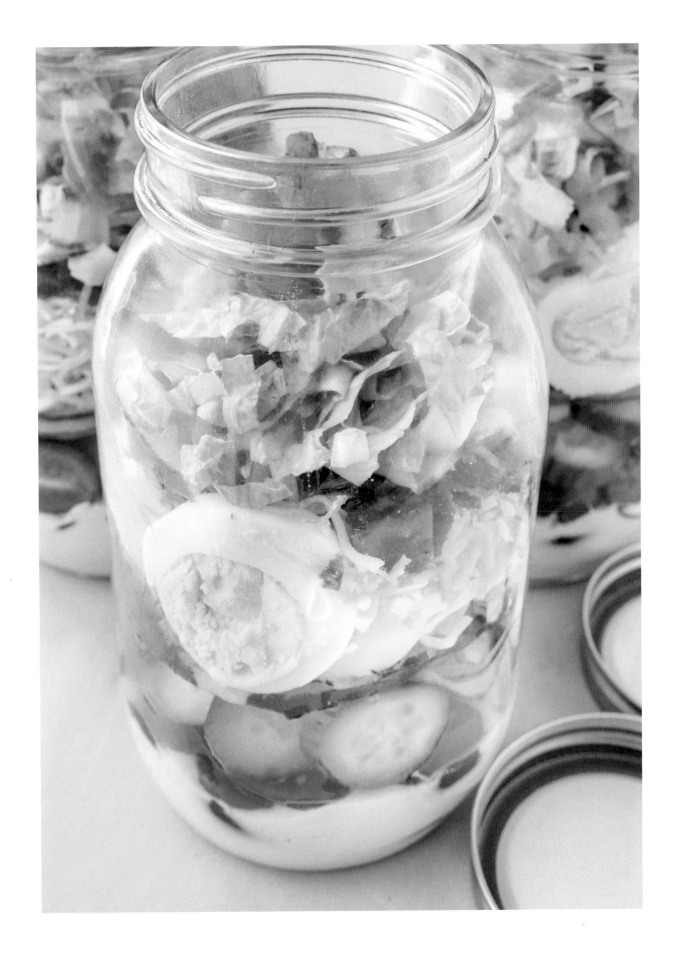

EGG SALAD WRAPS

Yield: 3 servings

Prep Time: 15 minutes

Cook Time: 11 minutes

6 large eggs

6 slices bacon

¼ cup mayonnaise

¾ teaspoon Dijon mustard

Salt and pepper

6 butter lettuce or romaine lettuce leaves

1 small Roma tomato, thinly sliced

Egg salad is yet another make-ahead staple that I often have on hand in my fridge. I like to add a scoop to butter lettuce wraps with bacon and tomato, which has a BLT feel, but with a little more substance.

1. Place the eggs in a large saucepan and cover with cold water. Bring to a boil, then cover with a lid, turn off the heat, and let the eggs stand in the hot water for 11 minutes. Immediately put the eggs in an ice bath.

2. While eggs are in the hot water, cook the bacon in a large skillet until crispy. Remove from the pan and chop into small pieces.

3. Once the eggs are cool, peel and chop the eggs and put them in a medium bowl. To the eggs, add the mayonnaise, mustard, and cooked bacon. Stir until the ingredients are well incorporated. Season with salt and pepper to taste and stir once more to combine.

4. Place 2 lettuce leaves on each serving plate and top with 1 or 2 tomato slices and one-third of the egg salad.

note If you prefer a tangier egg salad, add a splash of pickle juice!

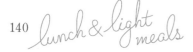

PER SERVING:

CALORIES **352** · FAT **30g** · PROTEIN **19g** · TOTAL CARBS **2g** · FIBER **1g** · NET CARBS **1g**

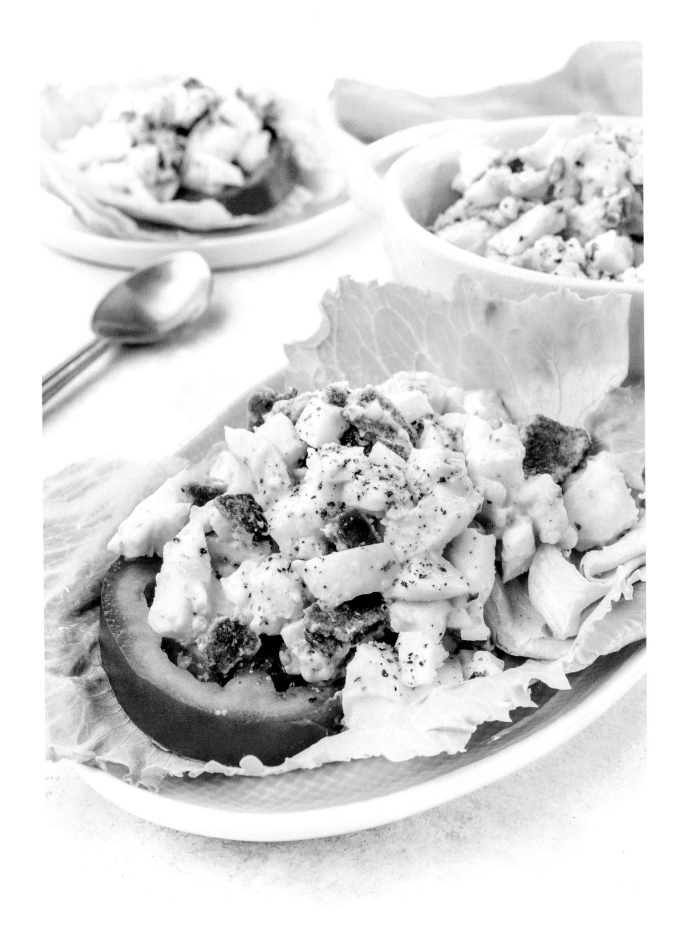

BROCCOLI CHEDDAR SOUP

Yield: 8 servings (1 cup per serving)

Prep Time: 10 minutes

Cook Time: 45 minutes

¼ cup (½ stick) unsalted butter

1 cup diced yellow onions

2 cloves garlic, minced

1 quart (32 ounces) vegetable broth or chicken broth

6 cups broccoli florets

1 cup half-and-half

1 (8-ounce) package cream cheese

2 cups shredded sharp cheddar cheese

1 tablespoon hot sauce (optional)

Salt and pepper

This is a classic creamy soup that your whole family will enjoy. Any leftovers will reheat really well, and oftentimes soups taste even better on the second day!

1. Melt the butter in a large pot or Dutch oven over medium-high heat, then add the onions and garlic and sauté until the onions are soft and the garlic is fragrant, about 5 minutes.

2. Pour in the broth and broccoli florets and simmer uncovered for 30 minutes.

3. Add the half-and-half, cream cheese, cheddar cheese, and hot sauce, if using. Continue cooking and stirring for about 10 minutes, until the cheese is melted and the soup has thickened. Season with salt and pepper to taste. Store leftovers in an airtight container in the refrigerator for up to 4 days or in the freezer for up to 2 months.

PER SERVING:
CALORIES **365** · FAT **28g** · PROTEIN **16g** · TOTAL CARBS **9g** · FIBER **3g** · NET CARBS **6g**

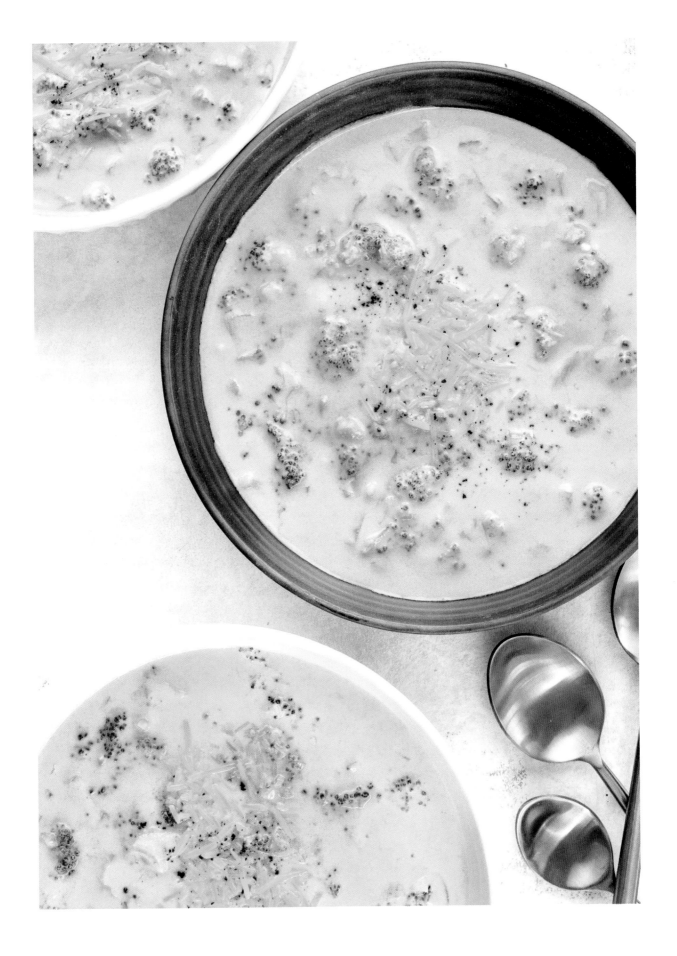

ITALIAN WEDDING SOUP

Yield: 8 servings (8 meatballs and 1½ cups soup per serving)

Prep Time: 30 minutes

Cook Time: 25 minutes

MEATBALLS

¼ medium-sized yellow onion, grated or finely diced

⅓ cup blanched almond flour

⅓ cup freshly grated Parmesan cheese

8 ounces ground beef

8 ounces ground pork

1 large egg

½ teaspoon salt

¼ teaspoon ground black pepper

SOUP

2 tablespoons olive oil

2 stalks celery

2 cloves garlic, minced

¾ medium-sized yellow onion, diced

3 quarts (96 ounces) chicken broth

4 cups spinach

½ cup chopped fresh parsley

Salt and pepper

Freshly grated Parmesan cheese, for garnish (optional)

This soup requires a little extra prep to make the meatballs, but the outcome is a really delicious soup that is always worth the effort!

MAKE THE MEATBALLS

1. Preheat the oven to 400°F. Line a rimmed baking sheet with parchment paper.

2. Place all the ingredients in a large bowl and mix well with your hands. Form into 1-inch meatballs and place on the prepared baking sheet. You should have about 64 meatballs.

3. Bake the meatballs for 20 minutes. While the meatballs are baking, prepare the soup.

MAKE THE SOUP

1. Heat the oil in a large pot or Dutch oven over medium-high heat. Add the celery, garlic, and onion and sauté until the onion is soft, about 5 minutes.

2. Pour in the broth and bring to a rolling boil. Lower the heat and simmer uncovered for 15 minutes.

3. Toss in the cooked meatballs, spinach, and parsley and simmer until the spinach is wilted. Season to taste with salt and pepper (remember that Parmesan cheese is salty, if using).

4. Ladle into bowls and garnish with Parmesan, if desired. Store leftovers in an airtight container in the refrigerator for up to 1 week or in the freezer for up to 1 month.

PER SERVING:
CALORIES **347** · FAT **23g** · PROTEIN **33g** · TOTAL CARBS **5g** · FIBER **1g** · NET CARBS **4g**

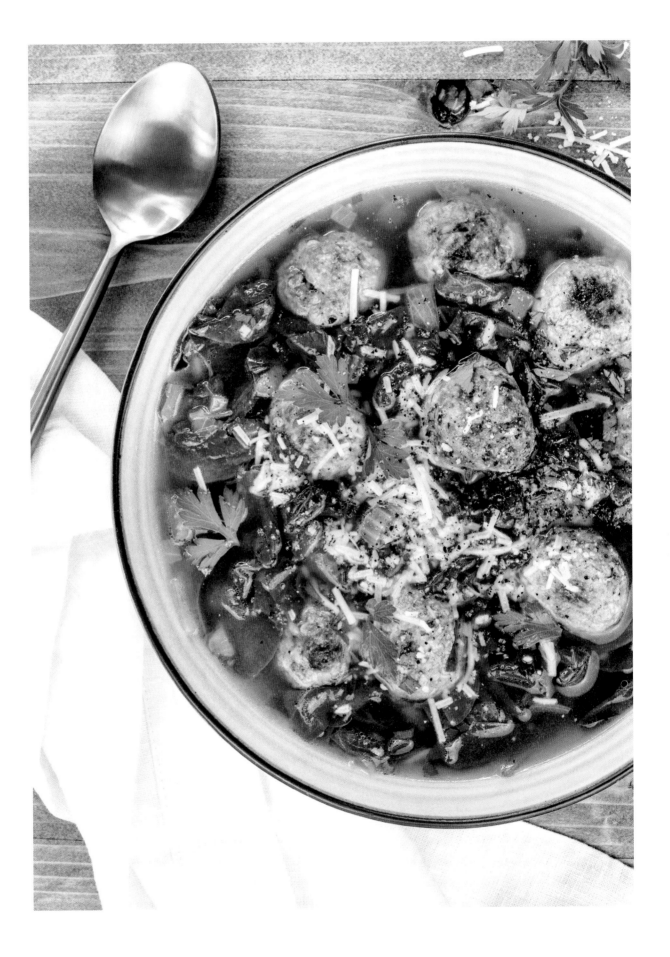

FRENCH ONION SOUP

Yield: 6 servings (about 1½ cups per serving)

Prep Time: 20 minutes

Cook Time: 1 hour 45 minutes

¼ cup (½ stick) unsalted butter

1 pound yellow onions, cut into ¼-inch slices

1 clove garlic, minced

½ teaspoon dried thyme leaves

¼ teaspoon ground black pepper

2 quarts (64 ounces) beef broth

Salt

6 slices provolone cheese

6 slices Swiss cheese

Special Equipment:
6 (12-ounce) oven-safe ceramic bowls or ramekins

French onion soup has always been one of my favorite soups. This flavorful broth is paired with caramelized onions and topped with melty, bubbly cheese. Yum!

1. Melt the butter in a Dutch oven or other large heavy-bottomed pot over medium-low heat. Add the sliced onions and cook until caramelized, 30 to 40 minutes.

2. Add the garlic, thyme, and pepper to the pot and cook for 1 minute.

3. Pour in the broth. Bring to a boil, then reduce the heat and simmer uncovered for 1 hour. Taste the soup and add salt to your liking.

4. Set the oven to the broil setting. Ladle the soup into six 12-ounce oven-safe ceramic bowls or ramekins. Top each bowl with a slice of provolone and a slice of Swiss cheese. Arrange the bowls on a rimmed baking sheet and place under the boiler for 3 to 5 minutes, until the cheese is melted and bubbly.

INSTANT POT METHOD:

Complete Steps 1 and 2 using the sauté setting. Pour in the broth, seal the lid, and set the Instant Pot to pressure cook for 20 minutes. Release the pressure and continue with Step 4.

PER SERVING:
CALORIES **336** · FAT **25g** · PROTEIN **19g** · TOTAL CARBS **8g** · FIBER **1g** · NET CARBS **7g**

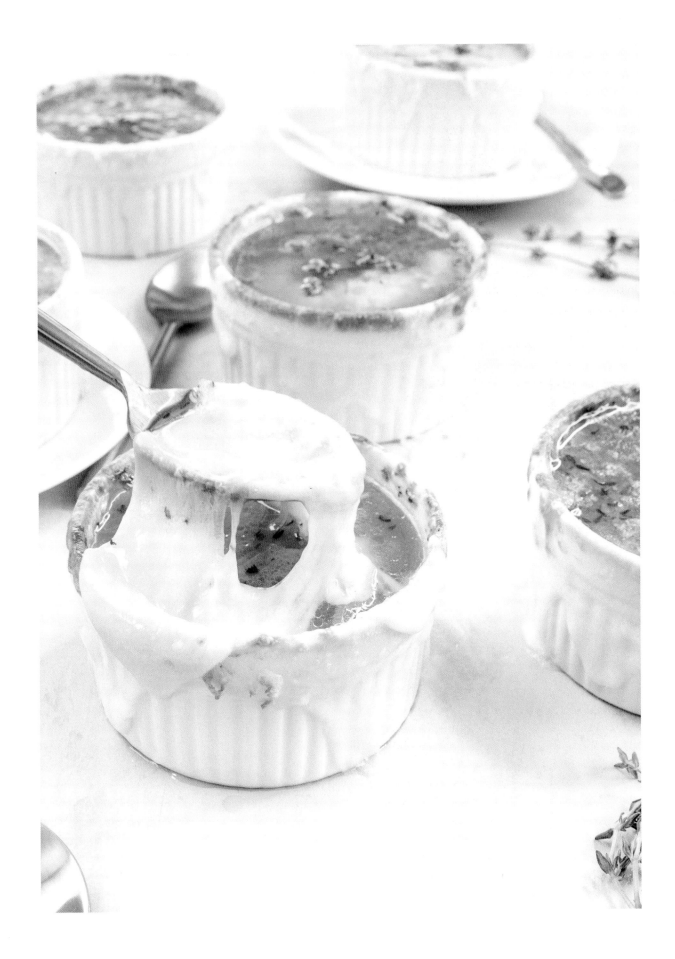

CREAM OF MUSHROOM SOUP

Yield: 6 servings (1 cup per serving)

Prep Time: 15 minutes

Cook Time: 40 minutes

1 tablespoon unsalted butter

½ cup diced yellow onions

2 pounds mushrooms, roughly chopped

2 cloves garlic, minced

½ teaspoon dried thyme leaves, or 1½ teaspoons fresh thyme leaves

1 quart (32 ounces) mushroom or vegetable broth

½ cup heavy whipping cream

1 (8-ounce) package cream cheese

¼ cup sherry or Madeira wine (optional)

With fewer than ten ingredients, this cream of mushroom soup is so easy to make, and it is a hearty and flavorful vegetarian option.

1. Melt the butter in a large pot over medium-high heat. Add the onions and sauté for 5 minutes. Add the mushrooms, garlic, and thyme and cook until the mushrooms are soft and fragrant, about 5 minutes. Reserve a bit of the mushroom mixture for garnishing the soup, if desired.

2. Pour in the broth and cream, then add the cream cheese. Bring to a simmer and continue to simmer uncovered for about 30 minutes, stirring occasionally to make sure the cream cheese is melted throughout the soup.

3. Blend the soup with an immersion blender, or use a regular blender to blend the soup in batches, until the desired consistency is reached.

4. Before serving, add the wine, if using, and stir to incorporate. Garnish with the reserved mushrooms and fresh thyme leaves, if desired. Store leftovers in an airtight container in the refrigerator for up to 4 days.

PER SERVING:
CALORIES **242** · FAT **21g** · PROTEIN **8g** · TOTAL CARBS **6g** · FIBER **1g** · NET CARBS **5g**

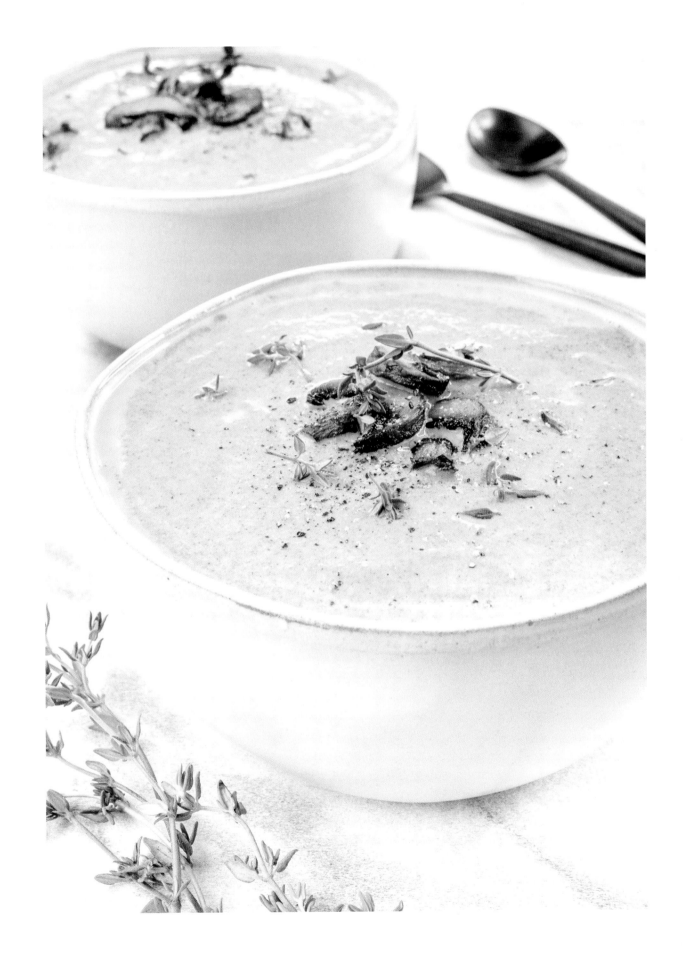

SHREDDED CHICKEN TACO SOUP

Yield: 6 servings (1 cup per serving)

Prep Time: 20 minutes

Cook Time: 8 hours

TACO SEASONING

(Makes ½ heaping cup)

¼ cup chili powder

2 tablespoons ground cumin

2 teaspoons onion powder

2 teaspoons smoked paprika

2 teaspoons dried oregano leaves

1½ teaspoons garlic powder

1 teaspoon salt

½ teaspoon ground black pepper

1 green bell pepper, chopped

½ large yellow onion, diced

1 pound boneless, skinless chicken breasts

1 quart (32 ounces) chicken broth

1 (10-ounce) can diced tomatoes and green chilies, with juices

3 tablespoons taco seasoning, from above or store-bought

¼ cup chopped fresh cilantro

Juice of ½ lime

SUGGESTED TOPPINGS

Fresh cilantro leaves

Diced avocado

Sliced jalapeño peppers

Taco 'bout an easy and delicious slow cooker recipe! When it comes to cooking, I love simple recipes, and this is about as easy as they come! Toss some fresh ingredients into the slow cooker at the start of a busy day and come home to a delicious and warm meal.

1. If using store-bought taco seasoning, skip to Step 2. To make the taco seasoning, put the ingredients in a small bowl and mix together until well blended. (You will use only 3 tablespoons for this recipe; store leftovers in an airtight container for up to a year.)

2. Place the bell pepper and onion in a 6-quart slow cooker. Place the chicken breasts on top, then pour the broth and tomatoes and green chilies (with the juices) over the chicken and vegetables. Add the taco seasoning and stir it into the broth.

3. Cover and cook on low for 6 to 8 hours, or until the internal temperature of the chicken reaches 165°F and the veggies are soft.

4. Remove the chicken from the slow cooker and shred the meat with 2 forks. Return the chicken to the slow cooker, add the chopped cilantro and lime juice, and stir to incorporate.

5. Serve warm. If desired, top the soup with cilantro leaves, diced avocado, and/or sliced jalapeños. Store leftovers in an airtight container in the refrigerator for up to 1 week or in the freezer for up to 6 months.

note This recipe uses my homemade taco seasoning. Of course, you can use store-bought, but homemade is always better! You'll end up with more than you need for this soup, but you'll find many uses for it (and it keeps a long time!). One of my favorite uses is making seasoned ground meat for tacos or taco salads. Use 2 tablespoons of taco seasoning and ¼ cup of water for every 1 pound of ground beef. After browning the meat, drain the fat and add the seasoning and water. Stir well and allow to simmer and reduce for 3 to 5 minutes.

PER SERVING:
CALORIES **145** · FAT **1g** · PROTEIN **21g** · TOTAL CARBS **6g** · FIBER **1g** · NET CARBS **5g**

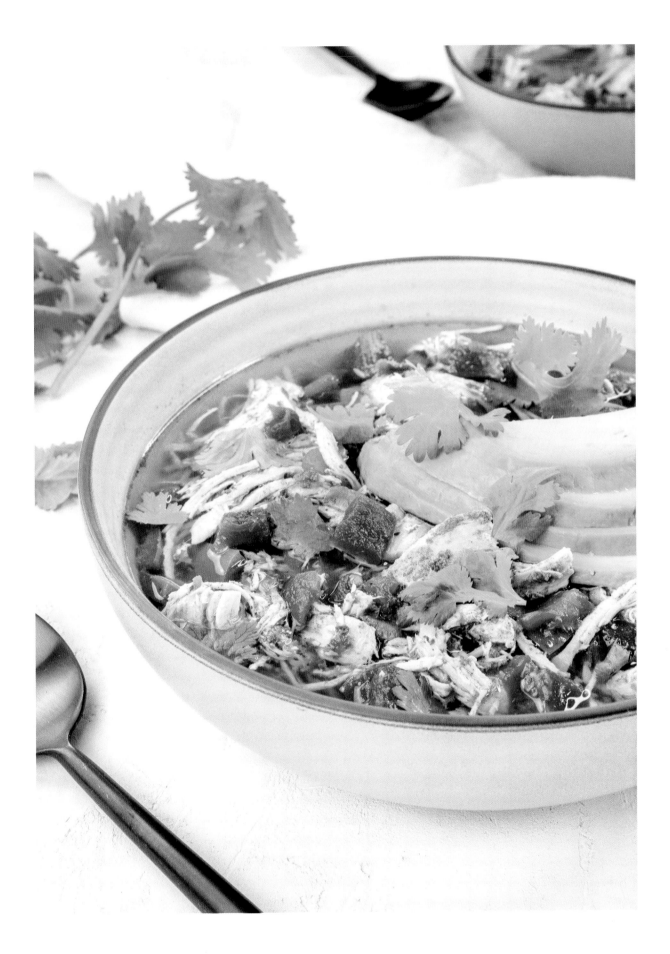

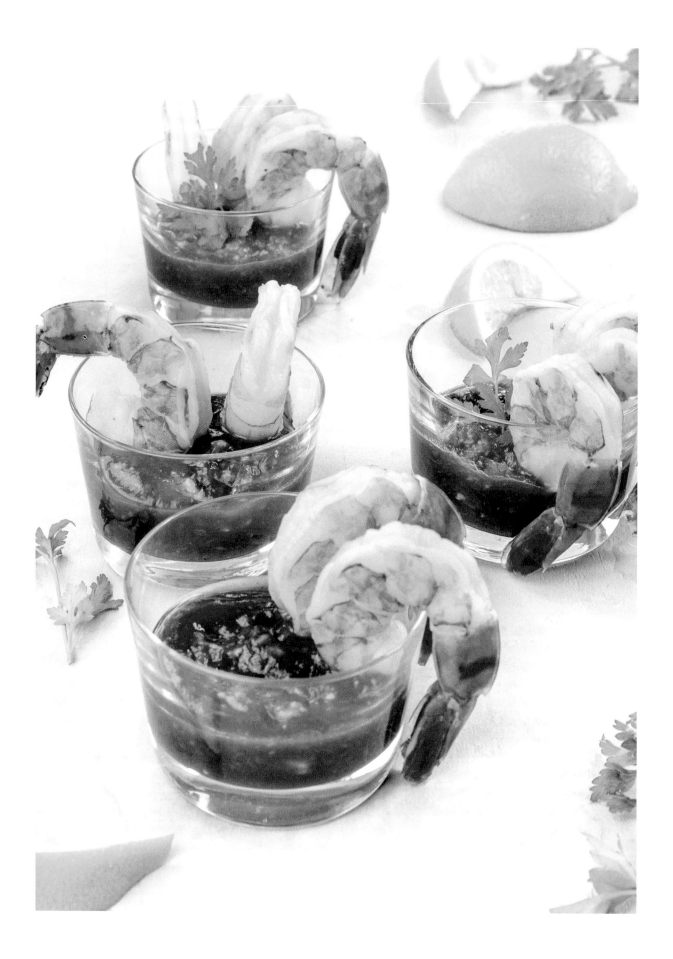

appetizers & snacks

LAMB FETA MEATBALLS WITH MINT YOGURT SAUCE

Yield: 8 servings (2 meatballs and 1 heaping tablespoon of sauce per serving)

Prep Time: 30 minutes, plus 30 minutes to chill sauce

Cook Time: 20 minutes

MINT YOGURT SAUCE

½ cup full-fat Greek yogurt

1 tablespoon fresh lemon juice

1 clove garlic, pressed

½ cup finely chopped fresh mint, plus more for garnish if desired

Salt and pepper, to taste

MEATBALLS

1 pound ground lamb

2 large eggs

1 tablespoon chopped fresh rosemary

1 clove garlic, minced

⅓ cup diced red onions

¼ cup blanched almond flour

1 tablespoon half-and-half

½ cup crumbled feta cheese

¼ teaspoon salt

¼ teaspoon ground black pepper

Pinch of red pepper flakes (optional)

Meatballs make the perfect keto appetizer, and there are so many different ways to prepare them. I love this recipe made with rich and flavorful lamb, paired with a light and tangy mint sauce.

1. Make the sauce: Place all the ingredients for the sauce in a small bowl and mix well. Refrigerate for at least 30 minutes before serving.

2. Make the meatballs: Preheat the oven to 400°F. Line a rimmed baking sheet with parchment paper.

3. Place all the ingredients for the meatballs in a large bowl and mix well with your hands. Form into 16 equal-sized balls, 1½ to 2 inches in diameter.

4. Place the meatballs on the prepared baking sheet and bake until fully cooked through, 18 to 20 minutes. Serve the meatballs on a bed of the sauce, or serve the sauce on the side for dipping. Garnish with additional chopped mint and/or small mint leaves, if desired.

AIR FRYER METHOD:

To make the meatballs in an air fryer, spray the air fryer basket with cooking spray. Cook the meatballs at 380°F for 12 minutes.

PER SERVING:
CALORIES **210** · FAT **15g** · PROTEIN **16g** · TOTAL CARBS **2g** · FIBER **0g** · NET CARBS **2g**

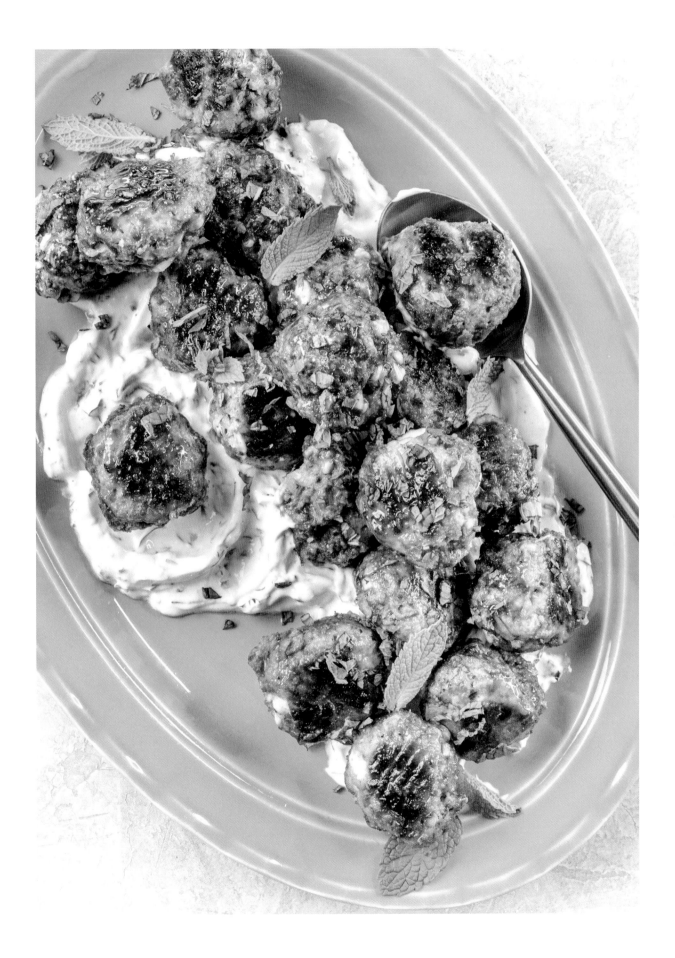

SPINACH ARTICHOKE DIP

Yield: 6 cups (¼ cup per serving)

Prep Time: 10 minutes

Cook Time: 2 hours

1 pound fresh spinach, finely chopped

1 (14-ounce) can quartered artichoke hearts, drained and coarsely chopped

⅓ cup finely chopped yellow onions

3 cloves garlic, minced

1 (8-ounce) package cream cheese, cut into 1-inch pieces

1 cup sour cream

2 cups shredded mozzarella cheese

½ cup freshly grated Parmesan cheese

1 teaspoon salt

1 teaspoon ground black pepper

Hot sauce, to taste (optional)

This versatile recipe is a real crowd-pleaser. For cookouts or parties, you can serve this dip straight from the slow cooker to keep it warm, or you can transfer it to a serving platter with celery sticks, cucumber slices, mushrooms, pork rinds, or keto crackers. If there are any leftovers, the dip can be spread over chicken and baked, stuffed into mushrooms, used in an omelet, or used as a topping for zucchini noodles.

Place all the ingredients in a 6-quart slow cooker and stir to combine. Cover and cook on high for 2 hours. Serve directly from the slow cooker, or transfer to a serving dish.

PER SERVING:

CALORIES **96** · FAT **7g** · PROTEIN **4g** · TOTAL CARBS **3g** · FIBER **1g** · NET CARBS **2g**

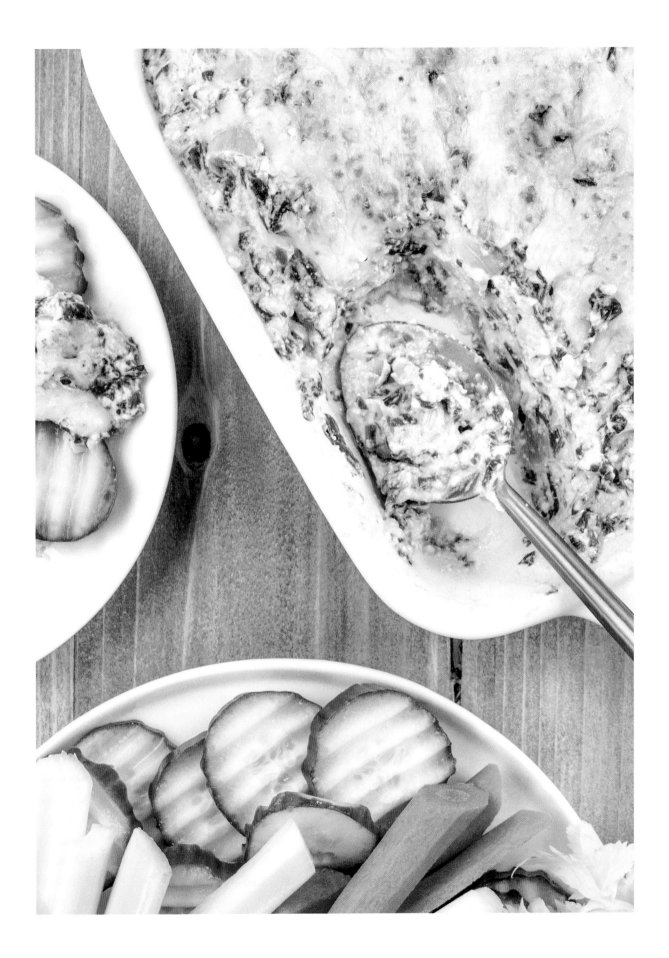

SALT AND VINEGAR WINGS

Yield: 5 servings (about 4 drums and/or flats per serving)

Prep Time: 10 minutes

Cook Time: 1 hour 5 minutes

WINGS

2 pounds chicken wings, drums and flats separated

1 tablespoon baking powder

¼ teaspoon garlic powder

Salt and pepper

SAUCE

¼ cup apple cider vinegar

¼ cup (½ stick) unsalted butter

2 teaspoons salt

Serving tip:
Serve with celery sticks and ranch dressing (page 86).

I have a strong affinity for all things salt and vinegar. These wings are cooked until perfectly golden and crisp without the mess of deep-frying, and then they are finished off in a buttery sauce with a perfect kick of vinegar.

1. Preheat the oven to 250°F. Set a wire rack on a rimmed baking sheet.

2. In a large bowl, toss the flats and drums with the baking powder and garlic powder. Shake off any excess powder and place the wings on the wire rack in single layer.

3. Bake for 30 minutes, then remove from the oven. Spray the chicken with cooking spray and sprinkle with salt and pepper. Flip the drums and flats over and repeat.

4. Put the pan back in the oven and raise the oven temperature to 425°F. Bake the chicken for an additional 30 minutes, until golden brown. Remove from the oven and let sit for 5 minutes.

5. While the wings are resting, prepare the sauce: Heat all the sauce ingredients in a small saucepan over medium-high heat until the butter is melted, then whisk to combine.

6. Place the chicken in a large bowl, pour the sauce over the chicken, and toss to coat.

PER SERVING:
CALORIES **388** · FAT **31g** · PROTEIN **28g** · TOTAL CARBS **0g** · FIBER **0g** · NET CARBS **0g**

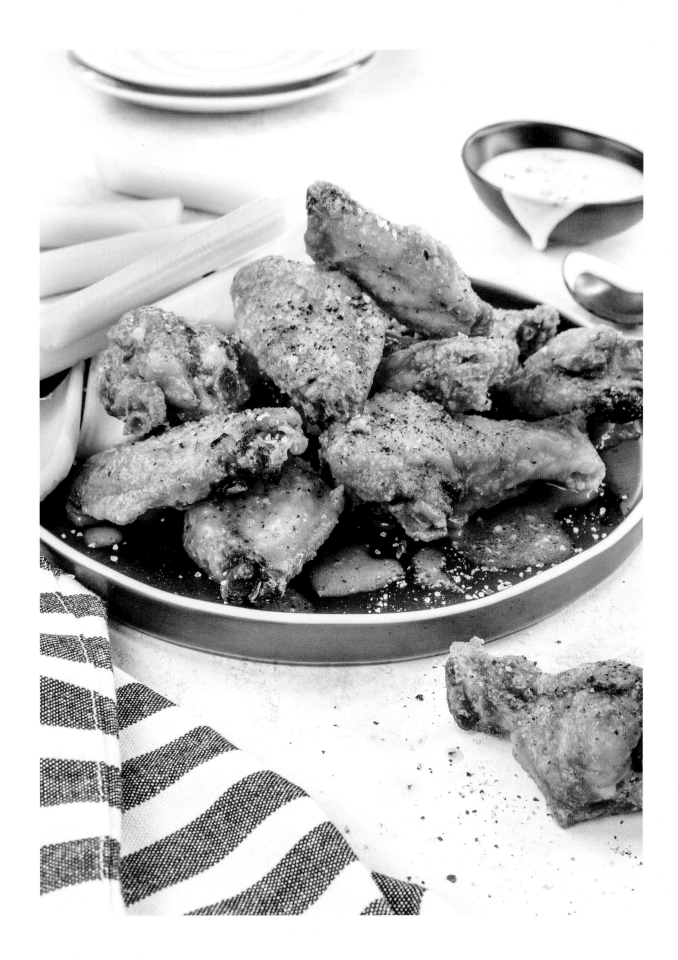

LOADED BACON CHEESE BALL

Yield: 12 servings (3 tablespoons per serving)

Prep Time: 15 minutes, plus 1 hour to chill (not including time to make seasoning mix or cook bacon)

1 (8-ounce) package cream cheese, softened

2 cups shredded cheddar cheese

1 tablespoon ranch herb mix, homemade (page 85) or store-bought

2 green onions, sliced

6 slices crispy cooked bacon, chopped

¾ cup chopped raw pecans

A retro appetizer with a modern flair that is always a hit at any party.

1. Mix the cream cheese, cheddar cheese, and ranch seasoning with an electric mixer until smooth. Fold in the green onions and bacon by hand until incorporated.

2. Place the mixture in the center of a large sheet of plastic wrap. Then cover with the plastic wrap and form into a ball. Refrigerate for at least 1 hour.

3. Put the pecans on a plate. Remove the cheese ball from the plastic wrap and roll in the pecans until well-coated. Store in the refrigerator in an airtight container for up to 1 week.

Serving tip:
Serve with celery sticks, cucumber slices, sliced bell peppers, or pork rinds.

PER SERVING:
CALORIES **222** · FAT **20g** · PROTEIN **9g** · TOTAL CARBS **3g** · FIBER **1g** · NET CARBS **2g**

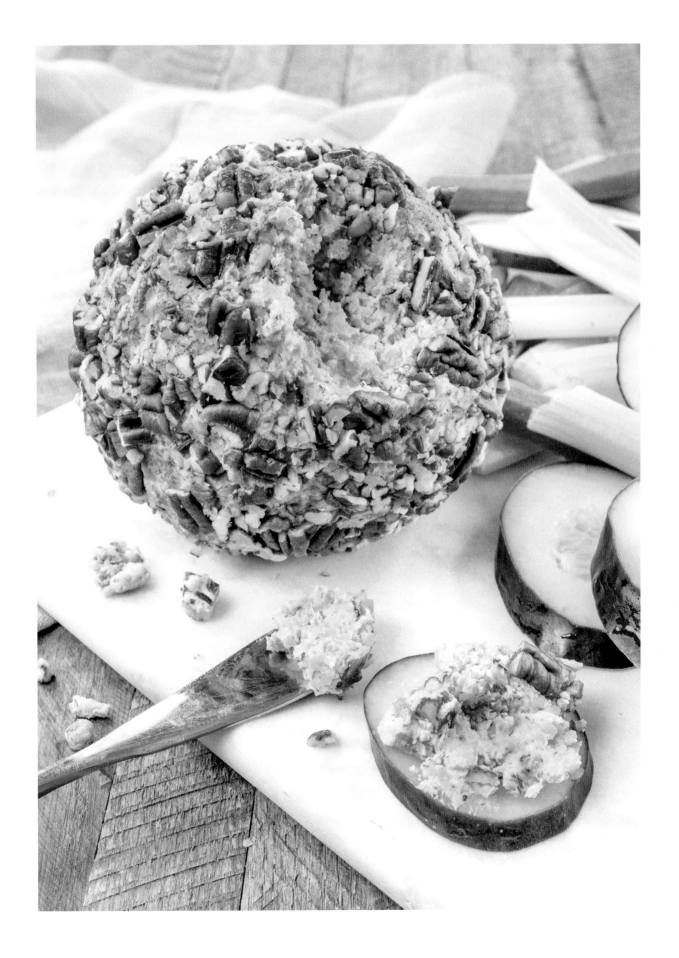

SHRIMP COCKTAIL

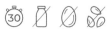

Yield: 5 servings (¼ pound shrimp and ¼ cup sauce per serving)

Prep Time: 5 minutes , plus 15 minutes to chill (not including time to make ketchup)

COCKTAIL SAUCE

1 cup sugar-free ketchup, homemade (page 87) or store-bought

¼ cup prepared horseradish

2 tablespoons fresh lemon juice

1¼ pounds precleaned and precooked large or jumbo shrimp

Fresh parsley sprigs, for garnish (optional)

To make things easier, I usually go to the seafood counter at my local grocery store and buy precleaned and precooked shrimp. It's thawed and ready to use. However, if you eat shrimp frequently, buying precooked frozen shrimp in bulk is often more cost-effective. To thaw frozen precooked shrimp, place the shrimp in a bowl and submerge them in cool water for 10 minutes, then empty the water and repeat this step a second time, allowing the shrimp to soak for another 5 to 10 minutes. Repeat, if needed, until the shrimp are thawed. Drain the water and place the thawed shrimp in the fridge for a few minutes to chill before serving.

1. Mix together all the cocktail sauce ingredients until well combined. Refrigerate for at least 15 minutes, or until ready to use.

2. Serve the chilled sauce in a cocktail glass with the shrimp alongside. Garnish with sprigs of parsley, if desired.

PER SERVING:
CALORIES **132** · FAT **1g** · PROTEIN **24g** · TOTAL CARBS **10g** · FIBER **1g** · ERYTHRITOL **3g** · NET CARBS **6g**

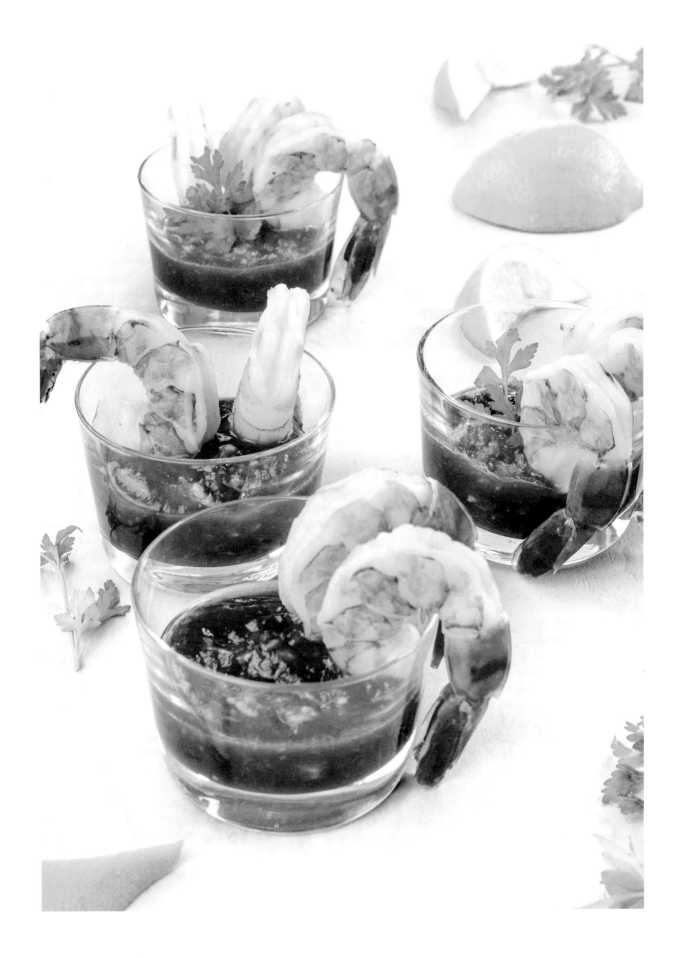

SAUSAGE-STUFFED MUSHROOMS

Yield: 32 mushrooms (4 per serving)

Prep Time: 10 minutes

Cook Time: 37 minutes

1 (8-ounce) package cream cheese, softened

32 large cremini mushrooms (about 2 inches in diameter)

1 pound bulk pork sausage, mild or hot

1 cup chopped fresh spinach

Chopped fresh parsley, for garnish (optional)

These stuffed mushrooms are my go-to recipe for any potluck. They're always a huge hit. As always, I like to keep things simple, so these are made with only four main ingredients! You can prep them in advance and then pop them in the oven (or air fryer) right before serving. I prefer to use cremini mushrooms because I find them to be more hearty, but white mushrooms work just as well.

1. Place one oven rack in the middle position and another rack in the top position. Preheat the oven to 350°F. Set a wire rack on a rimmed baking sheet.

2. Put the cream cheese in a large bowl and set aside.

3. Separate the mushroom stems from the caps. Chop 1 cup of the stems, then set them aside.

4. Brown the sausage in a large skillet over medium-high heat, stirring often to crumble, about 8 minutes. Drain the fat, then pour the warm sausage over the cream cheese.

5. Sauté the chopped mushroom stems in the same skillet until soft, about 5 minutes. Add the chopped spinach and sauté for another 1 to 2 minutes.

6. Add the spinach and mushroom mixture to the bowl with the sausage and cream cheese. Mix well to incorporate.

7. Stuff the mushroom caps generously with the sausage mixture. Place the mushrooms on the wire rack on the baking sheet.

8. Bake on the middle rack for 20 minutes, or until the mushrooms are soft and the tops are golden brown. Transfer the pan to the top rack in the oven and broil on high until bubbly and golden brown, 1 to 2 minutes. Serve warm or at room temperature. Garnish with parsley, if desired.

AIR FRYER METHOD:

To make the stuffed mushrooms in an air fryer, spray the air fryer basket with cooking spray. Cook the prepared mushrooms at 325°F for 16 to 18 minutes.

PER SERVING:
CALORIES **303** · FAT **25g** · PROTEIN **15g** · TOTAL CARBS **4g** · FIBER **1g** · NET CARBS **3g**

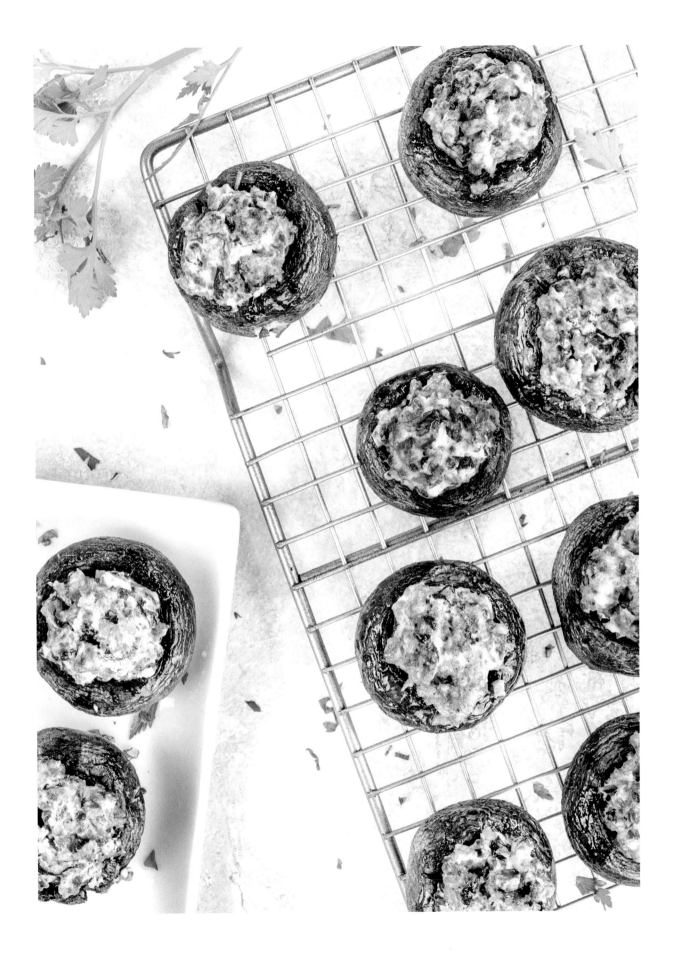

MINI SPINACH SOUFFLÉS

Yield: 12 soufflés (1 per serving)

Prep Time: 10 minutes

Cook Time: 20 minutes

2 (10-ounce) packages frozen chopped spinach, thawed

1 cup freshly grated Parmesan cheese

½ cup blanched almond flour

5 large eggs, lightly beaten

6 tablespoons (¾ stick) unsalted butter, melted and cooled

¼ cup heavy whipping cream

2 cloves garlic, minced

½ teaspoon salt

These delicious and easy soufflés can be served as an appetizer or side dish! I love to slice these in half and smear each side with salted butter.

1. Preheat the oven to 350°F. Coat a standard-size muffin pan with cooking spray.

2. Squeeze the spinach well in cheesecloth or paper towels to remove the excess liquid. Put the spinach along with the rest of the ingredients in a large bowl and stir to combine.

3. Divide the spinach mixture evenly among the muffin wells, using a little less than ¼ cup for each one.

4. Bake until lightly golden brown on top, about 20 minutes; a toothpick or knife inserted in the center should come out clean. Allow to cool in the pan for 5 minutes before transferring the soufflés to a serving dish. Store leftovers in an airtight container in the refrigerator for up to 3 days.

PER SERVING:

CALORIES **149** · FAT **12g** · PROTEIN **7g** · TOTAL CARBS **2g** · FIBER **1g** · NET CARBS **1g**

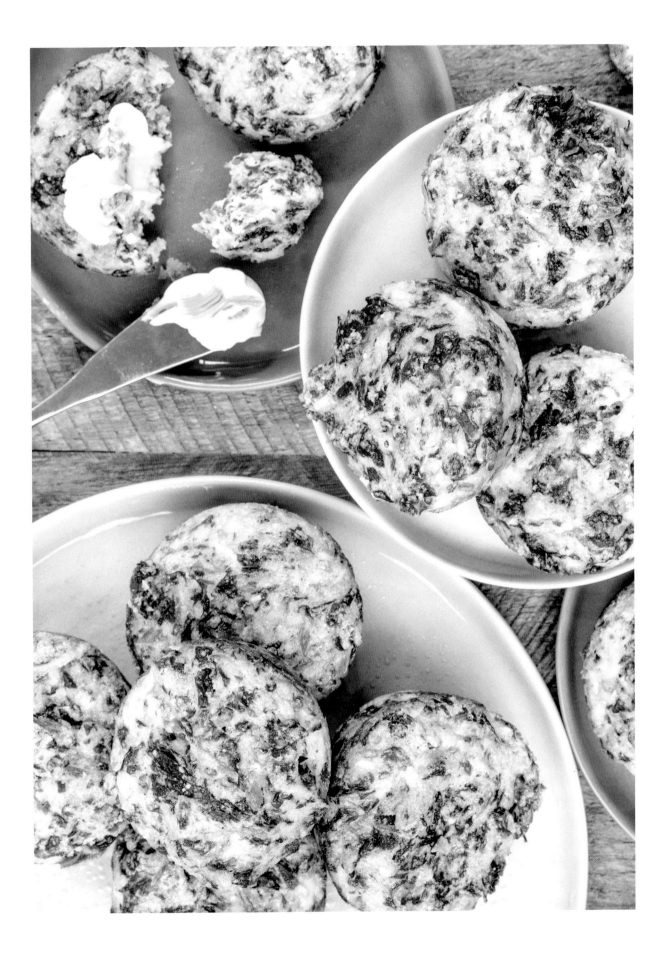

HERBED DEVILED EGGS

Yield: 12 deviled eggs (2 per serving)

Prep Time: 20 minutes

Cook Time: 11 minutes

6 large eggs

½ cup packed fresh parsley leaves

6 fresh basil leaves

1 clove garlic, peeled

1 green onion, coarsely chopped

3 tablespoons freshly grated Parmesan cheese

1 tablespoon fresh lemon juice

2 teaspoons Dijon mustard

1 teaspoon salt

½ teaspoon ground black pepper

Pinch of red pepper flakes

3 tablespoons olive oil

Chopped fresh parsley, for garnish (optional)

There are a million different ways to make deviled eggs, but I love this recipe because it is packed with flavor from the fresh herbs. If you're short on time, or if you like shortcuts like I do, look for packaged hard-boiled eggs at your local market.

1. Place the eggs in a large saucepan and cover with cold water. Bring to a boil, then cover with the lid, turn off the heat, and let the eggs stand in the hot water for 11 minutes. Immediately put the eggs in an ice bath to cool until ready to peel and use.

2. While the eggs are cooling, place the parsley, basil, garlic, green onion, Parmesan cheese, lemon juice, mustard, salt, black pepper, and red pepper flakes in a food processor. Turn it to high speed and drizzle the olive oil into the food processor until the mixture develops a pastelike consistency.

3. Peel the hard-boiled eggs and cut them in half. Scoop the yolks into a medium bowl and set the whites aside.

4. Add the herb mixture from the food processor to the bowl with the egg yolks and mash until the ingredients are well incorporated and there are no lumps. Transfer the yolk mixture to a zip-top plastic bag and cut off one corner of the bag.

5. Fill the egg white halves evenly with the yolk mixture. If desired, sprinkle with additional salt and pepper and garnish with parsley just before serving. Store covered in the refrigerator for up to 3 days.

PER SERVING:

CALORIES **144** · FAT **13g** · PROTEIN **7g** · TOTAL CARBS **1g** · FIBER **0g** · NET CARBS **1g**

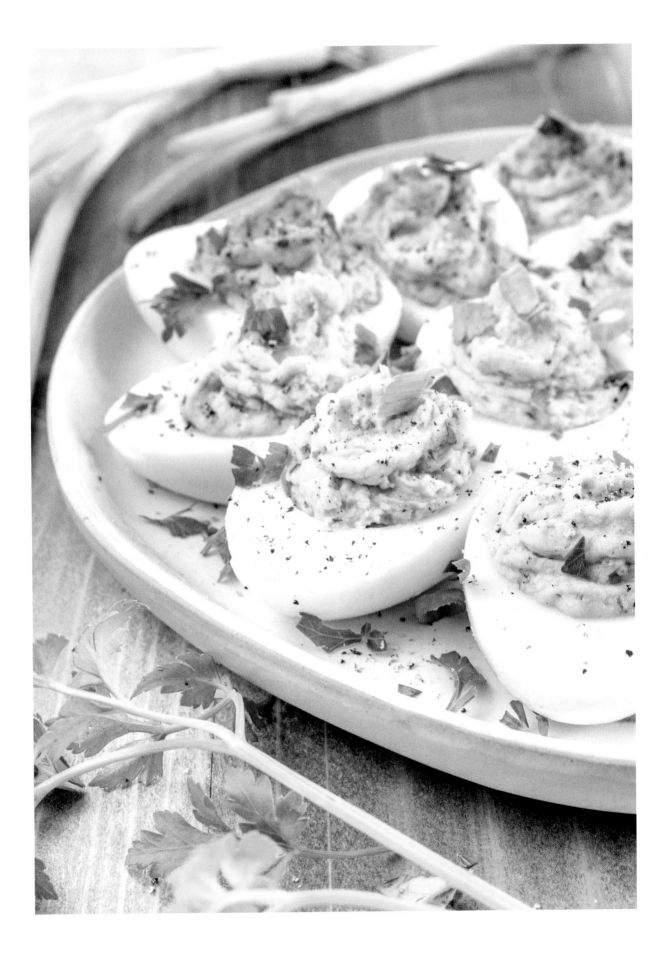

SHRIMP SALAD CUCUMBER ROUNDS

Yield: 15 rounds (3 per serving)

Prep Time: 15 minutes, plus 1 hour to chill

SHRIMP SALAD

8 ounces frozen precooked large shrimp, peeled and deveined (see note)

3 tablespoons mayonnaise

1½ tablespoons finely chopped red onions

¼ cup finely chopped celery (about 1 stalk)

1 teaspoon fresh lemon juice, plus more for the top if desired

½ teaspoon Old Bay seasoning, plus more for sprinkling (optional)

1 teaspoon chopped fresh dill, plus some small pieces for garnish

Salt and pepper to taste

½ medium cucumber (about 4 inches long), for serving

These rounds are a perfect finger food and can be served as an appetizer or a light snack. You can also use the shrimp salad to make a heartier meal for lunch or dinner. Try stuffing half of a pitted avocado with it or filling a lettuce wrap! You'll find this option in the meal plan on page 317.

1. If using frozen shrimp, thaw according to the package instructions.

2. Rinse the shrimp, then drain it very well and chop it into large pieces.

3. Place the chopped shrimp and the rest of the salad ingredients in a bowl and mix well. Cover and refrigerate for 1 hour.

4. Slice the cucumber crosswise into fifteen ¼-inch rounds and place them on a plate or serving tray.

5. Scoop about 1 tablespoon of shrimp salad onto each cucumber slice. Garnish with a small piece of dill. If desired, sprinkle the rounds with Old Bay seasoning and squeeze a little fresh lemon juice over the top.

note I often go to the seafood counter to buy already thawed shrimp. In that case, you need only 6 ounces, because thawed shrimp weighs less than frozen shrimp.

PER SERVING:

CALORIES 82 · FAT 8g · PROTEIN 9g · TOTAL CARBS 2g · FIBER 0g · NET CARBS 2g

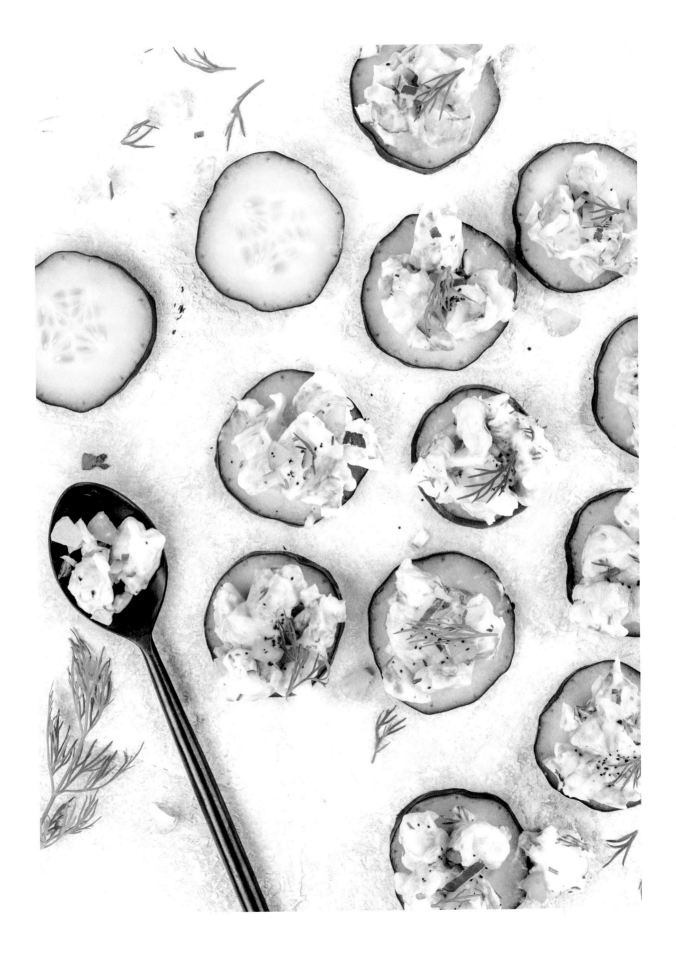

GRILLED EGGPLANT "BRUSCHETTA"

Yield: 5 servings (2 rounds per serving)

Prep Time: 15 minutes

Cook Time: 10 minutes

FOR THE GRILL

1 medium eggplant

Salt

1 medium Roma tomato

1 tablespoon olive oil

TOPPING

½ cup crumbled feta cheese

2 tablespoons chopped fresh basil

1½ teaspoons olive oil

Grilled tomato halves (from above)

Salt and pepper

In the summertime, I love to use the grill to make fresh and easy appetizers so I can avoid turning on the oven. These eggplant bites are grilled to perfection and very flavorful!

1. Slice the eggplant crosswise into 10 even rounds, about ½ inch thick. Lay the rounds on a rimmed baking sheet and sprinkle them with salt; the salt will cause excess water to be extracted. Cut the tomato in half lengthwise and set aside.

2. Preheat a grill or grill pan to medium-high heat.

3. Use a paper towel to soak up the excess liquid from the eggplant and wipe away the salt.

4. Coat the eggplant and tomato in the olive oil and place on the grill. Cook the eggplant slices for about 5 minutes on each side and the tomato halves for 2 to 3 minutes on each side. Remove the eggplant and tomato from the grill, placing the eggplant slices on a serving platter and the tomato halves on a cutting board.

5. Make the topping: Put the feta, basil, and olive oil in a small bowl and gently mix to combine. Once the tomato is cool enough to handle (but still warm), cut it into cubes and add them to the feta and basil mixture. Season with salt and pepper to taste and use a fork to gently combine the ingredients.

6. Spread the topping evenly over the grilled eggplant rounds and serve.

PER SERVING:

CALORIES **91** · FAT **7g** · PROTEIN **3g** · TOTAL CARBS **7g** · FIBER **3g** · NET CARBS **4g**

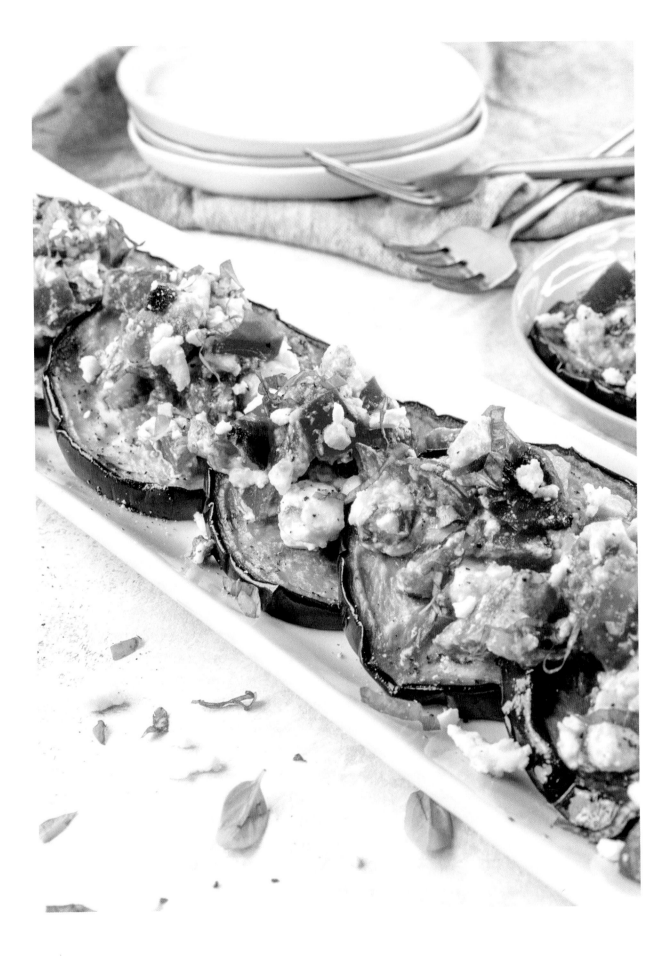

ANTIPASTO SKEWERS

Yield: 12 skewers (1 per serving)

Prep Time: 15 minutes

12 Kalamata olives, pitted

12 grape tomatoes

24 thin slices salami

12 small marinated mozzarella balls

12 marinated artichoke hearts

12 bite-size pieces roasted red pepper

2 tablespoons olive oil, for drizzling

Salt and pepper

These skewers are great to serve at a picnic or casual gathering. They are made with simple and fresh Mediterranean ingredients that everyone loves. When I serve them to guests, they are always one of the first appetizers to go!

1. Assemble the skewers by layering an olive, a tomato, a salami slice (folded in quarters), a mozzarella ball, an artichoke heart, a second salami slice (folded in quarters), and a roasted red pepper piece.

2. Drizzle the skewers with the olive oil and season with salt and pepper to taste. Serve right away or store in a covered container in the refrigerator for up to 2 days.

Special Equipment:
12 (6-inch) skewers

PER SERVING:
CALORIES **98** · FAT **8g** · PROTEIN **4g** · TOTAL CARBS **2g** · FIBER **0g** · NET CARBS **2g**

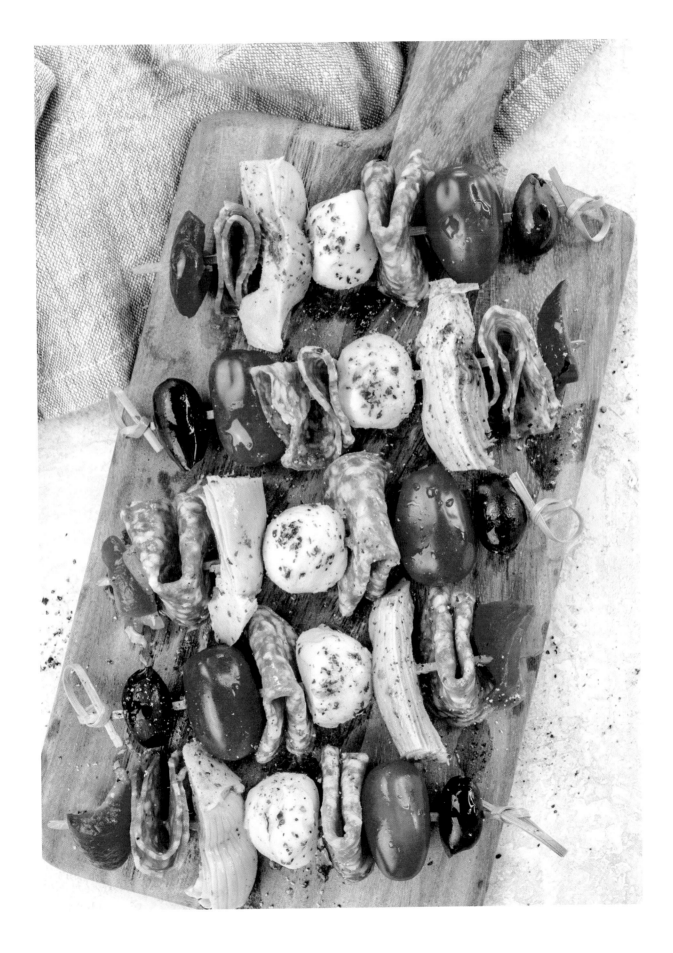

CAPRESE PIZZA CRISPS

Yield: 12 crisps (3 per serving)

Prep Time: 5 minutes

Cook Time: 12 minutes

¾ cup freshly grated Parmesan cheese

4 to 6 large fresh basil leaves, torn into 12 (1-inch) pieces

3 Roma tomato slices, quartered

½ teaspoon Italian seasoning

My daughter and husband both love pizza, so when they want a snack in a hurry, I like to make these pizza crisps. They have the perfect pizza flavor without the carbs!

1. Preheat the oven to 400°F.

2. Divide the Parmesan cheese evenly among the wells of a standard-size muffin pan, about 1 tablespoon per well. Place a piece of basil on top of the cheese in each well, then add one-quarter of a tomato slice and sprinkle with a pinch of Italian seasoning.

3. Bake for 8 to 12 minutes, until the cheese is golden brown and crisp throughout. Use a fork to transfer each crisp to a cooling rack and allow to cool for 5 minutes before eating.

Serving tip:
Eat as is or dip in no-sugar-added marinara sauce (see page 82 for my recipe, or use store-bought).

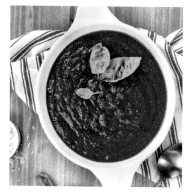

PER SERVING:
CALORIES **85** · FAT **5g** · PROTEIN **7g** · TOTAL CARBS **2g** · FIBER **0g** · NET CARBS **2g**

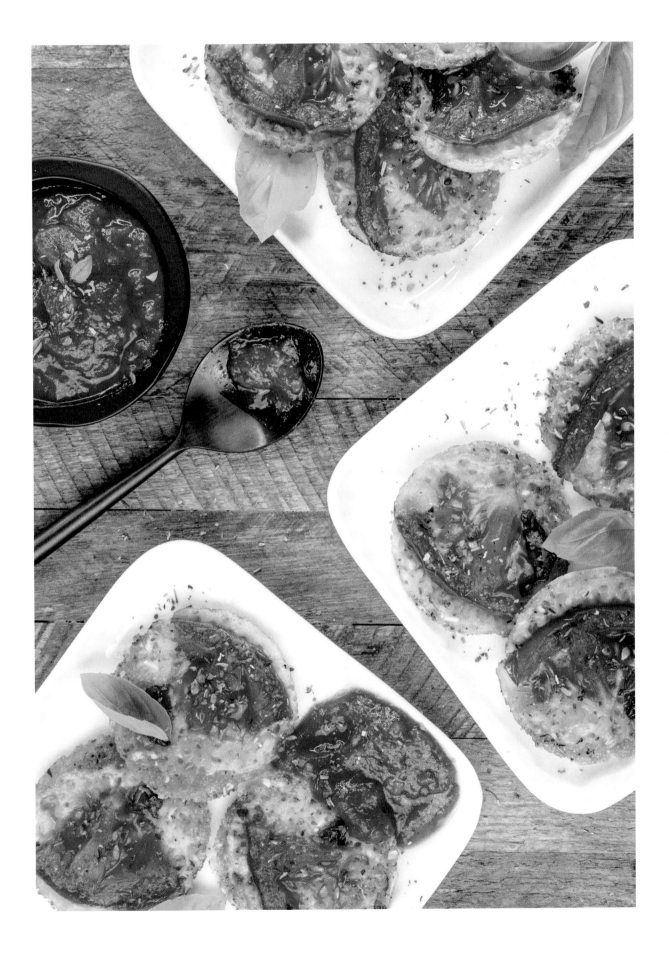

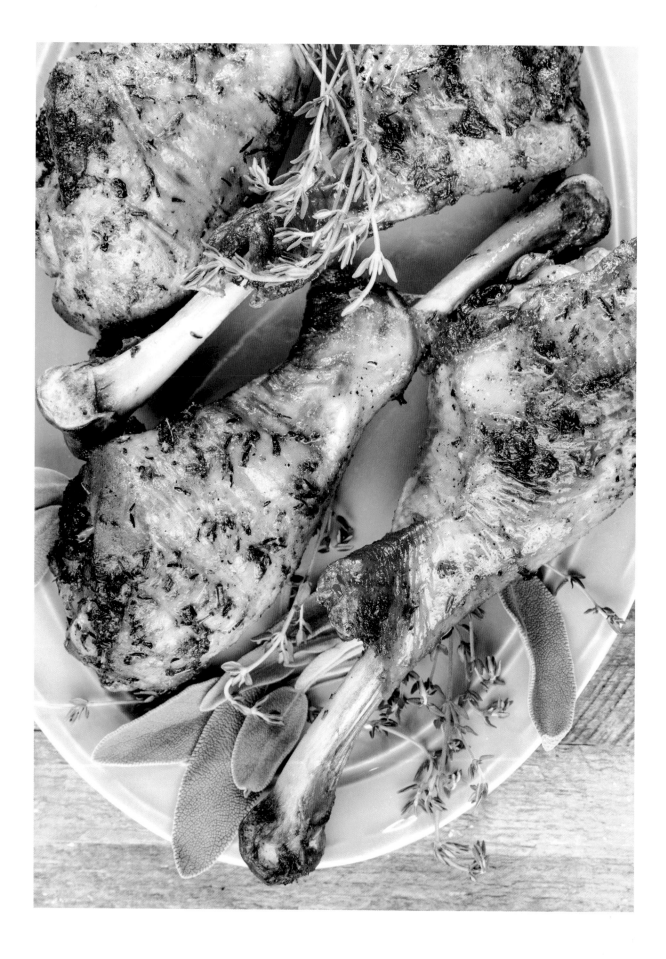

chicken & turkey

CHICKEN SATAY SKEWERS WITH PEANUT SAUCE

Yield: 8 skewers (2 skewers and 2 heaping tablespoons sauce per serving)

Prep Time: 10 minutes, plus 2 hours to marinate

Cook Time: 10 minutes

CHICKEN SATAY

⅓ cup full-fat coconut milk

1 tablespoon curry powder

½ teaspoon salt

1 clove garlic, minced

Juice of 1 lime

1¼ pounds chicken tenders

1 green onion, sliced, for garnish

SAUCE

¼ cup natural peanut butter (salted)

¼ cup full-fat coconut milk

1 tablespoon soy sauce or coconut aminos

½ teaspoon grated ginger, or ¼ teaspoon ginger powder

1 teaspoon toasted sesame oil

1 tablespoon Swerve confectioners'-style sweetener

1 to 2 teaspoons Sriracha sauce (optional)

Chopped peanuts, for garnish (optional)

Special Equipment:
8 (12-inch) skewers

Kids and adults alike enjoy these lightly spiced satay skewers, which are served with a quick and delicious peanut sauce. This dish pairs well with Thai Cucumber Salad (page 248), cauliflower rice, or a side salad.

1. Make the chicken satay: Whisk together the coconut milk, curry powder, salt, garlic, and lime juice in a small bowl.

2. Put the chicken in a gallon-sized zip-top plastic bag and pour the marinade over the chicken. Seal the bag and place in the refrigerator to chill for at least 2 hours or up to overnight, turning the bag occasionally.

3. Preheat a grill or grill pan to medium-high heat. If using wooden or bamboo skewers, soak them in water for about 15 minutes.

4. Remove the chicken from the marinade and discard the excess marinade. Thread the chicken evenly onto eight 12-inch skewers; you should be able to fit 2 or 3 pieces on each skewer.

5. Spray the grates of the grill or grill pan with cooking spray. Grill the skewers for about 5 minutes on one side, then flip them over and grill for another 5 minutes, until the chicken is cooked through and no longer pink.

6. While the chicken is cooking, make the peanut sauce: Place the peanut butter and coconut milk in a microwave-safe bowl and microwave for 20 seconds, or until the peanut butter is melted and mixes easily with coconut milk. Whisk to combine, then add the remaining ingredients for the sauce and whisk again until well incorporated.

7. Remove the chicken skewers from grill, top with the sliced green onion and some chopped peanuts, if desired, and serve with the peanut sauce for dipping.

PER SERVING:
CALORIES **322** · FAT **17g** · PROTEIN **38g** · TOTAL CARBS **8g** · FIBER **3g** · ERYTHRITOL **2g** · NET CARBS **3g**

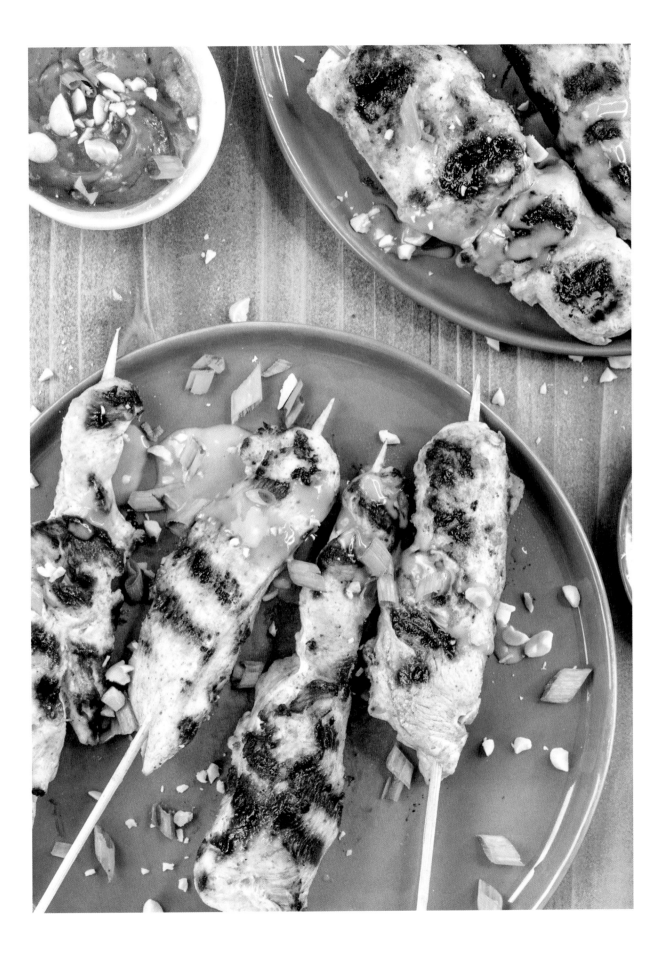

PROSCIUTTO-STUFFED CHICKEN

Yield: 6 servings

Prep Time: 15 minutes

Cook Time: 21 minutes

4 ounces sliced prosciutto, chopped

1 cup baby spinach, chopped

½ cup shredded Gruyère cheese

6 (3- to 4-ounce) bone-in chicken thighs, deboned with skin on

2 teaspoons Italian seasoning or poultry seasoning

Salt and pepper

2 tablespoons olive oil

Chicken thighs are a great option for a ketogenic diet because they have a higher fat content than other cuts of chicken, especially if you buy them with the skin on. While you're shopping, make things easier on yourself by asking the butcher to debone your skin-on chicken thighs; this will save you time when preparing dinner! However, you can always debone the thighs yourself if you prefer; there are plenty of YouTube videos that will walk you through the process.

1. Preheat the oven to 475°F.

2. In a bowl, combine the prosciutto, spinach, and cheese.

3. Pound the chicken thighs, skin side down, to an even thickness of ¼ to ½ inch. Sprinkle the Italian seasoning over the chicken.

4. Place one-sixth of the prosciutto filling in the center of each thigh. Tightly roll up the thighs and season the skin with salt and pepper.

5. Heat the oil in a large oven-safe sauté pan or cast-iron skillet over high heat. When the pan is good and hot, place the thighs in the pan skin side up. Sear the thighs for about 2 minutes, then flip them over and sear with the skin side down for an additional 2 minutes. Lower the heat to medium and cook until the fat is rendered, about 12 minutes.

6. Flip the chicken over one more time so that the skin is facing up again and place the pan in the oven for 5 minutes, to crisp the skin. Remove from the oven and serve.

note The easiest way to pound chicken is with a meat mallet. If you don't have one, you can use a rolling pin or heavy spoon to pound the chicken. As always, cover the meat with plastic wrap first.

PER SERVING:

CALORIES **338** · FAT **26g** · PROTEIN **24g** · TOTAL CARBS **1g** · FIBER **0g** · NET CARBS **1g**

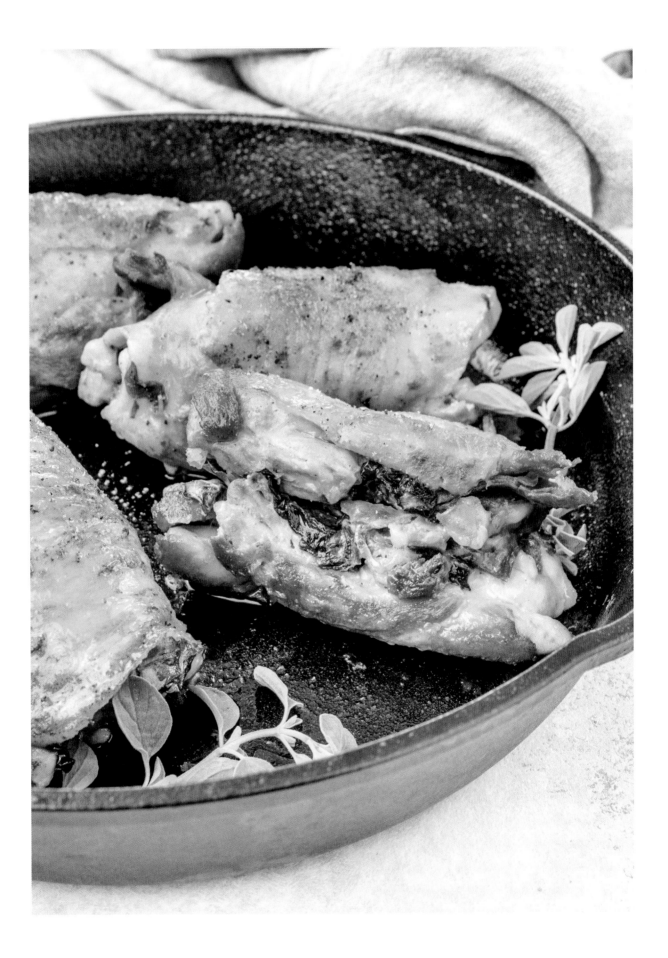

ROASTED TURKEY LEGS

Yield: 4 servings

Prep Time: 10 minutes

Cook Time: 50 minutes

4 (10-ounce) turkey legs

¼ cup (½ stick) unsalted butter, softened

1 teaspoon salt

1 teaspoon dried rosemary leaves

1 teaspoon dried rubbed sage

1 teaspoon dried thyme leaves

½ teaspoon ground black pepper

½ teaspoon garlic powder

Ready for your house to smell like Thanksgiving day? These turkey legs are so delicious with their moist dark meat and perfectly crispy skin. If you prefer, you can make this recipe with fresh herbs; substitute 1 tablespoon of fresh herbs for every 1 teaspoon of dried herbs.

1. Preheat the oven to 450°F. Have on hand a roasting pan with a roasting rack inside. If you don't have a roasting pan and rack, set a wire rack on a rimmed baking sheet.

2. Use paper towels to pat the turkey legs dry. In a bowl, combine the softened butter with the salt, herbs, and spices. Use your hands to cover each leg evenly with the butter and herb mixture. If you can, use your fingers to push some of the butter mixture under the skin as well.

3. Place the turkey legs on the rack and roast uncovered for 15 minutes. After 15 minutes, baste the legs with the melted butter that has collected at the bottom of the pan and turn each leg slightly so that the skin browns evenly.

4. Continue to roast for another 15 minutes, baste again, and then loosely cover the pan with aluminum foil to finish cooking for an additional 15 to 20 minutes. The legs are done when the internal temperature reaches 165°F.

5. Remove the roasted turkey legs from the oven and allow to rest, still covered with foil, for 10 minutes before serving.

PER SERVING:

CALORIES **555** · FAT **36g** · PROTEIN **55g** · TOTAL CARBS **1g** · FIBER **1g** · NET CARBS **0g**

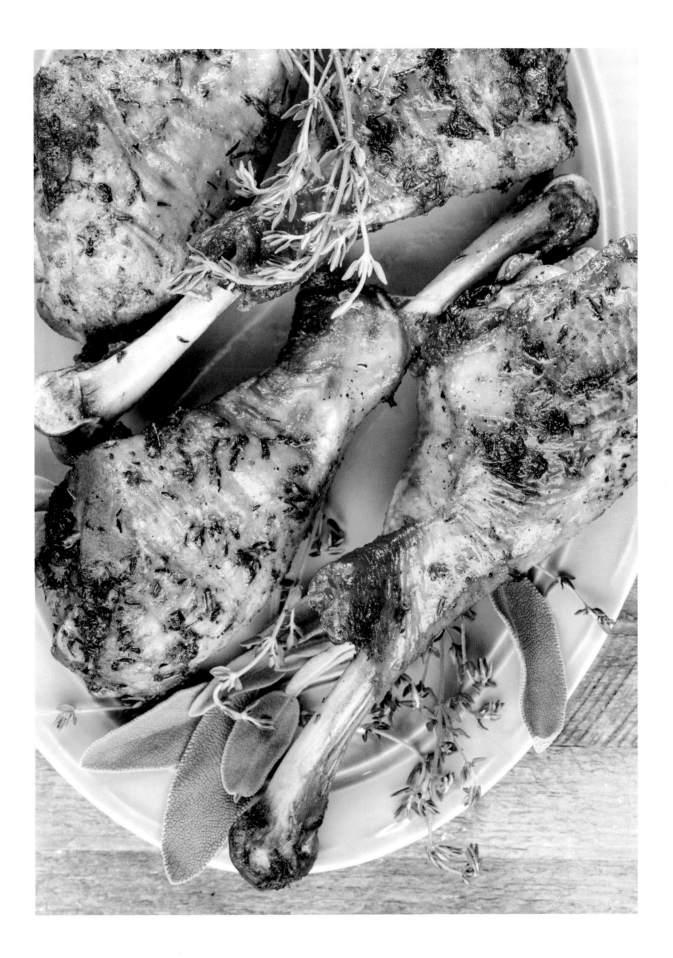

ZESTY RANCH TURKEY BURGERS

Yield: 6 burgers (1 per serving)

Prep Time: 10 minutes (not including time to make seasoning mix)

Cook Time: 10 minutes

2 pounds ground turkey (preferably dark meat)

2 cups shredded pepper Jack cheese or other shredded cheese of your choice

3 green onions, finely chopped

2 tablespoons ranch herb mix, homemade (page 85) or store-bought

2 tablespoons half-and-half

½ teaspoon salt

¼ teaspoon ground black pepper

These flavorful burgers are made with only a few simple ingredients and are ready in less than 30 minutes. They're best made with ground turkey thighs, but you can also use ground turkey breast. I've included three different cooking methods, which are all equally delicious!

1. Put all the ingredients in a bowl and use your hands to mix them together until everything is well incorporated. Form the meat mixture into 6 equal-sized patties, about ½ inch thick.

2. Cook the burgers using one of the three methods below:

To grill the burgers, preheat a grill or grill pan to medium-high heat, then spray the grate with cooking spray.

To pan-fry the burgers, heat a large skillet over medium-high heat, then spray it with cooking spray.

To broil the burgers, set an oven rack in the middle position and set the broil to high. Line a rimmed baking sheet with parchment paper and spray with cooking spray.

3. Arrange the burgers on the grill, in the skillet, or on the baking sheet. For all three methods, cook the burgers for 4 to 5 minutes per side, or until the internal temperature reaches 165°F. Season to taste with additional salt and pepper and serve.

Serving tip:
Wrap the burgers in lettuce leaves and top with your favorite low-carb burger toppings, or eat with a knife and fork with guacamole, sour cream, or Ranch Dip/Dressing (page 86).

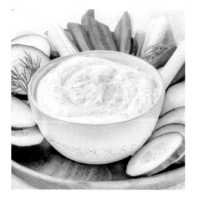

PER SERVING:
CALORIES **381** · FAT **24g** · PROTEIN **39g** · TOTAL CARBS **2g** · FIBER **0g** · NET CARBS **2g**

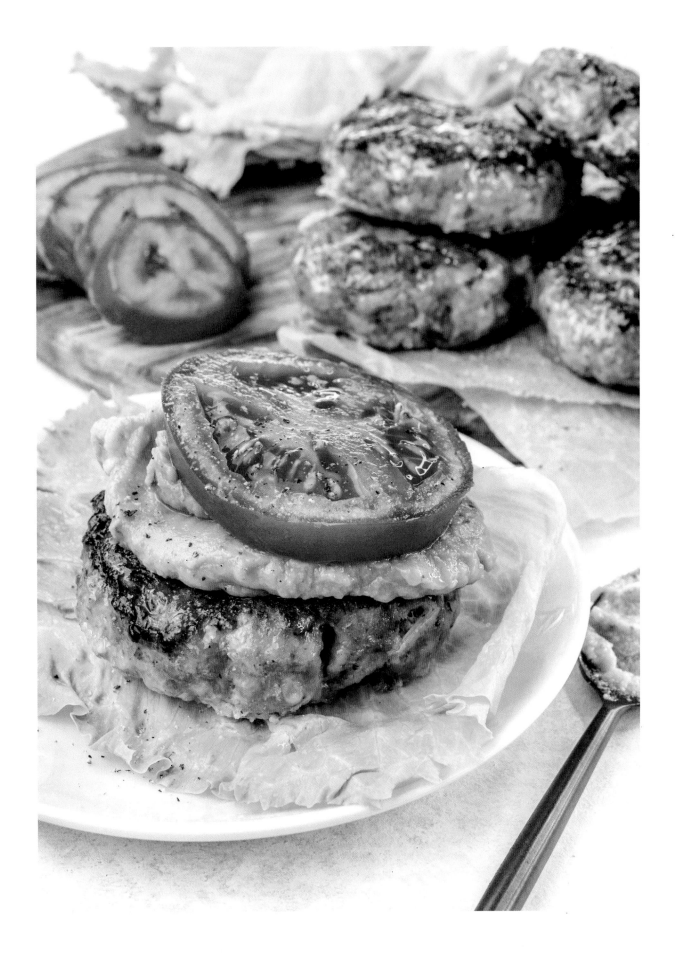

MUFFULETTA CHICKEN

Yield: 4 servings

Prep Time: 15 minutes

Cook Time: 22 minutes

OLIVE SALAD

¾ cup mixed olives, pitted and chopped

1 whole roasted red pepper from the jar, chopped

2 cloves garlic, minced

1 tablespoon capers, drained

1 tablespoon red wine vinegar

1 tablespoon olive oil

1 teaspoon dried oregano leaves

½ teaspoon ground black pepper

Pinch of red pepper flakes (optional)

CHICKEN

4 (6-ounce) boneless, skinless chicken breasts

2 tablespoons olive oil

4 slices provolone cheese

2 ounces sliced salami

2 ounces sliced capocollo (aka coppa or capicola)

4 ounces sliced ham

4 slices mozzarella cheese

Chopped fresh parsley, for garnish (optional)

A deconstructed New Orleans muffuletta sandwich, ditching the bread but keeping all the good stuff!

1. Combine all the olive salad ingredients in a bowl, cover, and put in the refrigerator until ready to use.

2. Prepare the chicken: Pound the chicken breasts to an even ½-inch thickness.

3. Heat the oil in a large oven-safe skillet over medium-high heat. Brown the chicken for 5 to 6 minutes per side.

4. Layer the provolone, salami, capocollo, ham, and mozzarella on top of the chicken. Turn the oven to the broil setting. Transfer the skillet to the oven and broil for 5 to 10 minutes, until the cheese is melted and the internal temperature of the chicken reaches 165°F.

5. Top each chicken breast with about ¼ cup of the olive salad before serving. Garnish with parsley, if desired.

note You can make the olive salad up to 3 days in advance.

PER SERVING:

CALORIES **584** · FAT **36g** · PROTEIN **59g** · TOTAL CARBS **3g** · FIBER **0g** · NET CARBS **3g**

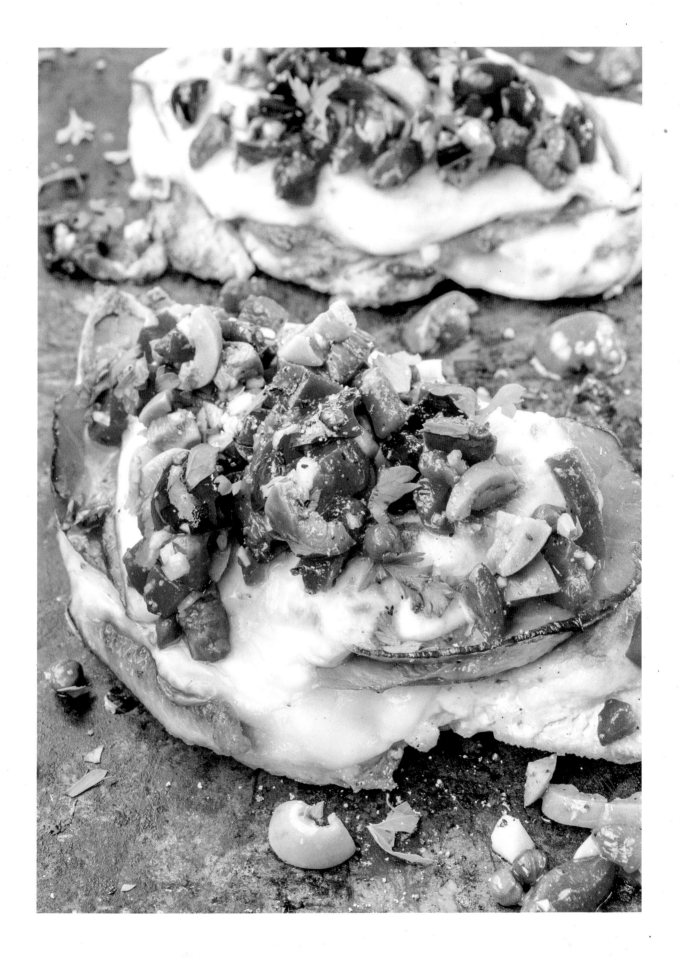

ONE-PAN CHICKEN FAJITAS

Yield: 6 servings

Prep Time: 10 minutes, plus 30 minutes to marinate

Cook Time: 20 minutes

FAJITAS

1¼ pounds boneless, skinless chicken breasts, sliced into ½-inch-thick strips

1 green bell pepper, sliced into strips

1 red bell pepper, sliced into strips

1 medium-sized yellow onion

2 cloves garlic, minced

2 tablespoons olive oil

1 tablespoon chili powder

1 teaspoon ground cumin

1 teaspoon smoked paprika

¼ teaspoon salt

¼ teaspoon ground black pepper

½ lime

¼ cup chopped fresh cilantro

SUGGESTED TOPPINGS

Sour cream (omit for dairy-free)

Shredded cheese (omit for dairy-free)

Jalapeño slices

Mexican food is one of my favorite cuisines, and I love this fajitas recipe because it is both easy to make and easy to clean up. You can serve the fajitas over cauliflower rice, wrapped in butter lettuce leaves, or over chopped romaine lettuce for a taco salad.

1. Preheat the oven to 400°F. Line a rimmed baking sheet with aluminum foil.

2. Place the ingredients for the fajitas, not including the lime and cilantro, in a gallon-sized zip-top plastic bag and toss until well coated. Place in the refrigerator to marinate for 30 minutes or up to 24 hours.

3. Spread the marinated chicken, peppers, and onion mixture evenly in a single layer on the prepared pan and bake for 10 minutes; discard the marinade.

4. Remove the pan from the oven and carefully pour off and discard any accumulated liquid. Use a spatula to toss the chicken and vegetables.

5. Return the pan to the oven for another 8 minutes, until the peppers and onions are soft, then broil for 1 to 2 minutes, until the veggies and chicken begin to brown around the edges.

6. Squeeze the lime juice over the fajitas and sprinkle with the cilantro. Serve with the toppings of your choice, if desired.

PER SERVING (WITHOUT TOPPINGS):
CALORIES **157** · FAT **7g** · PROTEIN **19g** · TOTAL CARBS **5g** · FIBER **2g** · NET CARBS **3g**

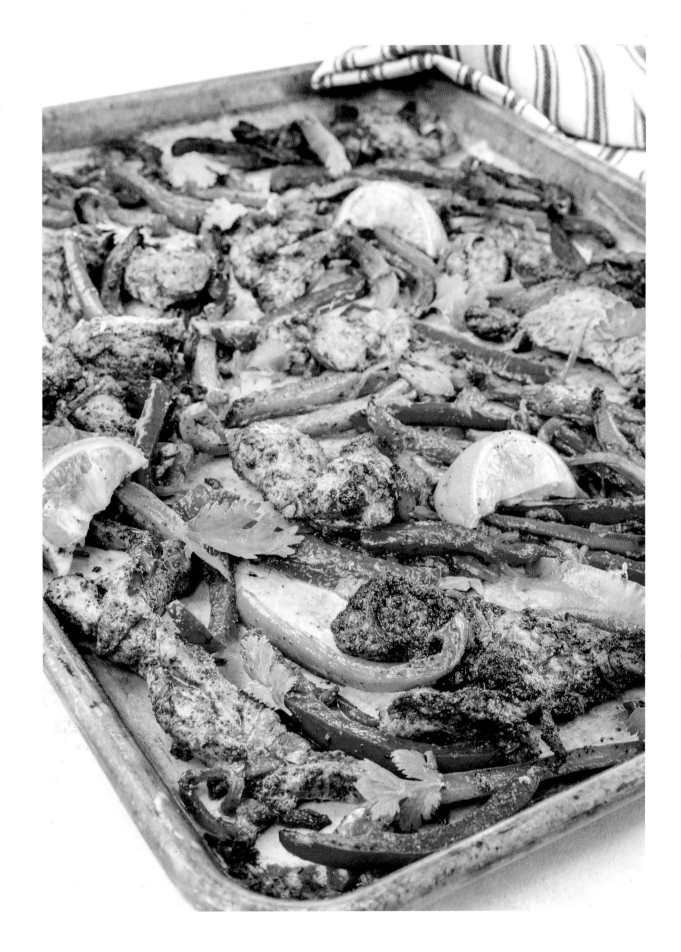

CAPRESE CHICKEN WITH PESTO FOR TWO

Yield: 2 servings

Prep Time: 10 minutes

Cook Time: 20 minutes

2 (5-ounce) boneless, skinless chicken breasts, pounded to an even thickness

2 tablespoons pesto

1 teaspoon salt

½ teaspoon ground black pepper

3 ounces fresh mozzarella cheese, cut into 2 slices

4 (¼-inch) slices Roma tomato (about ¾ tomato)

Italian seasoning, for sprinkling

Fresh basil, for garnish

This caprese chicken has so many amazing flavors, from the delicious pesto to the fresh tomatoes, and let's not forget the melted mozzarella cheese. And even better, cleanup is a breeze with this simple foil-pack baking method!

1. Preheat the oven to 375°F.

2. Tear off 2 sheets of aluminum foil, about 12 inches long. Place a chicken breast in the middle of each piece of foil and brush both sides of each breast with the pesto. Season with the salt and pepper.

3. Fold up all 4 sides of each foil packet to create "walls" around the chicken. Top each breast with a slice of mozzarella, 2 tomato slices, and a sprinkle of Italian seasoning.

4. Loosely fold the sides of the foil over the chicken, leaving some room over the top of the chicken so the cheese isn't touching the foil, then seal each packet closed.

5. Place the foil packets on a rimmed baking sheet and bake for 18 to 20 minutes, or until the internal temperature of the chicken reaches 165°F. Serve garnished with fresh basil.

PER SERVING:
CALORIES **337** · FAT **18g** · PROTEIN **38g** · TOTAL CARBS **5g** · FIBER **1g** · NET CARBS **4g**

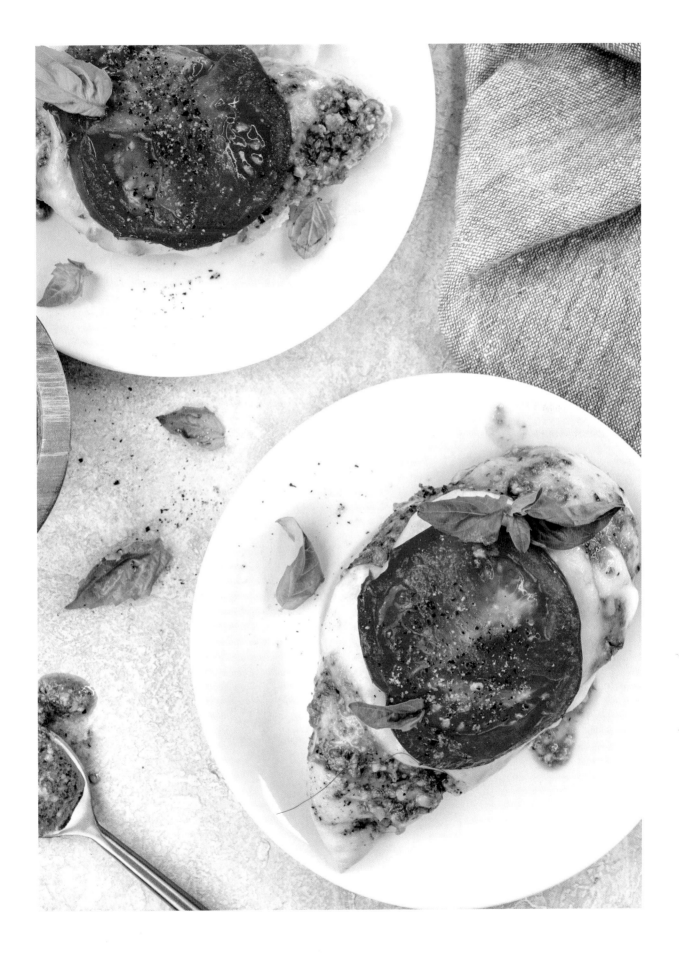

CRISPY BAKED CHICKEN THIGHS

Yield: 6 servings

Prep Time: 10 minutes

Cook Time: 18 minutes

6 (3- to 4-ounce) boneless, skinless chicken thighs

EGG WASH

2 large eggs

1 tablespoon heavy whipping cream

"BREADING"

¾ cup pork rinds (about 1½ ounces), crushed into powder

¾ cup freshly grated Parmesan cheese

1 teaspoon garlic powder

½ teaspoon paprika

½ teaspoon salt

½ teaspoon ground black pepper

Chopped fresh parsley, for garnish (optional)

Pork rinds make the most perfect coating. They have the texture of real breading without the added carbs! These baked chicken thighs are perfectly crispy and golden brown. Serve them with your favorite side and ranch dressing (page 86).

1. Preheat the oven to 400°F. Line a rimmed baking sheet with aluminum foil, then set a wire rack on the baking sheet. Spray the rack with cooking spray.

2. Pound the chicken thighs to an even thickness.

3. In a bowl, beat the eggs and cream until well mixed. In another bowl, stir together all the breading ingredients. Set aside.

4. One by one, dip each chicken thigh into the egg wash and then into the breading, coating the entire thigh, then lay them on the prepared rack.

5. Bake for 16 to 18 minutes, or until the internal temperature of the chicken reaches 165°F.

PER SERVING:

CALORIES **228** · FAT **11g** · PROTEIN **30g** · TOTAL CARBS **1g** · FIBER **0g** · NET CARBS **1g**

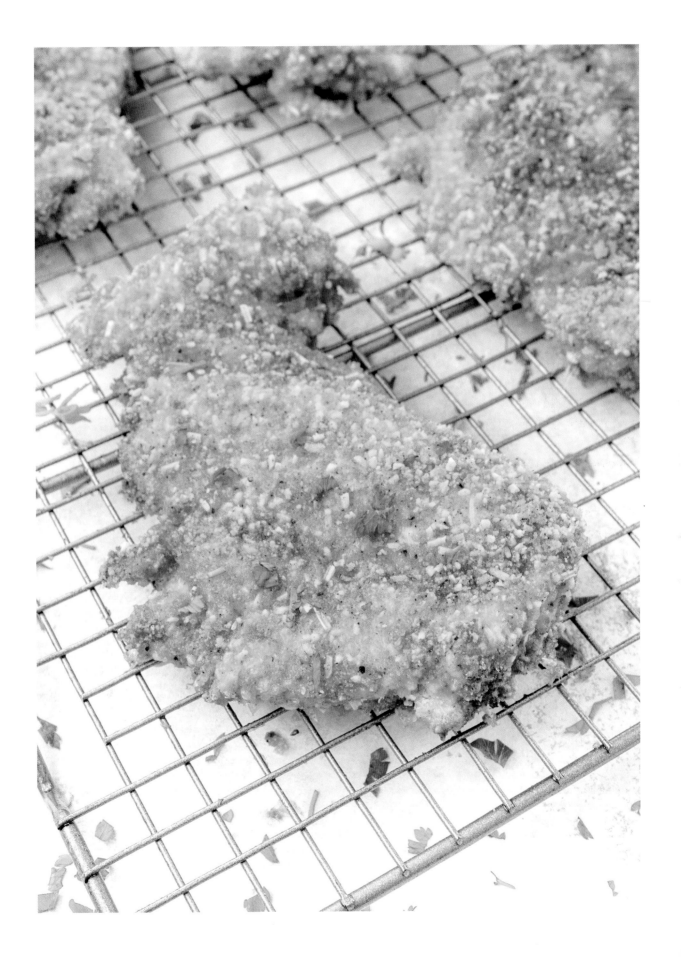

CREAMY SUN-DRIED TOMATO AND BASIL CHICKEN

Yield: 4 servings

Prep Time: 10 minutes

Cook Time: 17 minutes

2 large boneless, skinless chicken breasts (about 1½ pounds total)

½ teaspoon garlic powder

Salt and pepper

1 tablespoon olive oil

SAUCE

¼ cup dry white wine (such as Sauvignon Blanc)

¼ cup (½ stick) unsalted butter

⅓ cup heavy whipping cream

¼ cup chopped sun-dried tomatoes

¼ cup sliced fresh basil

½ teaspoon fresh lemon juice

A 30-minute, one-pan chicken dish with a creamy sauce featuring sun-dried tomatoes. Serve with a side of cauliflower mash (page 266) or zucchini noodles.

1. Cut each chicken breast in half horizontally to make 2 thinner pieces. Sprinkle the chicken all over with the garlic powder, then season them with salt and pepper.

2. Heat the olive oil in a large skillet over medium-high heat. When the oil is hot, add the chicken and cook for 4 to 5 minutes per side, or until it's nice and golden, then take the chicken out of the pan and set aside.

3. Pour the white wine into the pan and stir thoroughly. Add the butter to the pan and let it bubble for 2 minutes, then add the cream, sun-dried tomatoes, basil, and lemon juice and stir to combine.

4. Return the chicken to the pan and coat each breast in the cream sauce. Let simmer for another 5 minutes or so (turn the heat down if needed), until the chicken is cooked through and the sauce has thickened. Season with more salt and pepper, if needed.

PER SERVING:

CALORIES **347** · FAT **23g** · PROTEIN **27g** · TOTAL CARBS **2g** · FIBER **0g** · NET CARBS **2g**

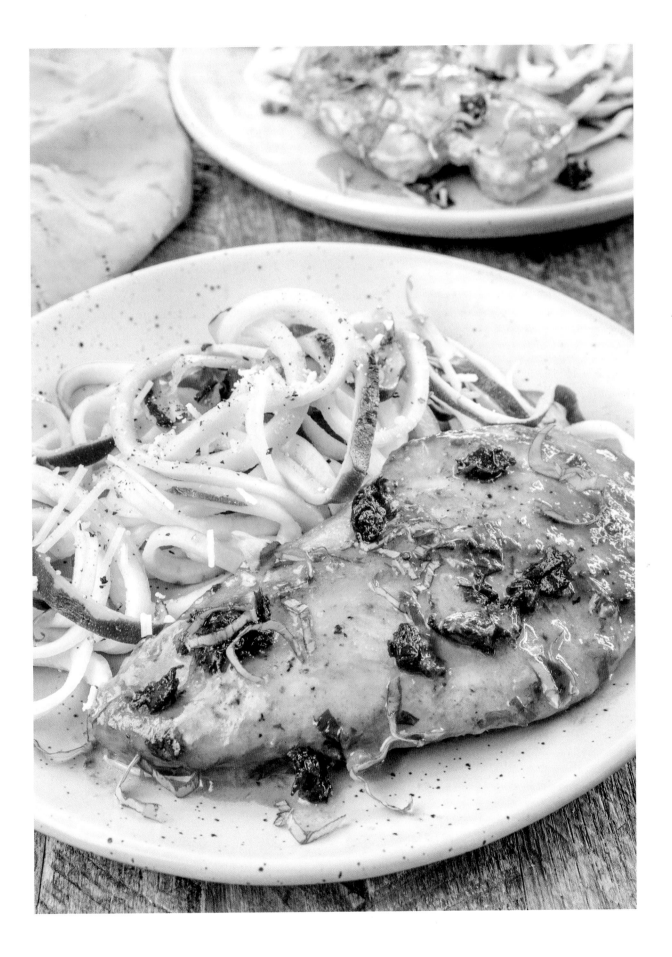

SHREDDED JALAPEÑO POPPER CHICKEN

Yield: 6 servings (¾ cup per serving)

Prep Time: 5 minutes (not including time to cook bacon)

Cook Time: 4 hours 15 minutes or 8 hours 15 minutes

2 pounds boneless, skinless chicken breasts

1 teaspoon garlic powder

1 (8-ounce) package cream cheese

¾ cup cooked and chopped bacon (about 8 slices), divided

1 (4-ounce) can diced jalapeños, drained

1 cup shredded cheddar cheese, divided

Salt and pepper

Sliced fresh jalapeño pepper, for garnish (optional)

Serving tip:
Serve as is or in butter lettuce wraps.

When I think of easy meals, I automatically think of using the slow cooker. Add a few ingredients to the pot, turn it on, and forget about it for hours until dinner time! This chicken is creamy, spicy, cheesy, AND has bacon to boot.

1. Put the chicken in a 4-quart slow cooker. Season the chicken with the garlic powder, then place the block of cream cheese on top.

2. Cover and cook until the chicken is cooked through, 3½ to 4 hours on high or 6 to 8 hours on low.

3. Shred the chicken with 2 forks in the slow cooker, then add ½ cup of the chopped bacon, the diced jalapeños, and ½ cup of the cheddar cheese. Mix until well blended, then season with salt and pepper to taste, keeping in mind that the bacon and cheese topping added in the next step will add a little saltiness.

4. Sprinkle the remaining ½ cup of cheddar cheese and ¼ cup of bacon on top, then place the lid back on and cook on high for 10 to 15 minutes more, or until the cheese is melted. Garnish with fresh jalapeño slices, if desired.

PER SERVING:

CALORIES **401** · FAT **23g** · PROTEIN **45g** · TOTAL CARBS **2g** · FIBER **0g** · NET CARBS **2g**

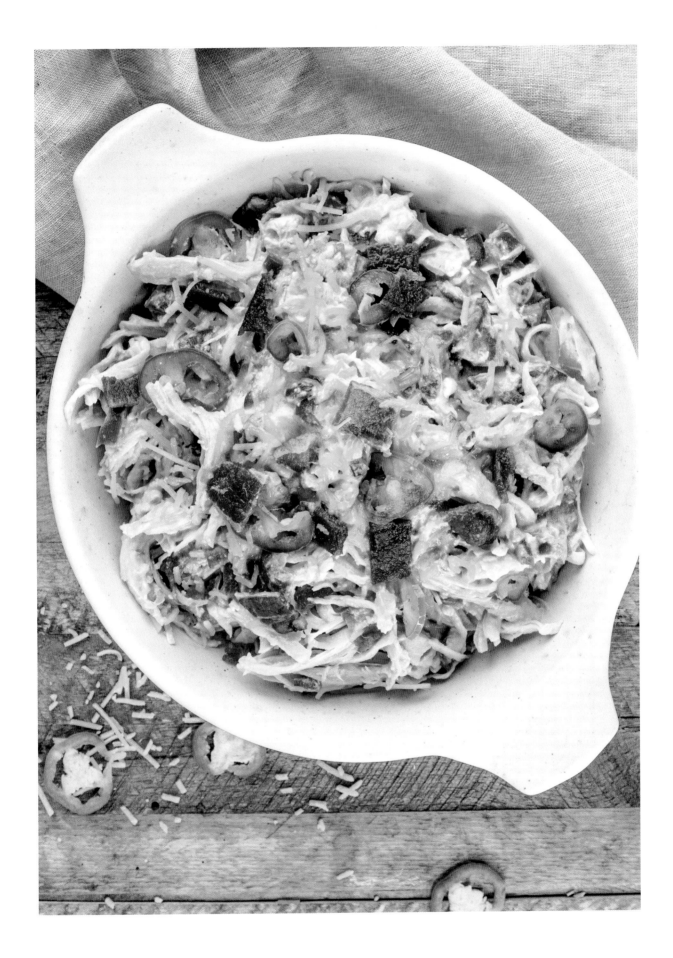

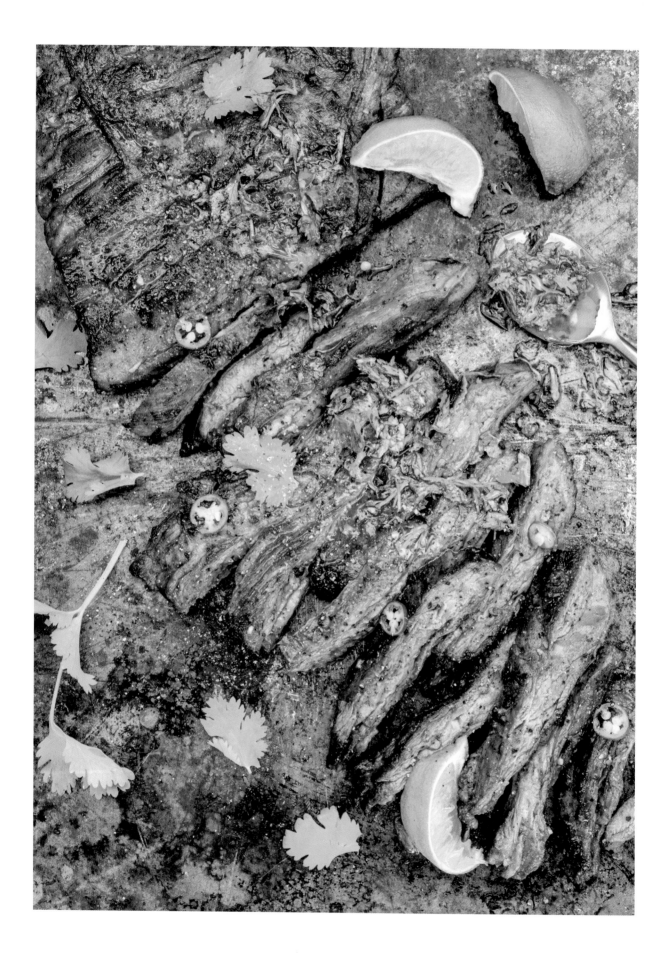

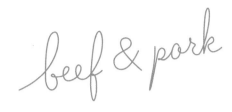

beef & pork

SKIRT STEAK KABOBS WITH CHIMICHURRI

Yield: 4 servings (1 kabob per serving)

Prep Time: 10 minutes, plus 15 minutes to marinate (not including time to make chimichurri)

Cook Time: 10 minutes

KABOBS

1 pound skirt steak, cut into 1 to 1½-inch pieces

5 cremini mushrooms, quartered

1 medium to large zucchini, sliced in half lengthwise and then crosswise into ¼-inch half-moons

½ large red onion, cut into 1-inch chunks

2 tablespoons olive oil

Juice of 1 lime

2 cloves garlic, pressed

1 teaspoon salt

½ teaspoon ground black pepper

¼ cup Chimichurri (page 88), for serving

Kabobs are one of my favorite fast and delicious meals to grill. If there are leftovers, I often remove the meat and veggies from the skewers, roughly chop the ingredients, and use them in salads or breakfast omelets.

1. Place all the ingredients for the kabobs in a gallon-sized zip-top plastic bag and shake the bag to fully coat the ingredients. Place in the refrigerator to marinate for at least 15 minutes.

2. Preheat a grill to medium-high heat. If using wooden or bamboo skewers, soak them in water for about 15 minutes.

3. Dump the kabob ingredients into a large bowl and discard the excess marinade. Thread the meat and vegetables onto four 12-inch skewers, alternating the ingredients. Each skewer should fit about 6 slices of beef, 5 mushroom quarters, and 5 red onion chunks.

4. Grill the kabobs for 3 to 5 minutes on each side, or until the beef is cooked to your liking and the veggies are tender.

5. Allow to rest for 3 to 5 minutes, then top each skewer with 1 tablespoon of chimichurri and serve. Store leftovers in an airtight container in the refrigerator for up to 4 days.

Special Equipment:
4 (12-inch) skewers

PER SERVING:
CALORIES **363** · FAT **27g** · PROTEIN **24g** · TOTAL CARBS **7g** · FIBER **1g** · NET CARBS **6g**

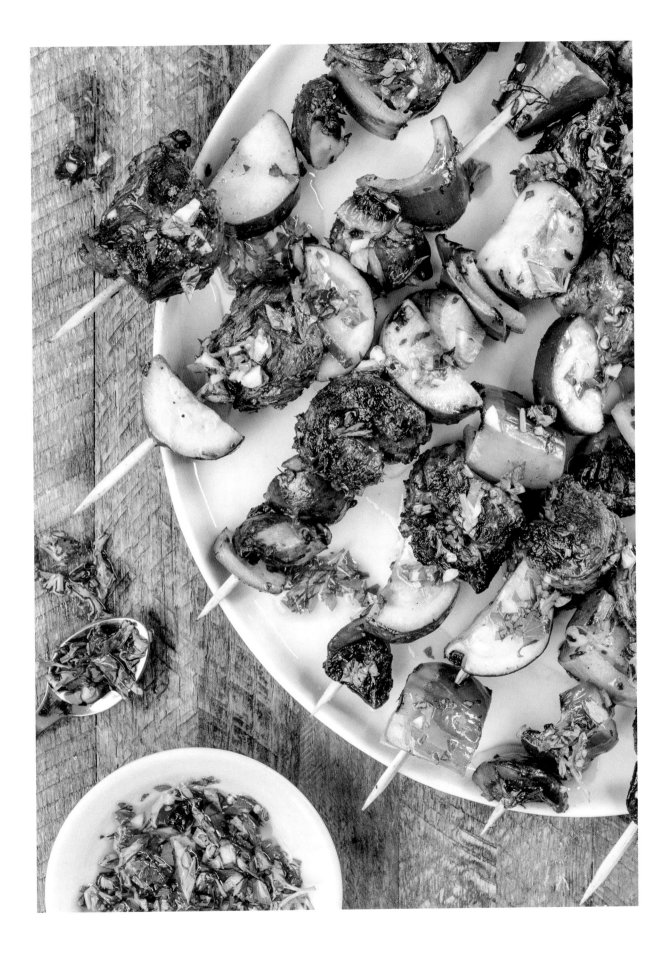

STUFFED BELL PEPPERS

Yield: 8 servings

Prep Time: 15 minutes (not including time to make marinara)

Cook Time: 43 minutes

1 tablespoon olive oil

1 pound ground beef

8 ounces bulk Italian sausage

½ cup diced yellow onions

1 cup riced cauliflower

4 bell peppers (any color)

2 cups no-sugar-added marinara sauce, homemade (page 82) or store-bought

8 ounces Parmesan cheese, freshly grated

8 ounces shredded Italian cheese blend, divided

Salt and pepper

Chopped fresh parsley, for garnish (optional)

You're going to love these hearty and flavorful stuffed peppers! Feel free to prepare the filling and stuff the peppers ahead of time, and bake them later when you're ready to eat. You can also throw them in an air fryer; see below.

1. Preheat the oven to 375°F.

2. Heat the oil in a large skillet over medium-high heat. When hot, add the ground beef and sausage and cook, breaking up the meat into crumbles, until browned, about 5 minutes.

3. Add the onions to the pan and cook for 5 minutes, until the onions are soft.

4. Drain the meat and onion mixture, then add the riced cauliflower and cook for 2 to 3 minutes, until the cauliflower begins to soften. Transfer the mixture to a large bowl to cool while you prepare the bell peppers.

5. Cut the bell peppers in half lengthwise. Remove the seeds, membranes, and stems.

6. Mix the marinara sauce and grated Parmesan cheese into the meat mixture, then fill each pepper half generously with the meat and cheese filling. Top each pepper with 1 ounce of shredded Italian blend cheese.

7. Place the stuffed peppers on a rimmed baking sheet and bake for 30 minutes, until the peppers are soft and the cheese is bubbly. Season to taste with salt and pepper and garnish with parsley, if desired.

AIR FRYER METHOD:

To make the stuffed peppers in an air fryer, coat the air fryer basket with cooking spray. Cook the stuffed peppers for 25 minutes at 350°F.

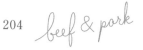

PER SERVING:

CALORIES 395 · FAT 27g · PROTEIN 33g · TOTAL CARBS 10g · FIBER 3g · NET CARBS 7g

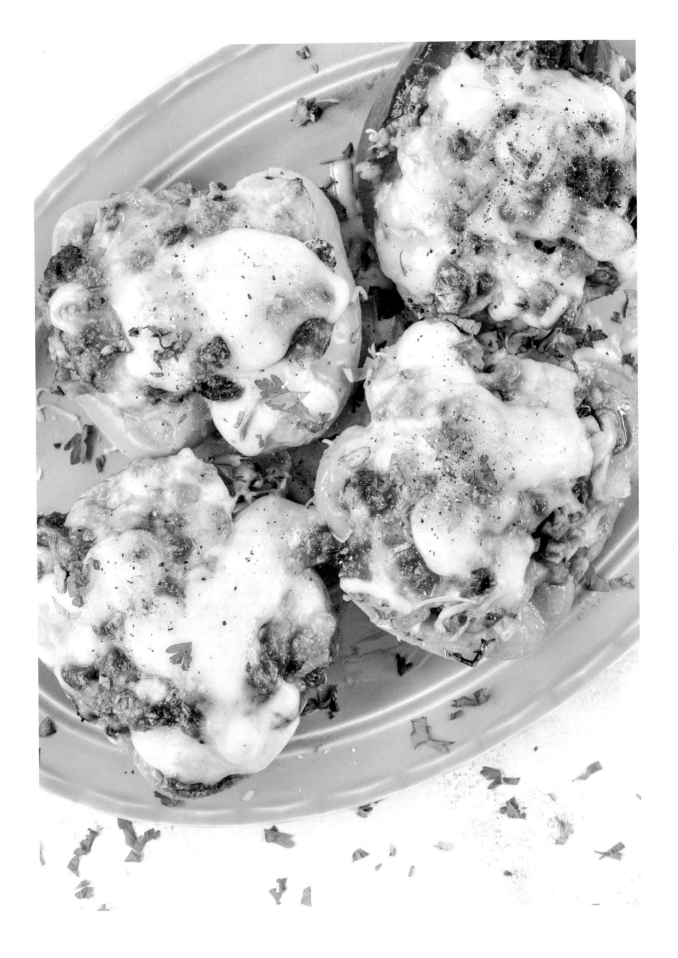

MEATLOAF MUFFINS

Yield: 12 muffins (2 per serving)

Prep Time: 10 minutes (not including time to make ketchup)

Cook Time: 25 minutes

1 pound ground bison or ground beef

1 stalk celery, diced

½ cup grated or minced yellow onions

1 clove garlic, minced

½ medium-sized green bell pepper, finely chopped

½ cup crushed tomatoes

1 large egg

½ cup blanched almond flour

½ cup freshly grated Parmesan cheese

¾ cup sugar-free ketchup, homemade (page 87) or store-bought

If you haven't tried ground bison, I encourage you to give it a try! It is deliciously tender and has a lighter flavor than ground beef. I usually serve these mini meatloaves for dinner with a green salad and Roasted Garlic Cauliflower Mash (page 266).

1. Preheat the oven to 400°F and coat a standard-size muffin pan with cooking spray.

2. Place all the ingredients, except the ketchup, in a large bowl. Using your hands, mix well to combine.

3. Scoop up about ¼ cup of the meat mixture, roll it into a ball, and drop it into one of the wells in the muffin pan. Repeat with the rest of the meatloaf mixture; you should have 12 balls in total. Top each muffin with 1 tablespoon of ketchup.

4. Bake for 20 to 25 minutes, until the ketchup is brown and caramelized and the meat is cooked through.

PER SERVING:
CALORIES **230** · FAT **13g** · PROTEIN **21g** · TOTAL CARBS **13g** · FIBER **2g** · ERYTHRITOL **5g** · NET CARBS **6g**

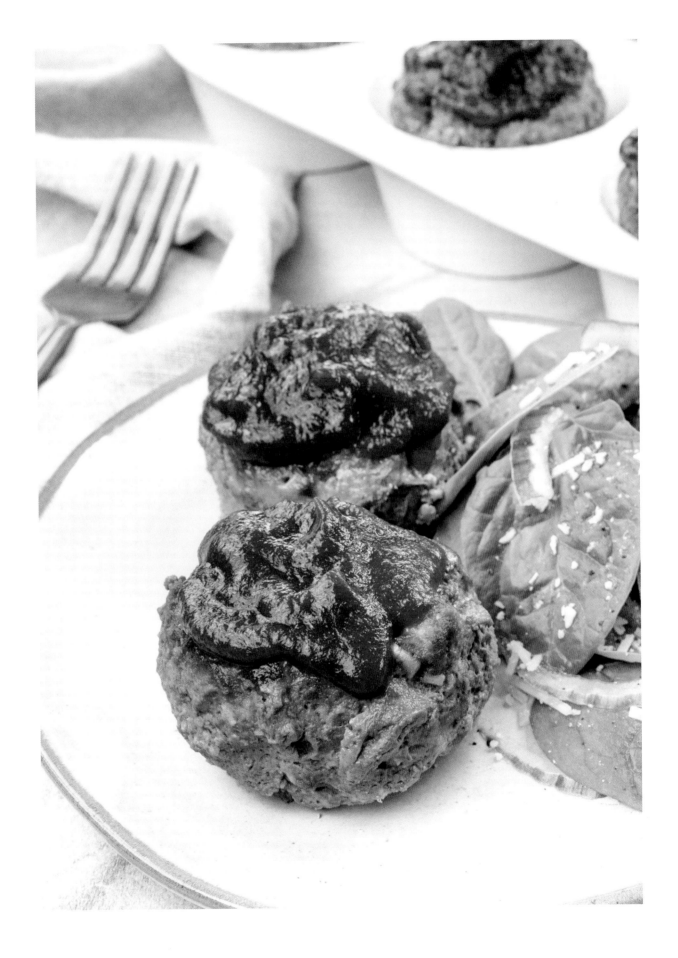

SHEPHERD'S PIE

Yield: 6 servings

Prep Time: 20 minutes

Cook Time: 1 hour

Shepherd's pie is a classic when it comes to comfort food, and it also happens to be one of my husband's favorites! Thanks to some trusty cauliflower mash, this traditional meat and potato dish is easily converted to a keto-friendly version.

CAULIFLOWER TOPPING

1 large head cauliflower (about 2 pounds), cored and separated into florets

2 tablespoons unsalted butter

2 tablespoons heavy whipping cream

1 cup shredded cheddar cheese, divided

2 large egg yolks

¼ teaspoon salt

¼ teaspoon ground black pepper

MEAT FILLING

2 tablespoons unsalted butter

2 stalks celery, chopped

½ cup chopped yellow onions

2 cloves garlic, minced

1 pound ground beef (see note)

¼ cup beef broth or red wine

1 small zucchini, diced

1 tablespoon fresh thyme leaves, chopped

2 tablespoons tomato paste

Salt and pepper

Chopped fresh parsley, for garnish (optional)

note Feel free to use any kind of ground meat you like. I used 80% lean ground beef, but lamb or turkey would work as well.

MAKE THE CAULIFLOWER TOPPING

1. Steam or boil the cauliflower florets until soft, 8 to 10 minutes. Drain the cauliflower and dry it as much as possible. Use a dish towel to squeeze out the excess liquid.

2. Transfer the cauliflower to a food processor. Add the butter, cream, ½ cup of the cheddar cheese, the egg yolks, salt, and pepper and process until smooth. Set aside.

MAKE THE MEAT FILLING

1. Heat the butter in a large skillet over medium-high heat. Add the celery, onions, and garlic to the pan and sauté until the onions are soft and translucent.

2. Add the ground beef to the pan and cook until browned, breaking up the meat into crumbles.

3. Pour in the beef broth to deglaze the pan, scraping the browned bits off the bottom of the pan.

4. Add the zucchini, thyme, and tomato paste and stir to incorporate. Reduce the heat to low and let simmer until all the liquid is cooked out, about 10 minutes. Season with salt and pepper to taste.

ASSEMBLE THE PIE

1. Preheat the oven to 400°F.

2. Place the meat filling in a 3-quart casserole dish or a 10-inch cast-iron skillet. Evenly spread the mashed cauliflower over the top, making sure it goes all the way to the sides of the dish. Top with the remaining ½ cup of cheddar cheese.

3. Bake for 30 minutes, until bubbling. Garnish with parsley, if desired.

PER SERVING:
CALORIES **401** · FAT **30g** · PROTEIN **27g** · TOTAL CARBS **8g** · FIBER **3g** · NET CARBS **5g**

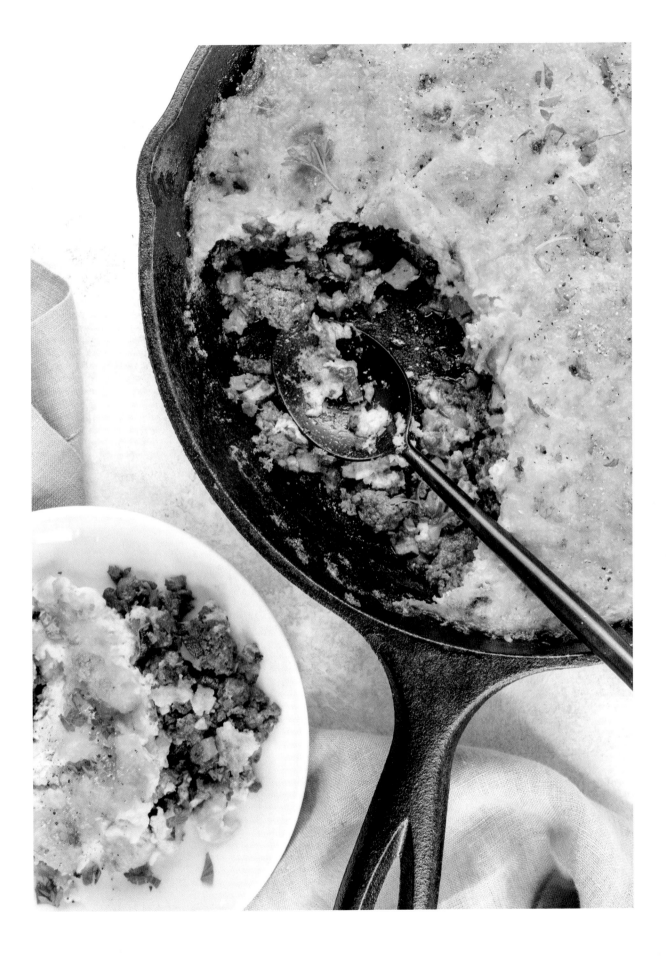

MIKE'S SPINACH SALAD WITH WARM BACON DRESSING

Yield: 2 servings

Prep Time: 10 minutes (not including time to cook eggs)

Cook Time: 18 minutes

4 slices thick-cut bacon

1 shallot

1 portobello mushroom cap

6 ounces baby spinach

2 hard-boiled eggs, sliced

Pepper

WARM BACON DRESSING

2 tablespoons bacon fat (from above)

2 tablespoons red wine vinegar

1 tablespoon Swerve confectioners'-style sweetener

½ teaspoon Dijon mustard

When we lived in Florida, we would often host small get-togethers at our house, and our best friend, Mike, could always be found in the kitchen making amazing food for everyone. In the spirit of the good ol' days, I asked him to create a recipe for this book. I hope you enjoy this delicious and flavorful salad. Cheers to good friends who are really more like family.

1. Fry the bacon in a skillet over medium-high heat until crispy, 8 to 10 minutes, then remove from the pan and set aside on a paper towel–lined plate to drain. Reserve 2 tablespoons of the bacon fat, leaving the rest (about 1 tablespoon) in the pan.

2. Thinly slice the shallot, then fry the shallot in the bacon fat until golden brown, 2 to 3 minutes. Remove from the pan and set on the paper towel with the fried bacon.

3. Slice the mushroom cap and sauté in the bacon fat until soft and tender, about 5 minutes, then remove to a bowl. Chop the cooled bacon.

4. Make the dressing: Put the reserved bacon fat in the same skillet you used to cook the bacon and vegetables and place the skillet over medium heat. Whisk in the vinegar, sweetener, and mustard and heat until warm.

5. To serve, divide the spinach, chopped bacon, and sautéed shallots and mushrooms between 2 plates. Arrange the sliced eggs on the top and drizzle each salad with about 2 tablespoons of the warm bacon dressing. Season with freshly ground black pepper.

PER SERVING:
CALORIES **416** · FAT **34g** · PROTEIN **18g** · TOTAL CARBS **13g** · FIBER **3g** · ERYTHRITOL **4.5g** · NET CARBS **5.5g**

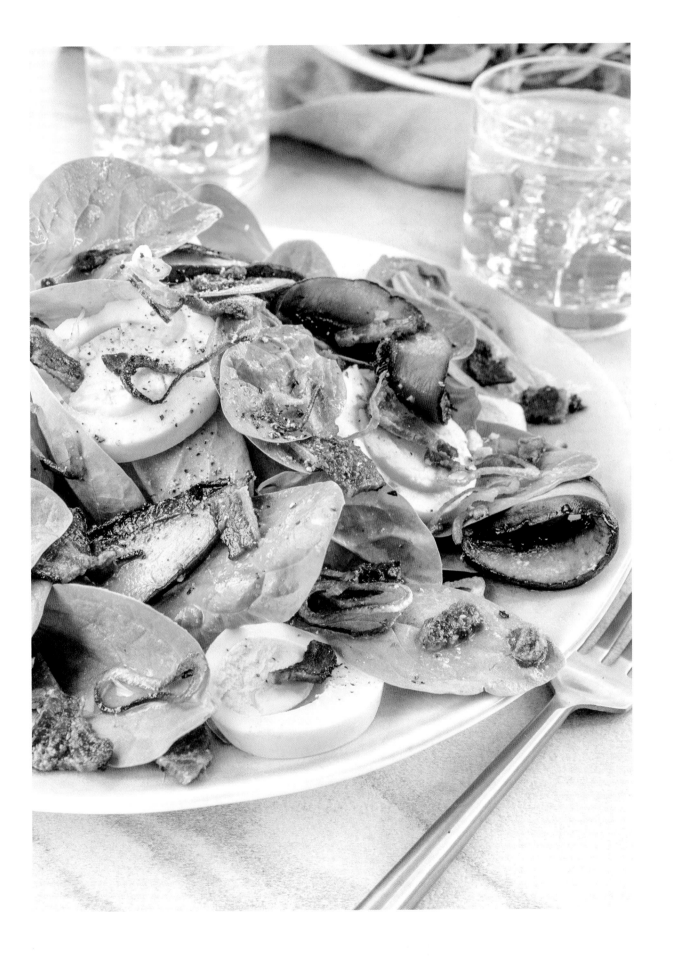

MAUI SHORT RIBS

Yield: 3 servings

Prep Time: 10 minutes, plus 6 hours to marinate

Cook Time: 10 minutes

MARINADE

1 cup soy sauce or coconut aminos

⅓ cup Swerve brown sugar

2 tablespoons grated ginger

2 cloves garlic, minced

2 teaspoons toasted sesame oil

Pinch of red pepper flakes (optional)

6 flanken short ribs, ½ inch thick

1 green onion, chopped, for garnish

You are going to love this delicious marinade-to-grill recipe. Flanken short ribs are cut thin, so they cook fast over high heat, yet stay tender from the marinade and get a nice caramelization on the outside. These sweet and spicy ribs will be a hit at any BBQ!

1. Place the ingredients for the marinade in a bowl and whisk to combine.

2. Place the short ribs in a gallon-sized zip-top plastic bag and pour the marinade over the top. Marinate the ribs for at least 6 hours; overnight is best.

3. When ready to cook, preheat a grill or grill pan to medium-high heat. Remove the ribs from the marinade and place on the grill. Pour the excess marinade into a small saucepan and bring to a boil over medium-high heat, stirring periodically as the ribs cook, to make a sauce.

4. Grill the ribs for 4 to 5 minutes per side, until they reach the desired doneness (4 minutes for pink in the middle and 5 minutes for more well-done ribs). Brush with the prepared sauce and top with the chopped green onion.

PER SERVING:

CALORIES 158 · FAT 11g · PROTEIN 15g · TOTAL CARBS 6g · FIBER 0g · ERYTHRITOL 4g · NET CARBS 2g

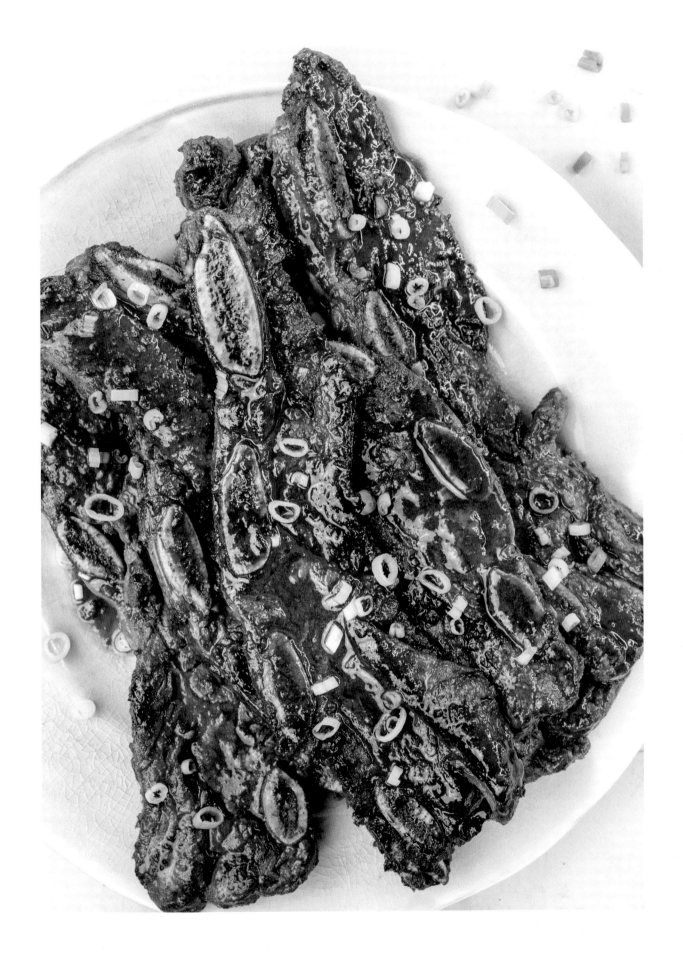

SLOW COOKER MISSISSIPPI POT ROAST

Yield: 6 servings (about 1 cup per serving)

Prep Time: 10 minutes

Cook Time: 8 hours

8 tablespoons (1 stick) unsalted butter, divided

1 (3-pound) chuck roast, cut in half lengthwise

1 tablespoon dried minced onions

1 tablespoon garlic powder

1 teaspoon dried dill weed

1 teaspoon ground black pepper

½ cup beef broth

½ cup pepperoncini juice (from the jar of pepperoncini)

12 pepperoncini

Chopped fresh parsley, for garnish (optional)

This is a classic slow cooker meal, made with unprocessed ingredients and low in carbs. I opted out of using prepackaged seasonings to avoid any unnecessary added ingredients.

1. Heat 2 tablespoons of the butter in a large skillet over high heat. Once hot, brown the beef for about 3 minutes per side.

2. Transfer the beef to a 6-quart slow cooker. Add the remaining 6 tablespoons of butter and the rest of the ingredients.

3. Cover and cook on low for 8 hours, or until the beef is fork-tender. Shred the meat with 2 forks and serve hot. Garnish with parsley, if desired.

beef & pork

PER SERVING:
CALORIES **429** · FAT **25g** · PROTEIN **48g** · TOTAL CARBS **3g** · FIBER **1g** · NET CARBS **2g**

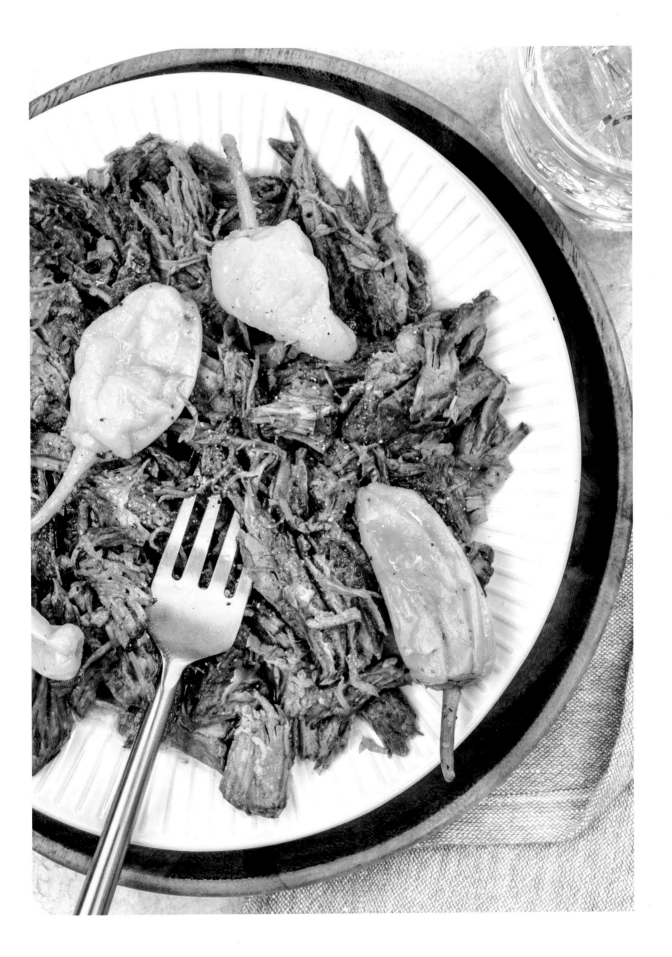

CARNE ASADA

Yield: 6 servings

Prep Time: 10 minutes, plus 2 hours to marinate

Cook Time: 14 minutes

MARINADE

⅓ cup chopped fresh cilantro

1 jalapeño pepper, seeded and minced

4 cloves garlic, minced

Juice of 3 limes

⅓ cup olive oil

½ teaspoon ground cumin

½ teaspoon salt

¼ teaspoon ground black pepper

2 pounds skirt steak

Serving tip:
Great with Chimichurri (page 88)!

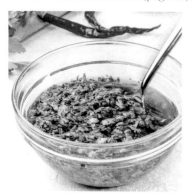

Pair this authentic Mexican grilled steak with Grilled Avocado with Cilantro Lime Sour Cream (page 252) for a delicious and easy meal!

1. In a small bowl, whisk together all the marinade ingredients.

2. Pound the steak to ½-inch thickness, then place the steak in a gallon-sized zip-top plastic bag. Pour the marinade into the bag and seal it, removing as much air from the bag as possible. Make sure all of the steak is coated with the marinade. Place in the refrigerator for a minimum of 2 hours or up to overnight.

3. Preheat a grill to high heat. Remove the steak from the marinade; discard the marinade. Cook for 5 to 7 minutes on each side for medium doneness. Remove the steak to a cutting board and let rest for 5 minutes.

4. Using a sharp knife, slice the steak at an angle against the grain. From there, you can further chop the carne asada into smaller pieces.

PER SERVING:
CALORIES **422** · FAT **32g** · PROTEIN **31g** · TOTAL CARBS **2g** · FIBER **0g** · NET CARBS **2g**

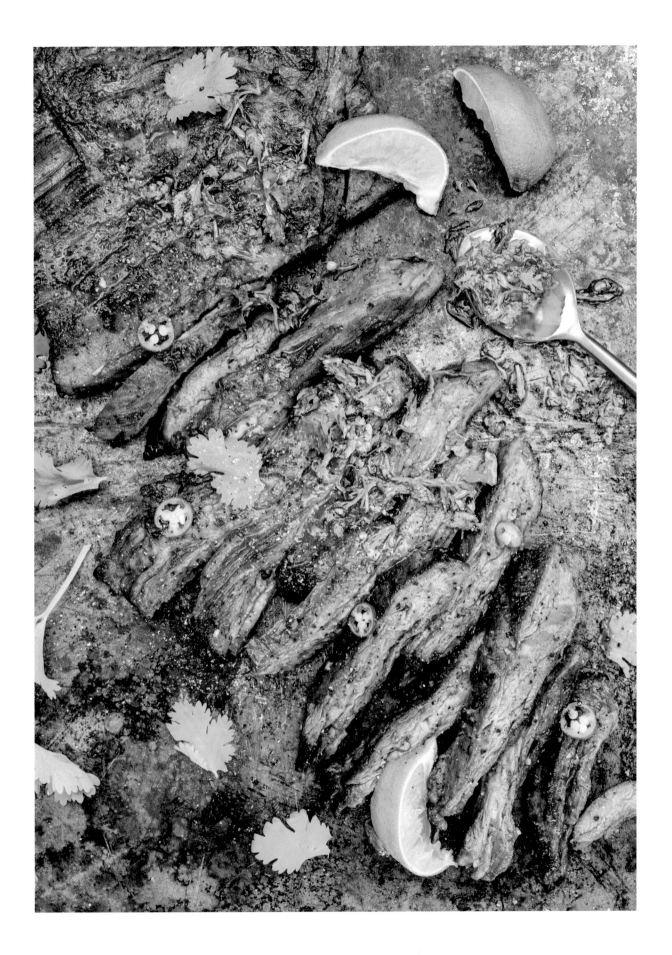

GRILLED "HONEY" MUSTARD PORK CHOPS

Yield: 4 servings

Prep Time: 5 minutes

Cook Time: 30 minutes

"HONEY" MUSTARD

½ cup mayonnaise

2 tablespoons Swerve confectioners'-style sweetener

2 tablespoons prepared yellow mustard

1 tablespoon Dijon mustard

4 bone-in pork chops (about 1 inch thick)

¼ teaspoon garlic powder

Pinch of salt

Pinch of ground black pepper

1½ teaspoons olive oil

Before starting keto, I ordered honey mustard with a lot of my meals, so I had high expectations for creating a keto-friendly honey mustard. After making a few batches, I used some of the honey mustard as a marinade for pork chops, and they were delicious! Enjoy!

1. Make the "honey" mustard: Place all the ingredients in a small bowl and stir until smooth and well blended. Transfer ¼ cup of the "honey" mustard to a separate bowl for glazing the pork chops; reserve the rest to serve as a dipping sauce.

2. Preheat a grill to medium-high heat.

3. Season the pork chops on both sides with the garlic powder, salt, and pepper. Then rub them with the oil.

4. Once the grill is nice and hot, spray the grate with cooking spray and set the seasoned pork chops on the grill. Cook for 10 to 15 minutes per side, or until the internal temperature reaches 145°F. When the chops are almost done, use a pastry brush to glaze the tops and sides with the reserved "honey" mustard, then flip the chops over and glaze the other side, using about 1 tablespoon of "honey" mustard for each chop.

5. Remove the pork chops from the grill and enjoy with the remaining "honey" mustard.

PER SERVING:
CALORIES **535** · FAT **32g** · PROTEIN **51g** · TOTAL CARBS **10g** · FIBER **3g** · ERYTHRITOL **4.5g** · NET CARBS **2.5g**

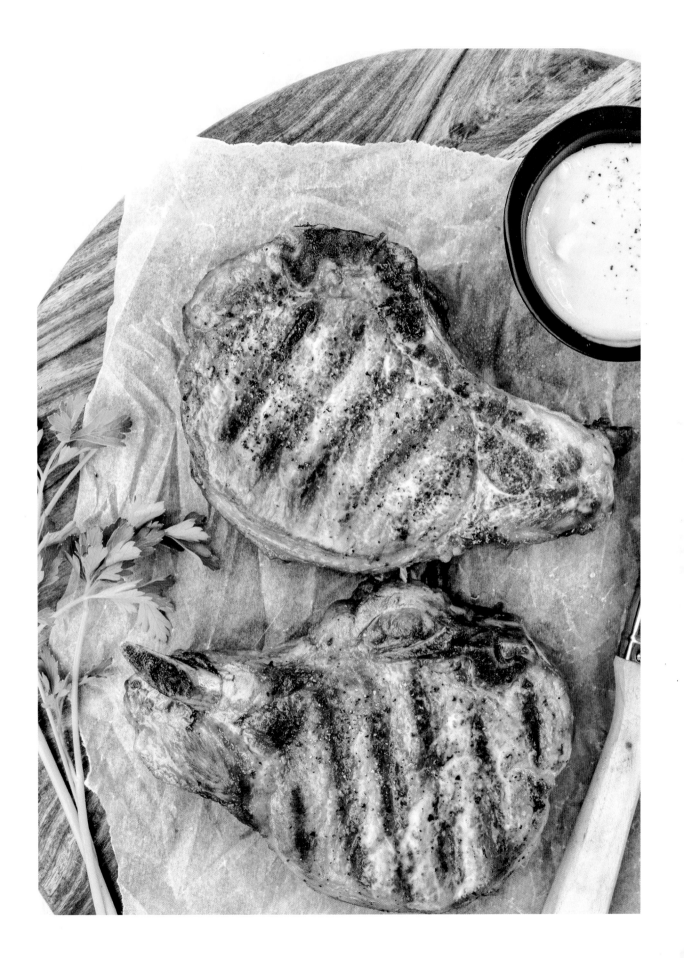

BEEF AND BROCCOLI

Yield: 4 servings

Prep Time: 10 minutes, plus 30 minutes to marinate

Cook Time: 9 minutes

SAUCE

¼ cup soy sauce or coconut aminos

¼ cup beef broth

1 tablespoon toasted sesame oil

1 tablespoon fish sauce

1 tablespoon Swerve brown sugar

2 teaspoons grated ginger

1 pound flank steak

1 tablespoon coconut oil, avocado oil, or olive oil

6 cups broccoli florets

3 cloves garlic, minced

2 green onions, sliced (about ¼ cup)

2 teaspoons sesame seeds

Beef and broccoli is a staple menu item found in most Chinese restaurants. By cooking this dish at home you are able to avoid unwanted sugars and corn starch that are often used in Chinese restaurant sauces.

1. Make the sauce: Place the ingredients for the sauce in a small bowl and whisk to combine. You can also put everything in a mason jar, seal the lid, and shake.

2. Thinly slice the beef across the grain into bite-sized pieces, then put them in a gallon-sized zip-top bag along with 2 tablespoons of the sauce. Allow to marinate for 30 minutes to 1 hour. Set the rest of the sauce in the refrigerator for later.

3. In a large skillet over high heat, heat the oil until it's nice and hot. Place the beef in the skillet in a single layer and cook for about 1 minute on each side, then remove to a plate.

4. Put the broccoli, garlic, and reserved sauce in the skillet and cook until the broccoli is nearly crisp-tender, about 5 minutes. When the broccoli is almost done cooking, stir in the green onions and cook for 1 to 2 minutes. Add the sesame seeds and cooked beef, toss, and serve.

PER SERVING:

CALORIES **316** · FAT **17g** · PROTEIN **28g** · TOTAL CARBS **12g** · FIBER **5g** · ERYTHRITOL **2g** · NET CARBS **5g**

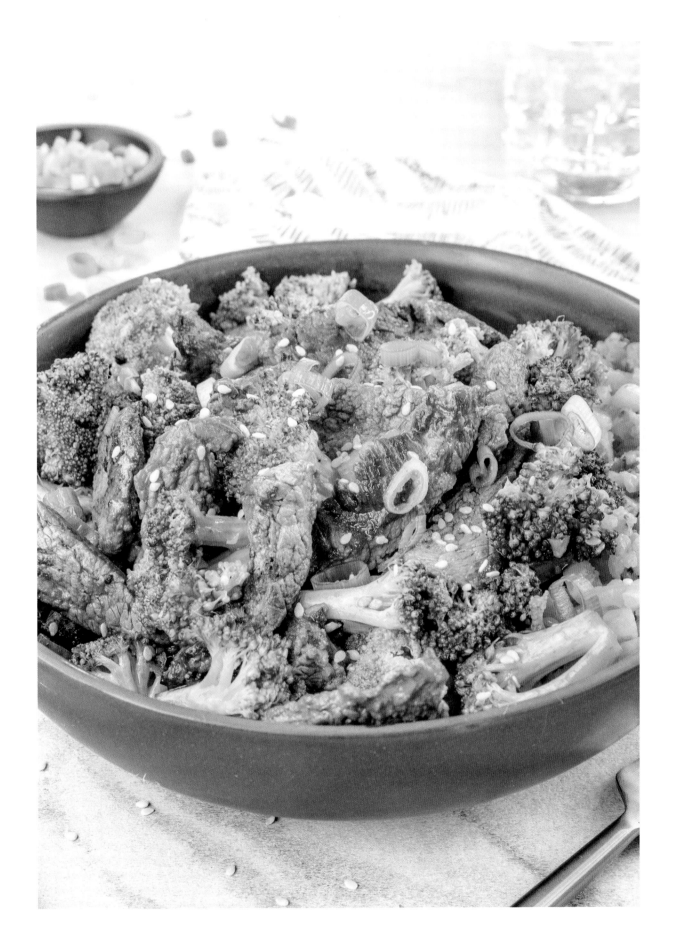

ITALIAN SAUSAGE WITH PEPPERS

Yield: 4 servings

Prep Time: 10 minutes

Cook Time: 28 minutes

2 tablespoons olive oil, divided

1 pound mild Italian sausage links

1 medium-sized yellow onion, sliced

2 cloves garlic, pressed

1 red bell pepper, sliced

1 (14½-ounce) can diced tomatoes

1 teaspoon dried oregano leaves

½ teaspoon salt

¼ cup chopped fresh basil

Freshly grated Parmesan cheese, for topping (optional; omit for dairy-free)

A simple and delicious meal that the whole family will love!

1. Heat 1 tablespoon of the olive oil in a large skillet over medium heat. Add the sausages and cook until browned on all sides and nearly cooked through. Transfer the sausages to a cutting board to rest.

2. Add the remaining 1 tablespoon of olive oil to the same pan along with the onion and garlic and sauté until the onion slices are soft and fragrant, 3 to 4 minutes. Then add the sliced bell pepper and sauté for 3 to 4 minutes. Next, add the tomatoes, oregano, and salt and mix well. Increase the heat to medium-high heat and simmer vigorously for 3 to 5 minutes to reduce the sauce.

3. Meanwhile, slice the sausages into ½-inch pieces. Add the sausage and basil to the sauce. Use a spatula to mix the sauce and coat all the sausage pieces.

4. Simmer over medium-low heat for 8 to 10 minutes, or until the sausage is fully cooked and the sauce is thick. Serve as is if dairy-free, or top with grated Parmesan cheese, if desired.

PER SERVING (WITHOUT CHEESE):
CALORIES **411** · FAT **33g** · PROTEIN **17g** · TOTAL CARBS **11g** · FIBER **3g** · NET CARBS **8g**

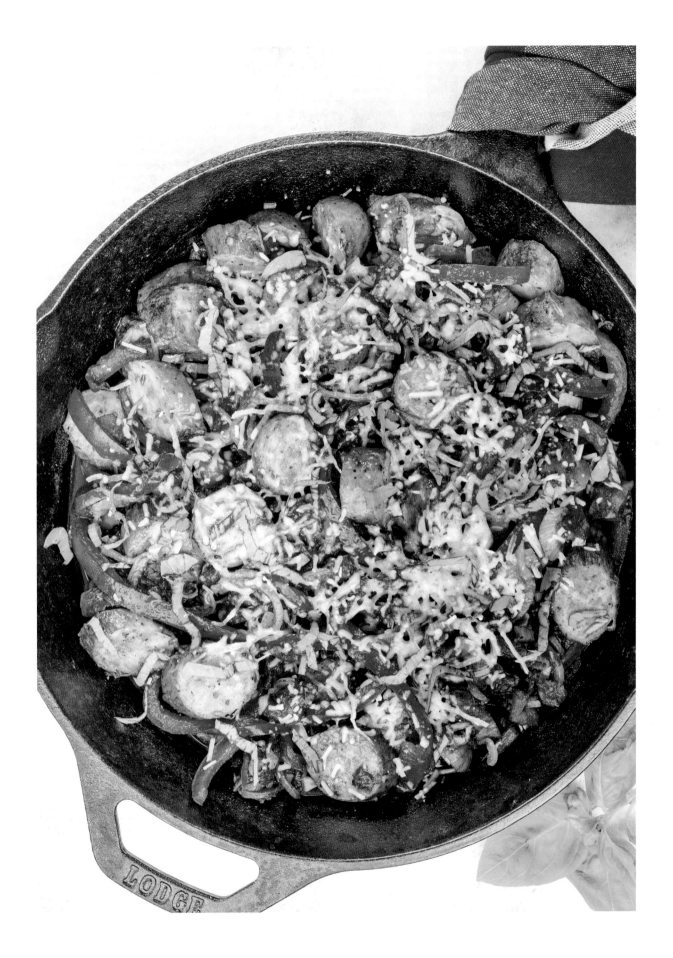

CALLIE'S KETO LASAGNA

Yield: 5 servings

Prep Time: 15 minutes (not including time to make marinara)

Cook Time: 45 minutes

2 medium zucchini

MEAT SAUCE

1 pound bulk mild Italian sausage or ground beef

1½ cups no-sugar-added marinara sauce, homemade (page 82) or store-bought

RICOTTA FILLING

¾ cup whole-milk ricotta (see note)

⅓ cup freshly grated Parmesan cheese

1 large egg

¼ cup sliced fresh basil

½ teaspoon garlic powder

½ teaspoon ground black pepper

¼ teaspoon salt

1 cup shredded mozzarella cheese

note Be sure to purchase a lower-carb ricotta. The carb amount should be around 1 gram per 2 tablespoons.

My lifelong best friend, Callie, created this recipe for this book. Callie and her husband, Robert, love keto lasagna so much that they even mentioned it in their wedding vows! This lasagna is hearty and delicious, with layers of Italian sausage, marinara sauce, ricotta, and mozzarella cheese.

1. Preheat the oven to 350°F.

2. Use a mandoline or knife to slice the zucchini lengthwise into long, thin planks and set aside.

3. Brown the sausage in a large sauté pan over high heat, breaking up the meat into crumbles, then add the marinara sauce and let simmer for 3 to 5 minutes.

4. In a medium bowl, mix together all the ricotta filling ingredients, not including the mozzarella.

5. In a 9 by 5-inch loaf pan, layer the ingredients as follows:

⅔ cup meat sauce

One-third of the ricotta filling

A single layer of zucchini slices

⅔ cup meat sauce

One-third of the ricotta filling

⅓ cup shredded mozzarella

A single layer of zucchini slices

⅔ cup meat sauce

One-third of the ricotta filling

A single layer of zucchini slices

⅔ cup shredded mozzarella

6. Bake for 30 minutes, until the cheese is melted and the zucchini is tender, then broil for 1 to 2 minutes, until the cheese starts to bubble and brown, watching carefully so the lasagna doesn't burn.

PER SERVING:

CALORIES **336** · FAT **23g** · PROTEIN **28g** · TOTAL CARBS **6g** · FIBER **2g** · NET CARBS **4g**

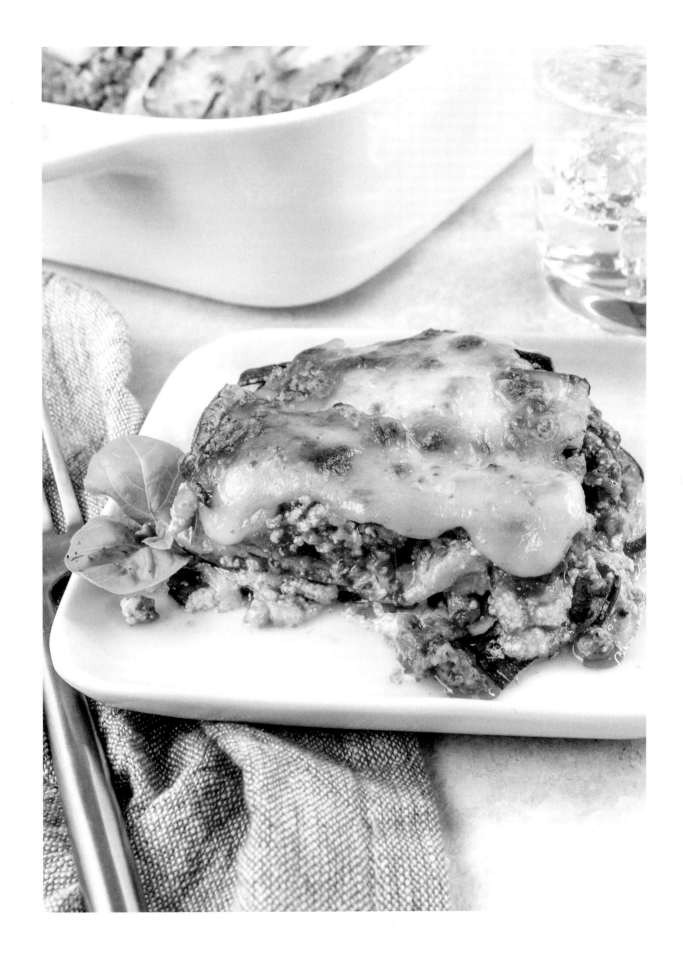

EGG ROLL IN A BOWL

Yield: 4 servings

Prep Time: 5 minutes

Cook Time: 15 minutes

1 tablespoon avocado oil

1 pound ground pork

2 cloves garlic, minced

1 teaspoon ginger powder

¼ teaspoon salt

¼ teaspoon ground black pepper

2 teaspoons toasted sesame oil

2 large eggs

1 (14-ounce) bag coleslaw mix

½ cup chopped green onions

¼ cup soy sauce or coconut aminos

FOR SERVING

1 tablespoon toasted sesame seeds

Keto Yum Yum Sauce (page 89) or Sriracha sauce, to taste (optional)

I'm all about this easy one-skillet recipe that is ready in only 20 minutes. This is a weekly staple in my house. I hope you enjoy it as much as we do!

1. Heat the avocado oil in a large skillet over medium-high heat. Add the ground pork, garlic, ginger, salt, and pepper and cook until the meat is browned, 7 to 10 minutes.

2. Make a well in the middle of the meat. Pour the sesame oil and then crack the eggs into the well and immediately start scrambling the eggs until they are firm and curds have formed.

3. Toss in the coleslaw mix, green onions, and soy sauce and cook, stirring occasionally, until the vegetables are tender and coated in oil but still crisp, about 3 minutes.

4. To serve, divide among 4 bowls and top with the toasted sesame seeds. Drizzle with the sauce, if desired.

note This dish can easily get too salty. Be sure to taste first before adding additional salt or soy sauce.

PER SERVING:

CALORIES **480** · FAT **33g** · PROTEIN **36g** · TOTAL CARBS **8g** · FIBER **3g** · NET CARBS **5g**

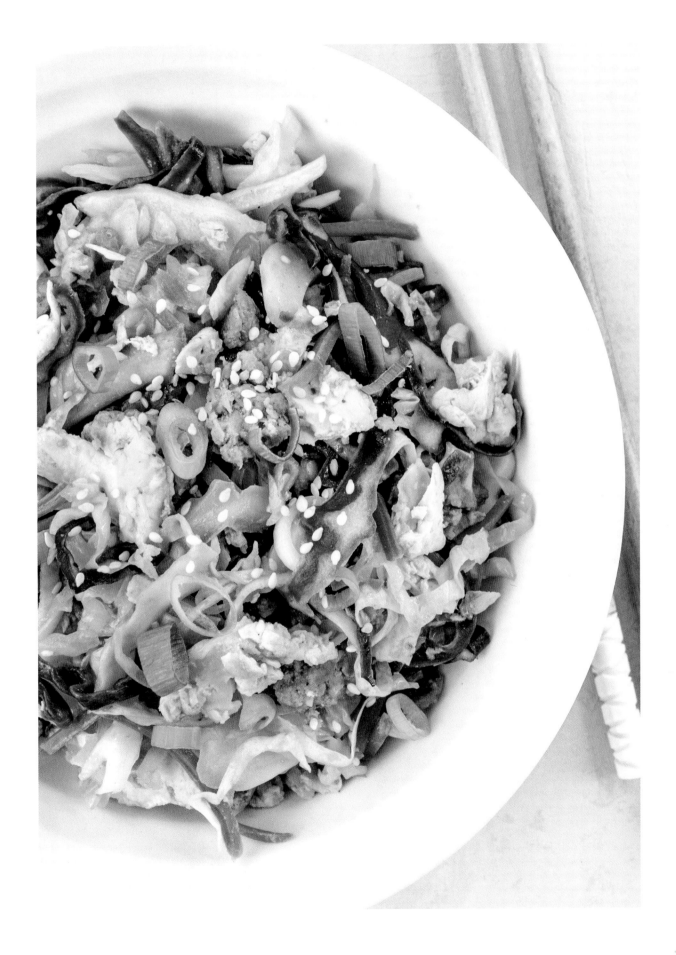

REUBEN CASSEROLE

Yield: 8 servings

Prep Time: 10 minutes (not including time to make dressing)

Cook Time: 40 minutes

1 pound sauerkraut

1 pound cooked corned beef or pastrami

¾ cup Sugar-Free Thousand Island Dressing (page 83)

½ cup sour cream

3 large eggs

8 ounces Swiss cheese, shredded or sliced

1 teaspoon caraway seeds (optional)

This warm and hearty casserole has all the components of a classic Reuben, and it's so delicious that you won't even miss the bread.

1. Preheat the oven to 350°F. Spray a 9 by 13-inch casserole dish with cooking spray.

2. Drain the sauerkraut and squeeze any extra liquid from it using a paper towel or cheesecloth. Layer the sauerkraut evenly in the bottom of the casserole dish.

3. Chop or coarsely shred the corned beef into about ½-inch pieces. Evenly spread the corned beef over the sauerkraut.

4. In a separate bowl, whisk together the Thousand Island dressing, sour cream, and eggs. Pour the mixture over the sauerkraut and corned beef.

5. Top the casserole with the Swiss cheese and caraway seeds, if using. Cover with aluminum foil and bake for 40 minutes, until bubbly.

PER SERVING:

CALORIES 372 · FAT 23g · PROTEIN 19g · TOTAL CARBS 3g · FIBER 1g · NET CARBS 2g

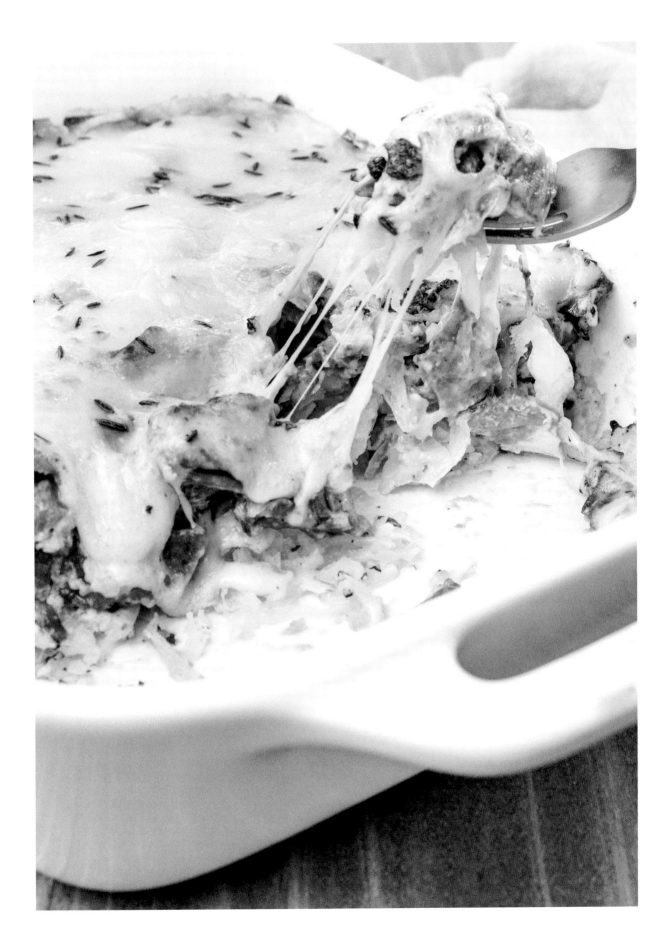

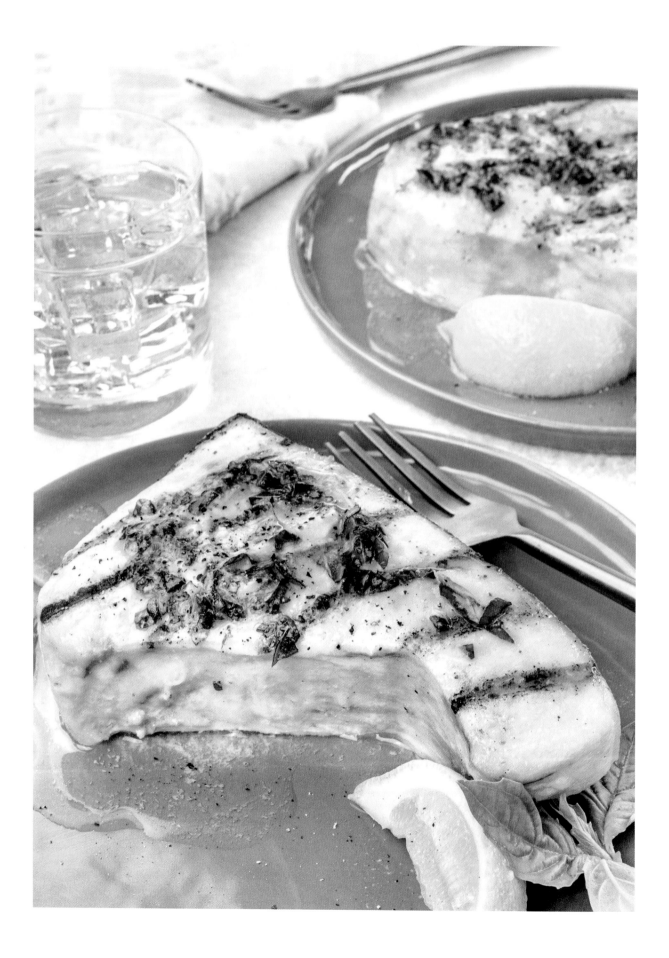

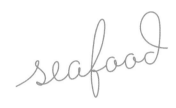

seafood

CAJUN SHRIMP AND "GRITS"

Yield: 4 servings

Prep Time: 15 minutes

Cook Time: 20 minutes

CAULIFLOWER "GRITS"

1 large head cauliflower

1 tablespoon unsalted butter

½ cup chicken broth

½ cup heavy whipping cream

1 cup shredded cheddar cheese

Salt and pepper

CAJUN SHRIMP

2 tablespoons olive oil

½ red bell pepper, diced

1 stalk celery, diced

¼ cup chicken broth

1 pound large or extra-large shrimp, peeled and deveined

2 teaspoons Cajun seasoning

1 green onion, chopped, for garnish

note Use 4 cups of packaged riced cauliflower to save time!

Shrimp and grits may be one of my top ten favorite foods. It is perfect for breakfast, lunch, or dinner and is easy to prepare. With a little cauliflower magic, I came up with creamy and cheesy "grits" to go with the spicy shrimp, giving this rendition the same texture and flavors of the classic Southern dish.

MAKE THE "GRITS"

1. Core the head of cauliflower and grate the cauliflower florets with a cheese grater or food processor to make cauliflower "rice." Chop up any large pieces that may not have gone through the grater. One large head of cauliflower should yield about 1 pound of riced cauliflower.

2. Melt the butter in a medium saucepan over medium-high heat, then add the cauliflower and sauté for 5 minutes. Add the chicken broth and cook over medium heat for about 5 more minutes, until most of the liquid is cooked out.

3. Slowly add the cream and cheese, stirring well to incorporate, until smooth and creamy.

Add salt and pepper to taste. Keep over very low heat while preparing the shrimp.

MAKE THE CAJUN SHRIMP

1. In a large skillet, heat the olive oil over medium-high heat. Sauté the bell pepper and celery for about 2 minutes. Add the chicken broth, stirring with a wooden spoon to scrape off the browned bits at the bottom of the pan.

2. Place the shrimp in the pan in a single layer and sprinkle with the Cajun seasoning. Lower the heat to medium and cook for 2 minutes per side, until the shrimp is pink.

3. To serve, spoon about 1 cup of the prepared "grits" into a shallow bowl and top with one-quarter of the Cajun shrimp. Repeat with the remaining grits and shrimp. Garnish with chopped green onions.

PER SERVING:

CALORIES **390** · FAT **29g** · PROTEIN **36g** · TOTAL CARBS **8g** · FIBER **3g** · NET CARBS **5g**

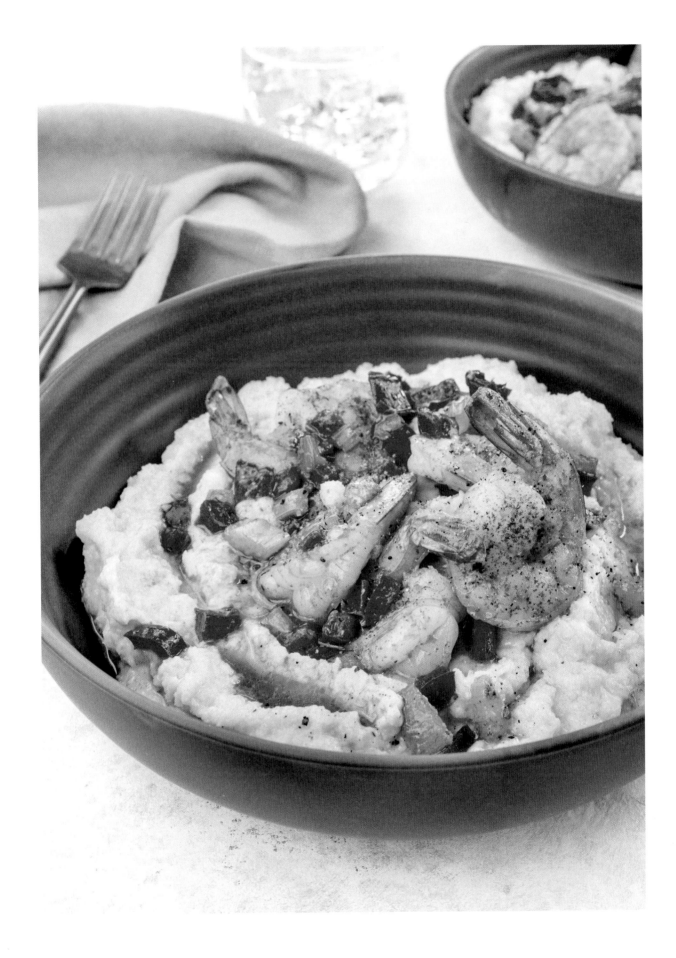

SHRIMP SCAMPI WITH ZUCCHINI NOODLES

Yield: 4 servings

Prep Time: 5 minutes

Cook Time: 9 minutes

4 tablespoons (½ stick) unsalted butter, divided

4 cloves garlic, minced

1 pound large shrimp, peeled and deveined

Salt and pepper

¼ cup dry white wine

½ teaspoon red pepper flakes (optional)

2 tablespoons fresh lemon juice

2 large zucchini, spiral-sliced (see note)

¼ cup chopped fresh parsley

When you want something fast, shrimp is always a great option. This entire dish took me less than 15 minutes to make, and uses minimal ingredients. I love using zucchini noodles in this dish to soak up all the delicious buttery garlic sauce.

1. Melt 2 tablespoons of the butter in a large sauté pan over medium-high heat. Add the garlic and sauté until fragrant, about 1 minute.

2. Add the shrimp in a single layer and season with salt and pepper. Cook for 1 to 2 minutes per side, until the shrimp just begin to turn pink.

3. Pour in the wine and add the red pepper flakes, if using. Bring to a simmer and cook for an additional 1 to 2 minutes, until the wine is reduced and the shrimp are cooked through.

4. Stir in the remaining 2 tablespoons of butter and the lemon juice. Add the zucchini noodles and parsley and toss until the butter is melted and the zucchini turns soft, 1 to 2 minutes.

note If you don't have a spiralizer, you can use a vegetable peeler and peel the zucchini into long strips to use as your "noodles."

PER SERVING:

CALORIES **232** · FAT **12g** · PROTEIN **24g** · TOTAL CARBS **5g** · FIBER **2g** · NET CARBS **3g**

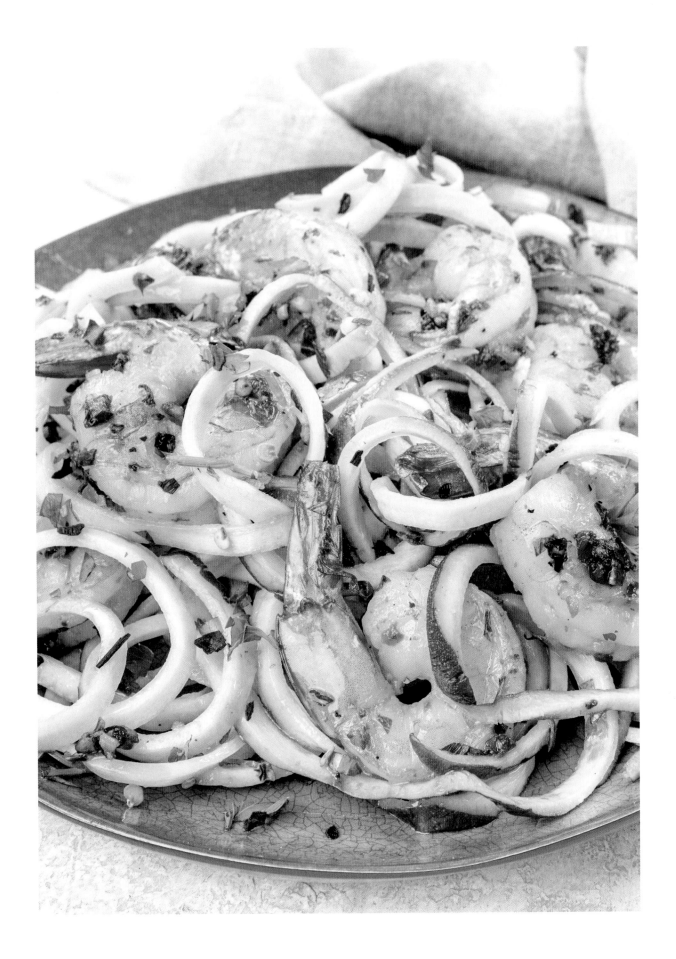

BACON-WRAPPED SCALLOPS

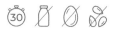

Yield: 16 bacon-wrapped scallops (4 per serving)

Prep Time: 5 minutes

Cook Time: 25 minutes

8 slices bacon, cut in half crosswise

16 large sea scallops (about 1 pound)

Salt and pepper

2 teaspoons olive oil, plus more for drizzling

Chopped fresh parsley, for garnish

Bite-sized surf and turf! Pair these scallops with a basic cauli-mash and some asparagus for the perfect 30-minute meal. This is also a great appetizer option!

1. Preheat the oven to 425°F. Line a rimmed baking sheet with parchment paper.

2. Place the bacon on the prepared baking sheet and bake for 6 to 8 minutes, until cooked but still slightly pliable.

3. Pat the scallops dry with a paper towel, then season lightly with salt and pepper. Wrap each scallop in a half slice of bacon and secure with a toothpick. Place on the prepared baking sheet.

4. Drizzle the olive oil over the scallops and bake for 15 to 17 minutes, until the scallops are opaque and the bacon is cooked through. Serve hot, drizzled with more olive oil and sprinkled with more freshly ground pepper. Garnish with parsley.

PER SERVING:
CALORIES **228** · FAT **12g** · PROTEIN **32g** · TOTAL CARBS **0g** · FIBER **0g** · NET CARBS **0g**

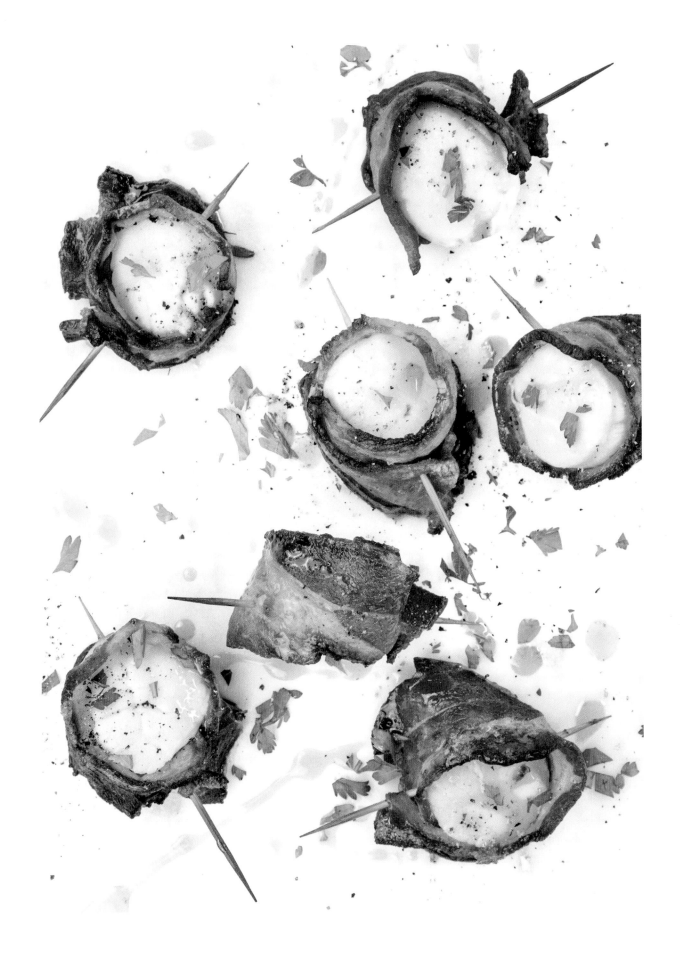

COD VERACRUZ

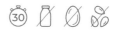

Yield: 4 servings

Prep Time: 10 minutes

Cook Time: 20 minutes

VERACRUZ SAUCE

2 tablespoons olive oil

½ red bell pepper, thinly sliced

½ medium-sized yellow onion, thinly sliced

2 cloves garlic, minced

1 (14½-ounce) can diced tomatoes

½ cup mixed olives, pitted and halved

½ jalapeño pepper, seeded and minced

1 tablespoon capers, drained

1 tablespoon dried oregano leaves

Salt and pepper

4 (4- to 6-ounce) cod fillets

Chopped fresh parsley, for garnish

Veracruz is a light and colorful sauce from Mexico that is full of tender cooked vegetables and spices. What I love about this particular recipe is that the fish is cooked right in the sauce, so you need only one pan! Alternatively, if you are not a fan of seafood, you can make the sauce (just complete Steps 1 and 2) and serve it with grilled chicken or pork tenderloin.

1. Heat the oil in a large skillet over medium-high heat. Add the bell pepper and onion slices and sauté until soft, 7 to 9 minutes.

2. Add the garlic, tomatoes, olives, jalapeño, capers, and oregano and stir to combine. Reduce the heat to medium-low and let simmer for about 5 minutes. Season with salt and pepper to taste.

3. Lightly season the cod fillets with salt and pepper and place over the veggies in the skillet. Spoon some of the sauce on top of the fish. Cover with the lid and cook over medium heat for 5 to 6 minutes, or until the fish flakes easily with a fork. Garnish with parsley and serve.

PER SERVING:
CALORIES **201** · FAT **6g** · PROTEIN **27g** · TOTAL CARBS **9g** · FIBER **3g** · NET CARBS **6g**

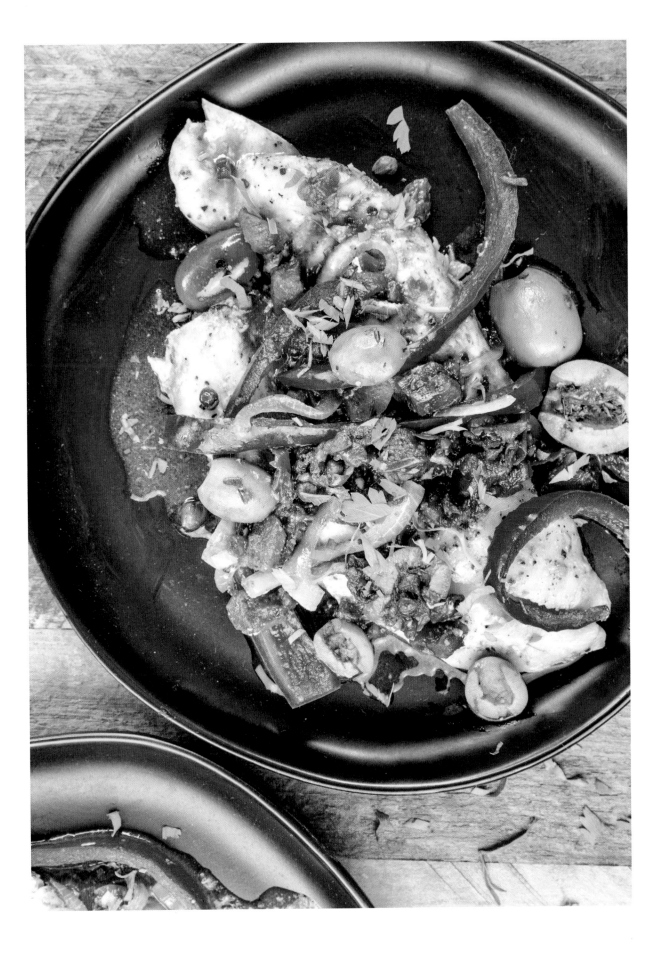

SRIRACHA LIME SALMON

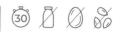

Yield: 4 servings

Prep Time: 5 minutes

Cook Time: 15 minutes

Grated zest of ½ lime

Juice of ½ lime

1 tablespoon Swerve brown sugar

1½ teaspoons Sriracha sauce

4 (4- to 6-ounce) salmon fillets

2 tablespoons chopped fresh cilantro, for garnish

A spicy, sweet, and sour trifecta! This salmon dish requires only six ingredients and takes just 20 minutes to make.

1. Preheat the oven to 400°F. Line a 9 by 13-inch baking dish with parchment paper.

2. In a bowl, whisk together the lime zest, lime juice, sweetener, and Sriracha.

3. Place the salmon in the prepared baking dish and pour the lime mixture over the top.

4. Bake the salmon until cooked through and flaky, about 15 minutes. Sprinkle with the cilantro and serve.

PER SERVING:
CALORIES **200** · FAT **6g** · PROTEIN **35g** · TOTAL CARBS **3g** · FIBER **0g** · ERYTHRITOL **3g** · NET CARBS **0g**

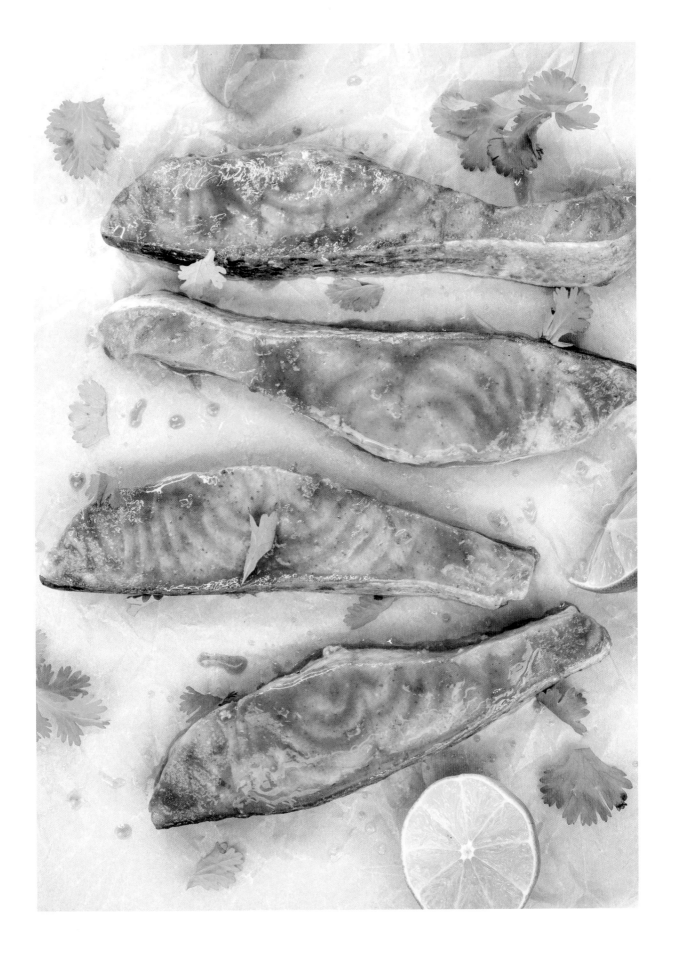

GRILLED SWORDFISH WITH BASIL BUTTER

Yield: 4 servings

Prep Time: 5 minutes

Cook Time: 6 minutes

4 (5- to 6-ounce) swordfish steaks

1 tablespoon olive oil

Salt and pepper

Lemon wedges, for garnish

BASIL BUTTER

¼ cup (½ stick) salted butter, softened

Grated zest of ½ lemon

2 tablespoons chopped fresh basil

⅛ teaspoon garlic powder

A melt-in-your-mouth mild-tasting fish with a delightful basil butter.

1. Preheat a grill to medium-high heat.

2. Brush the swordfish steaks with the oil and season them with salt and pepper. Grill the steaks until just cooked through, about 3 minutes per side.

3. While the fish is cooking, mix together the ingredients for the basil butter until combined.

4. Once the swordfish steaks are cooked, remove them from the grill, place on serving plates, and immediately top each steak with 1 tablespoon of the basil butter. Allow the butter to melt for 2 to 3 minutes, then garnish with lemon wedges and serve.

PER SERVING:
CALORIES **377** · FAT **26g** · PROTEIN **34g** · TOTAL CARBS **0g** · FIBER **0g** · NET CARBS **0g**

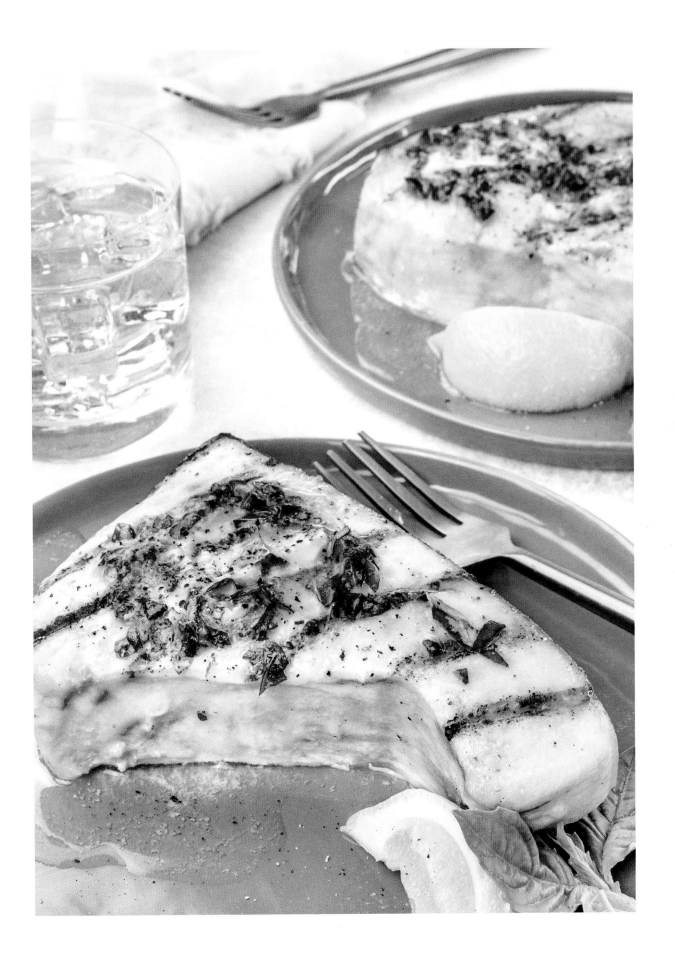

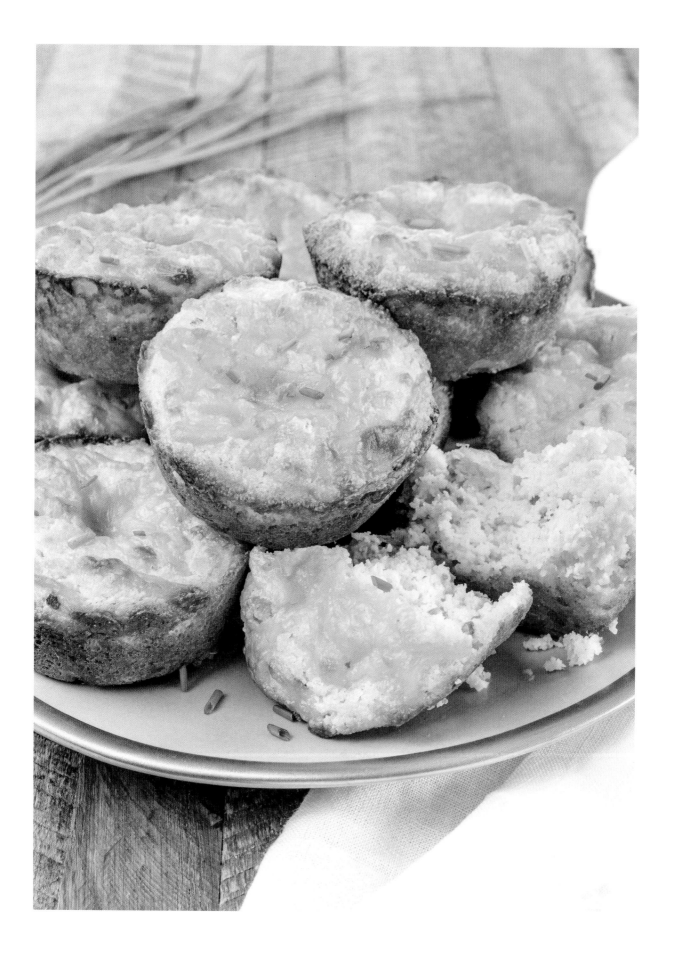

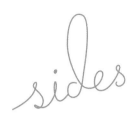

sides

BAKED SPINACH CHIPS **/ 246**

THAI CUCUMBER SALAD **/ 248**

STRAWBERRY SPINACH SALAD WITH
CANDIED PECANS **/ 250**

GRILLED AVOCADO WITH
CILANTRO LIME SOUR CREAM **/ 252**

ROASTED RAINBOW VEGGIES **/ 254**

COLESLAW **/ 256**

BROILED PARMESAN TOMATOES **/ 258**

CHEESY BROCCOLI BAKE **/ 260**

LEMON PARMESAN ASPARAGUS **/ 262**

THREE-CHEESE ZUCCHINI AU GRATIN **/ 264**

ROASTED GARLIC CAULIFLOWER MASH **/ 266**

CHEDDAR CHIVE BISCUITS **/ 268**

BAKED SPINACH CHIPS

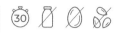

Yield: 2 servings

Prep Time: 3 minutes

Cook Time: 15 minutes

2½ ounces fresh spinach

Cooking spray

Salt and pepper

When you find yourself craving salty and crunchy chips, you can whip up a batch of these. Feel free to experiment with different seasonings, like a sprinkle of grated Parmesan cheese, taco seasoning (page 150), or Ranch Herb Mix (page 85)…the options are limitless!

1. Preheat the oven to 325°F. Line a rimmed baking sheet with parchment paper or a silicone baking mat.

2. Lay the spinach in a single layer on the prepared baking sheet. Lightly spray the spinach with cooking spray and season with salt and pepper. Bake for 10 minutes, then turn off the oven and leave the spinach in the oven for an additional 5 minutes, or until the chips are dry and crisp.

PER SERVING:
CALORIES **30** · FAT **2g** · PROTEIN **1g** · TOTAL CARBS **1.5g** · FIBER **1g** · NET CARBS **0.5g**

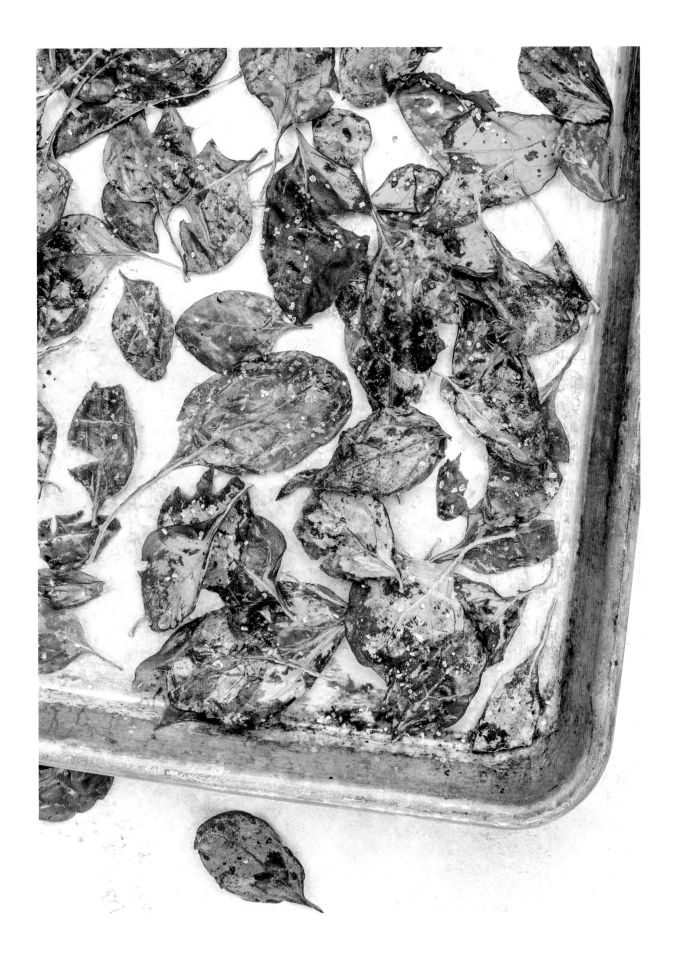

THAI CUCUMBER SALAD

Yield: 2 servings

Prep Time: 10 minutes, plus 10 minutes to chill

1 large cucumber

¼ cup thinly sliced red onions

¼ cup chopped fresh cilantro

¼ cup white vinegar

2 (1-gram) packets powdered stevia

1 teaspoon salt

Chopped peanuts, for garnish (optional; omit for nut-free)

Only six ingredients and 10 minutes are all you need to make this salty and sweet Thai salad. If you're feeling fancy, you can spiral-slice the cucumber for this salad.

1. Peel the cucumber, cut it in half lengthwise, and then seed it and slice it into half-moons.

2. Put the chopped cucumber in a large bowl along with the rest of the ingredients. Mix to combine. Place in the refrigerator to chill for at least 10 minutes. Serve cold, garnished with chopped peanuts, if desired.

PER SERVING (WITHOUT PEANUTS):
CALORIES **37** · FAT **0g** · PROTEIN **2g** · TOTAL CARBS **6g** · FIBER **2g** · NET CARBS **4g**

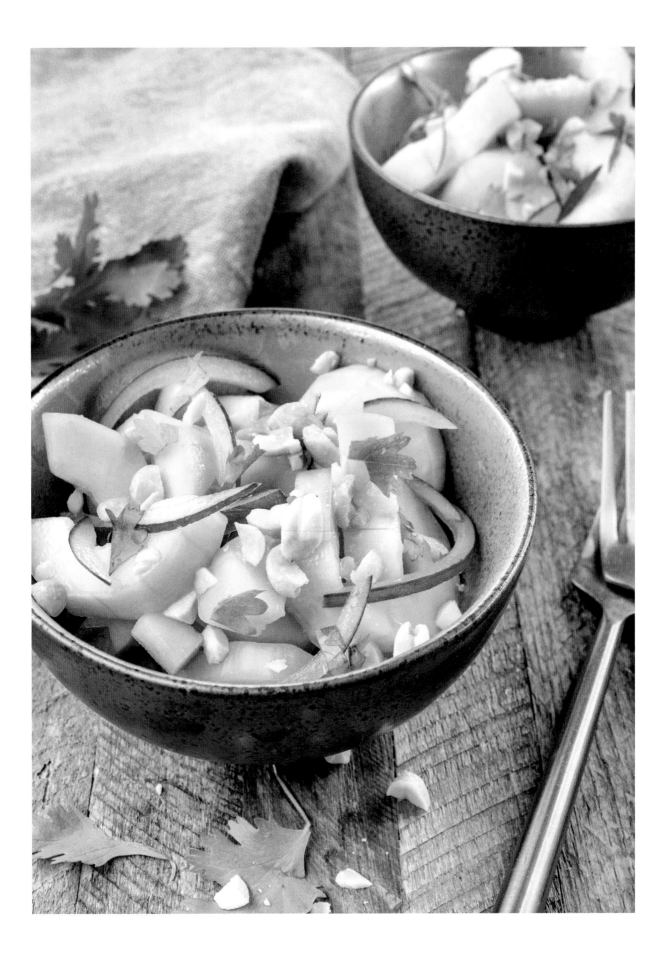

STRAWBERRY SPINACH SALAD WITH CANDIED PECANS

Yield: 4 servings

Prep Time: 5 minutes (not including time to make candied pecans or dressing)

6 ounces baby spinach

6 fresh strawberries, sliced

⅓ cup crumbled goat cheese

⅓ cup Tina's Candied Pecans (page 280), chopped

¼ to ½ cup Simple Vinaigrette (page 84) or other keto-friendly salad dressing of choice

Berries are a great keto option, but they need to be eaten in moderation. That is why I love to add just a few to a salad to brighten it up, like in this fresh spinach salad that also features creamy goat cheese, crunchy candied pecans, and a vinegary dressing. It is a perfect no-cook summertime side.

Toss the spinach, strawberries, goat cheese, and pecans together in a large salad bowl. Divide among 4 serving plates. Dress each salad with 1 to 2 tablespoons of the vinaigrette or other dressing of your choice.

note For a change, feel free to dress this salad with your favorite salad dressing. Make it a full meal by adding grilled chicken.

PER SERVING (WITH 2 T. SIMPLE VINAIGRETTE):
CALORIES 333 · FAT 33g · PROTEIN 5g · TOTAL CARBS 16g · FIBER 5g · ERYTHRITOL 8g · NET CARBS 3g

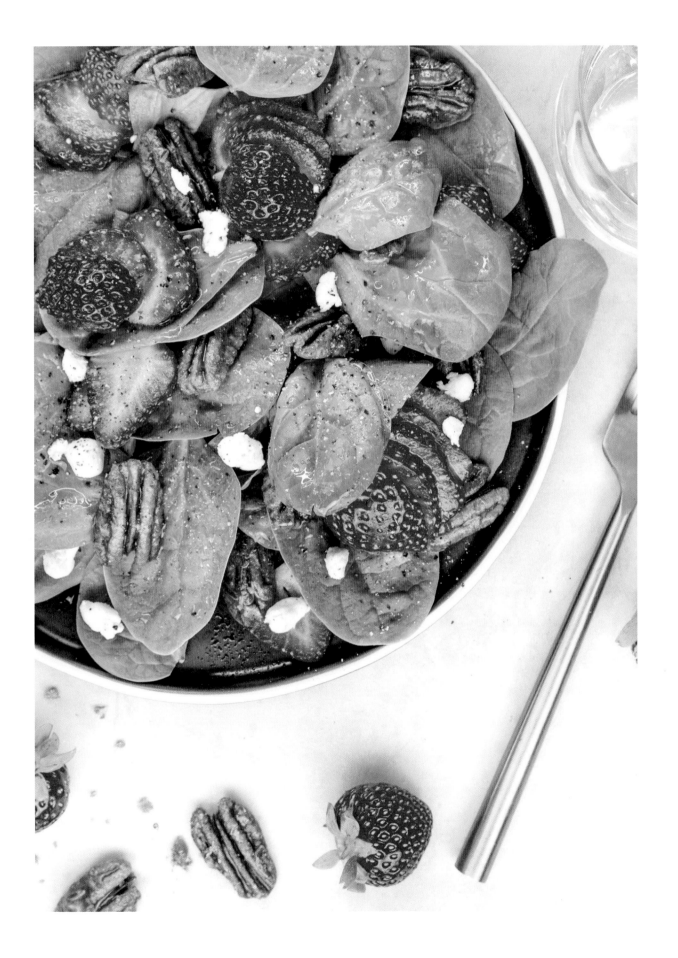

GRILLED AVOCADO WITH CILANTRO LIME SOUR CREAM

Yield: 2 servings

Prep Time: 10 minutes, plus 30 minutes to chill sauce

Cook Time: 5 minutes

SAUCE

¼ cup sour cream

Grated zest of ¼ lime

1 teaspoon fresh lime juice

1 tablespoon finely chopped fresh cilantro

⅛ teaspoon garlic powder

Small pinch of salt

1 avocado

1 teaspoon olive oil

Pinch of salt

Pinch of ground black pepper

Avocados are well loved in the keto community, but generally I didn't really love them cooked . . . until I tried a grilled one! This is a simple and delicious recipe that pairs perfectly with a variety of options, like pork chops, chicken, steak, or seafood.

1. In a small bowl, mix together all the ingredients for the sauce. Place in the refrigerator to chill for at least 30 minutes.

2. Preheat a grill to high heat.

3. Cut the avocado in half and remove the pit. Brush the flesh with the oil and season it with the salt and pepper.

4. Grill the avocado halves cut side down for about 5 minutes, or until they have even grill marks.

5. Remove the avocados from the grill and spoon the sauce over them, or put the sauce in a zip-top plastic bag, cut off one corner, and drizzle the sauce over the avocados.

PER SERVING:
CALORIES **199** · FAT **18g** · PROTEIN **2g** · TOTAL CARBS **8g** · FIBER **5g** · NET CARBS **3g**

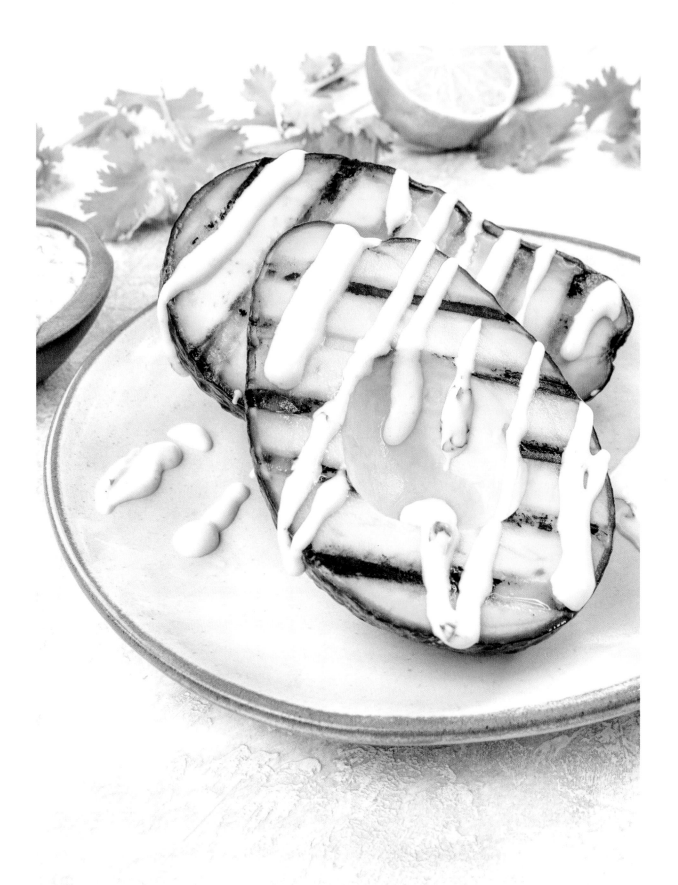

ROASTED RAINBOW VEGGIES

Yield: 8 servings (about 1 cup per serving)

Prep Time: 15 minutes

Cook Time: 25 minutes

7 ounces button mushrooms

1 orange bell pepper

20 radishes

2 small yellow squash

1 large head broccoli, separated into florets

1 medium-sized red onion

3 tablespoons olive oil

2 teaspoons salt

1 teaspoon ground black pepper

1 teaspoon garlic powder

A side that is as beautiful as it is delicious! Mushrooms tend to cook faster and shrink more than the other vegetables, so no need to chop them when prepping this side.

1. Preheat the oven to 400°F.

2. Put the mushrooms in a large mixing bowl. Cut the bell pepper in half lengthwise and remove the seeds, membranes, and stem. Chop the bell pepper, squash, broccoli, and onion into bite-sized pieces and add them to the bowl with the mushrooms.

3. Pour the olive oil over the vegetables and toss to coat evenly, then season with the salt, pepper, and garlic powder.

4. Evenly distribute the veggies on a rimmed baking sheet and bake for 25 minutes, flipping the veggies over halfway through cooking.

PER SERVING:
CALORIES **83** · FAT **5g** · PROTEIN **2g** · TOTAL CARBS **8g** · FIBER **3g** · NET CARBS **5g**

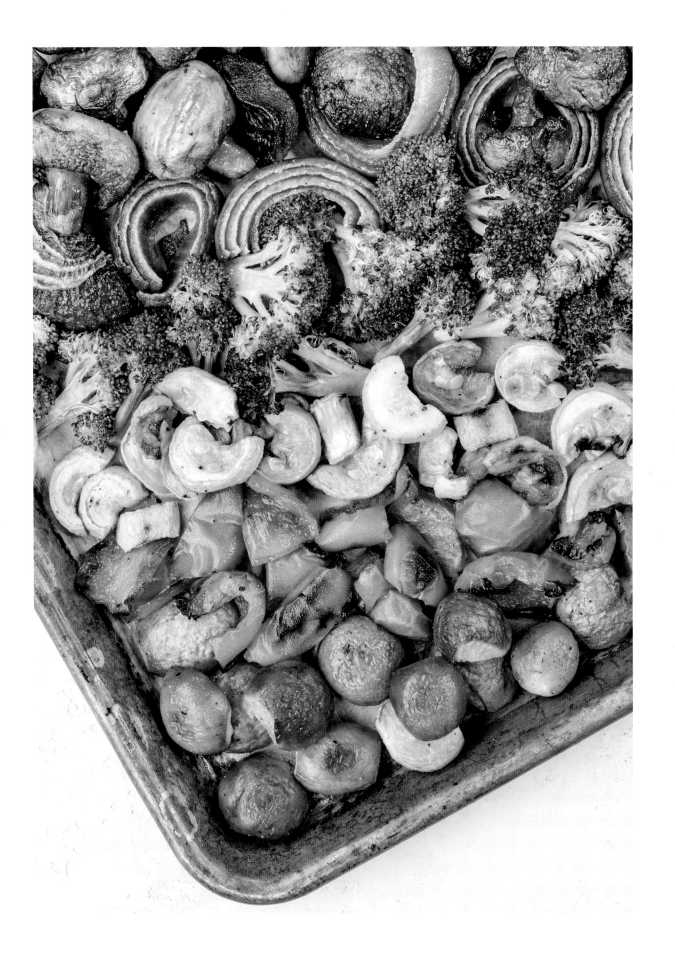

COLESLAW

Yield: 8 servings

Prep Time: 10 minutes

4 cups shredded green cabbage

2 cups shredded red cabbage

½ cup shredded carrots

DRESSING

⅓ cup mayonnaise

1 tablespoon apple cider vinegar

1 tablespoon Swerve confectioners'-style sweetener

1 teaspoon poppy seeds (optional)

¼ teaspoon salt

¼ teaspoon ground black pepper

Traditional coleslaw is one of those sides that is so close to being keto, yet most restaurants add a lot of sugar or honey to it. Luckily, this classic dish is super easy to make at home using a keto-friendly sweetener and simple ingredients.

Put the cabbage and carrots in a large bowl. In a small bowl, whisk together the ingredients for the dressing. Pour the dressing over the cabbage and toss together. Store leftovers in the refrigerator for up to 3 days.

PER SERVING:
CALORIES **51** · FAT **3g** · PROTEIN **1g** · TOTAL CARBS **6g** · FIBER **2g** · ERYTHRITOL **1g** · NET CARBS **3g**

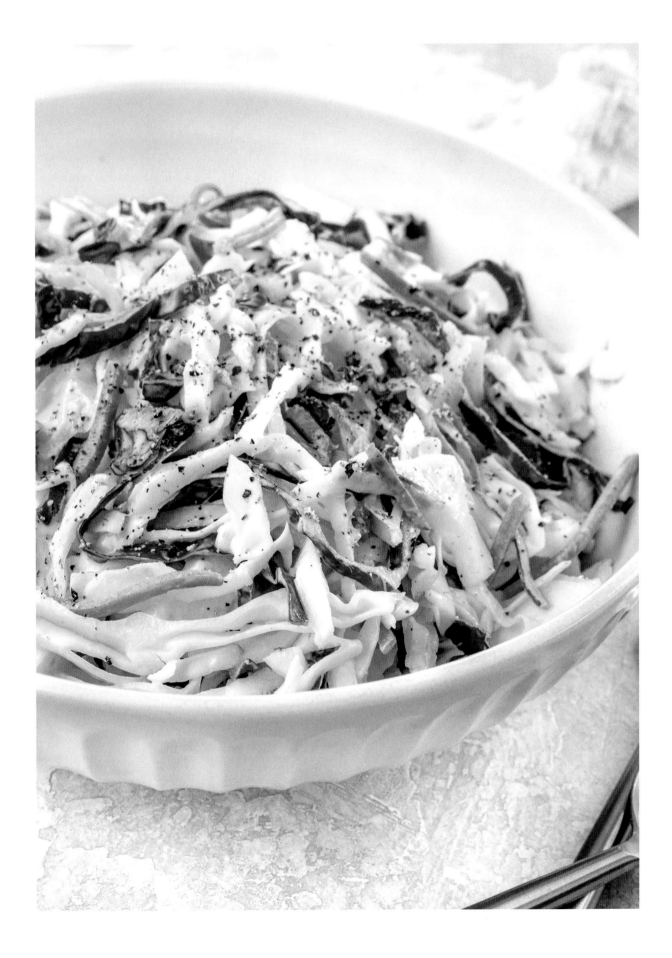

BROILED PARMESAN TOMATOES

Yield: 4 servings

Prep Time: 5 minutes

Cook Time: 6 minutes

2 Roma tomatoes

¼ teaspoon garlic powder

¼ cup freshly grated Parmesan cheese

2 tablespoons mayonnaise

1 tablespoon chopped fresh basil

Pinch of salt

Pinch of ground black pepper

I like tomatoes when they are raw, but I love them even more when they are broiled with cheese! These tomatoes are perfect as a side dish for breakfast, lunch, or dinner.

1. Cut the tomatoes in half lengthwise. Sprinkle the halves with the garlic powder.

2. Place the Parmesan cheese, mayonnaise, basil, salt, and pepper in a small bowl and mix well to combine. Spread the mixture evenly over the tomato halves.

3. Broil on high for 5 to 6 minutes, until the cheese is bubbling.

PER SERVING:
CALORIES **77** · FAT **6g** · PROTEIN **3g** · TOTAL CARBS **2g** · FIBER **1g** · NET CARBS **1g**

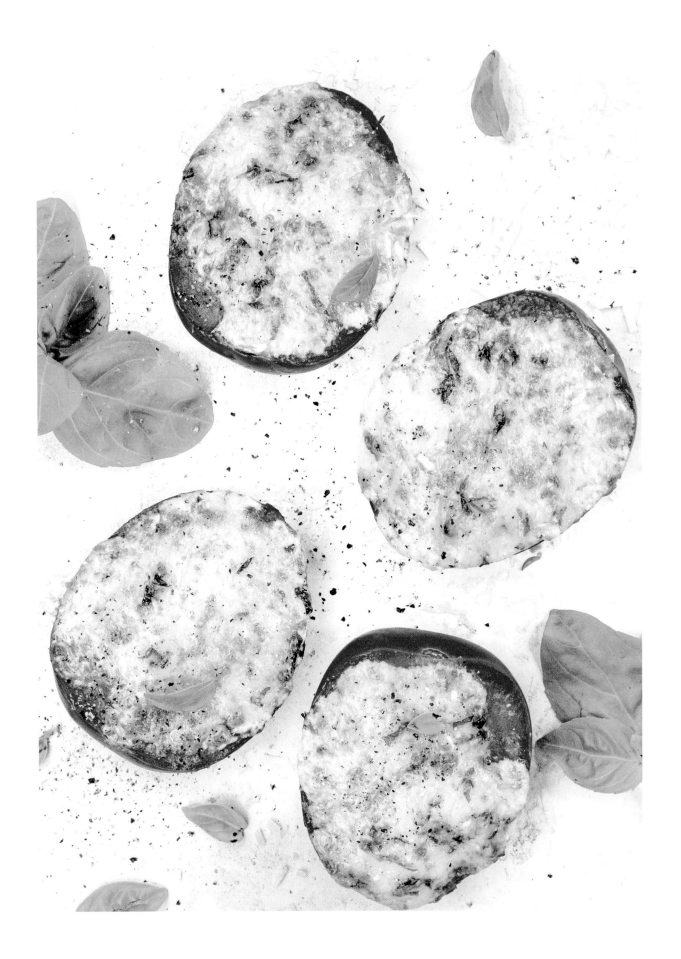

CHEESY BROCCOLI BAKE

Yield: 6 servings

Prep Time: 15 minutes (not including time to cook bacon)

Cook Time: 18 minutes

1 pound broccoli florets (from about 2 heads of broccoli), chopped into bite-sized pieces

6 slices chopped thick-cut bacon, cooked until crispy

2 cups shredded cheddar cheese, divided

½ cup sour cream

1 large or 2 small cloves garlic, pressed

Pinch of salt

Pinch of ground black pepper

As a parent, I'm always looking for ways to make veggies delicious and desirable for my little one, who is sometimes a picky eater. It's always a good feeling when Olivia asks for a broccoli bake with dinner—plus, we adults always enjoy it, too!

1. Preheat the oven to 350°F.

2. In a large pot of salted boiling water, blanch the broccoli florets for 3 minutes. Remove with a slotted spoon and put in a large bowl.

3. To the bowl with the broccoli, add the bacon, 1½ cups of the cheddar cheese, the sour cream, garlic, salt, and pepper. Mix together until well incorporated.

4. Pour the mixture into a 9-inch square casserole dish and top with the remaining ½ cup of cheddar cheese. Bake for 10 to 15 minutes, until the cheese is melted.

PER SERVING:
CALORIES **240** · FAT **20g** · PROTEIN **14g** · TOTAL CARBS **6g** · FIBER **2g** · NET CARBS **4g**

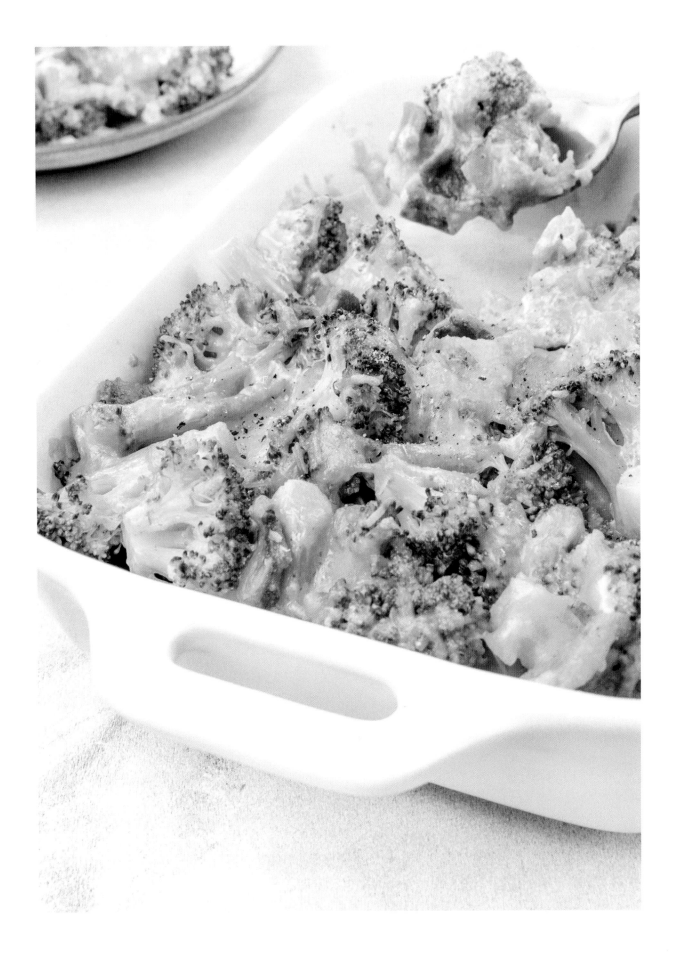

LEMON PARMESAN ASPARAGUS

Yield: 6 servings

Prep Time: 5 minutes

Cook Time: 12 minutes

1 pound asparagus, tough ends trimmed

3 tablespoons coconut oil, melted

Juice of ½ lemon

1 clove garlic, pressed

¼ teaspoon salt

¼ teaspoon ground black pepper

¾ cup freshly grated Parmesan cheese, divided

This is one of my favorite ways to prepare and cook asparagus, and my go-to for a quick yet flavorful side.

1. Preheat the oven to 425°F.

2. Put the asparagus, coconut oil, lemon juice, garlic, salt, pepper, and half of the cheese in a gallon-sized zip-top plastic bag. Shake until the asparagus is well coated.

3. Spread the asparagus evenly on a rimmed baking sheet. Bake for 10 to 12 minutes, until fork-tender but still crisp. Top with the remaining cheese before serving.

note To save time on cleanup, line the baking sheet with aluminum foil.

PER SERVING:
CALORIES **102** · FAT **9g** · PROTEIN **4g** · TOTAL CARBS **3g** · FIBER **2g** · NET CARBS **1g**

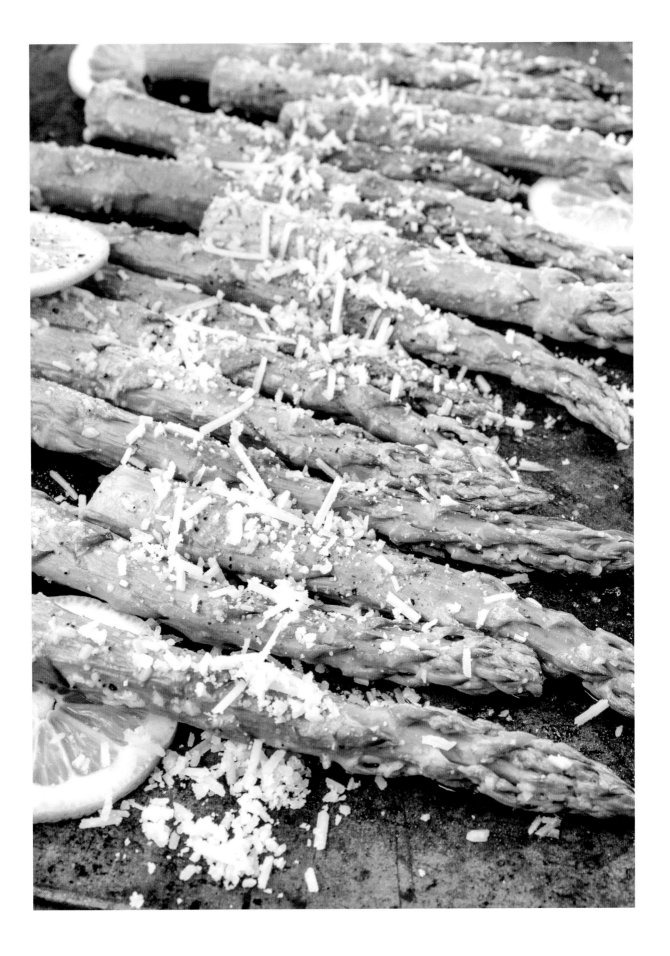

THREE-CHEESE ZUCCHINI AU GRATIN

Yield: 4 servings

Prep Time: 10 minutes

Cook Time: 30 minutes

2 to 3 medium or 4 small zucchini

1 cup shredded cheddar cheese

1 cup freshly grated Parmesan cheese

⅓ cup whipped cream cheese

⅓ cup half-and-half

½ teaspoon salt

¼ teaspoon ground black pepper

¼ teaspoon garlic powder

This squash casserole is loaded with cheeses and baked to perfection.

1. Preheat the oven to 400°F.

2. Using a mandoline or knife, slice the zucchini into thin rounds. Arrange a layer of the zucchini slices in a 8-inch square or similar-sized baking dish. (The dish pictured is 7½ by 6 inches.)

3. In a bowl, mix together the remaining ingredients.

4. Spread half of the cheese mixture over the layer of zucchini, then add a second layer of zucchini slices and top with the remaining cheese mixture.

5. Bake for 30 minutes, or until the zucchini is tender and the cheese is bubbly. Allow to cool for 5 minutes before serving.

note This recipe is easily doubled. Simply add two more layers and increase the baking time as needed.

PER SERVING:

CALORIES **215** · FAT **16g** · PROTEIN **14g** · TOTAL CARBS **8g** · FIBER **2g** · NET CARBS **6g**

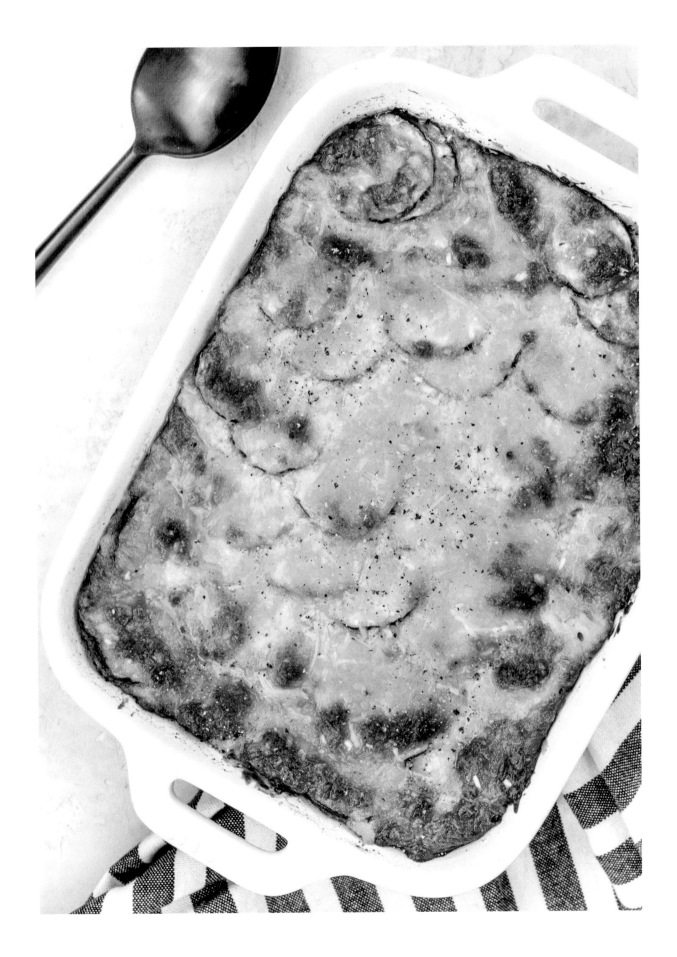

ROASTED GARLIC CAULIFLOWER MASH

Yield: 6 servings (½ cup per serving)

Prep Time: 10 minutes

Cook Time: 40 minutes

ROASTED GARLIC

1 bulb garlic

1 teaspoon olive oil, plus more for storage

CAULIFLOWER MASH

1 large head cauliflower

6 cloves roasted garlic (from above)

2 tablespoons olive oil

¼ cup unsweetened almond milk

1 teaspoon dried parsley, or 1 tablespoon chopped fresh parsley

½ teaspoon salt

½ teaspoon ground black pepper

Chopped fresh parsley, for garnish

note This recipe will leave you with extra roasted garlic. You can use it to make aioli, mix it with butter to spread over veggies, steak, or chicken, or chop it and add it to a salad dressing. Place the leftover cloves in an airtight container and cover them with olive oil. Store in the refrigerator for up to 2 weeks.

These are my classic "faux-tatoes" from *Simply Keto,* revamped and now dairy-free! When roasted, garlic becomes sweet, creamy, and so delicious. It makes a great addition to cauli mash.

MAKE THE ROASTED GARLIC

1. Preheat the oven to 400°F.

2. Cut the top off the bulb of garlic, about one-third of the way down, exposing the insides of most of the cloves. Place the bulb on a piece of aluminum foil, drizzle the olive oil over the top, and loosely wrap with the foil.

3. Roast for 40 minutes, until the cloves are golden brown and tender. When the garlic has been in the oven for 20 minutes, begin preparing the cauliflower mash.

4. Use a small spoon to gently scoop out the roasted garlic. Set aside 6 cloves for use in this recipe.

MAKE THE CAULIFLOWER MASH

1. Core the cauliflower and chop the florets into small pieces.

2. Bring a large pot of salted water to a boil. Add the cauliflower and cook until tender, about 20 minutes. Drain, then set on a paper towel and pat dry.

3. Put the cooked cauliflower along with the rest of the ingredients in a high-powered blender or food processor and blend just until smooth. Garnish with parsley.

INSTANT POT METHOD:

Core the cauliflower and cut the florets into 3 or 4 large sections. Pour 1 cup of water into the Instant Pot and place the cauliflower inside. Lock the lid, then turn the steam knob to the "sealed" setting. Press the vegetable steam button. Once complete, transfer the steamed cauliflower to a colander to drain, then set on a paper towel to dry. Complete Step 3 above for the mash.

PER SERVING:

CALORIES **71** · FAT **5g** · PROTEIN **2g** · TOTAL CARBS **6g** · FIBER **3g** · NET CARBS **3g**

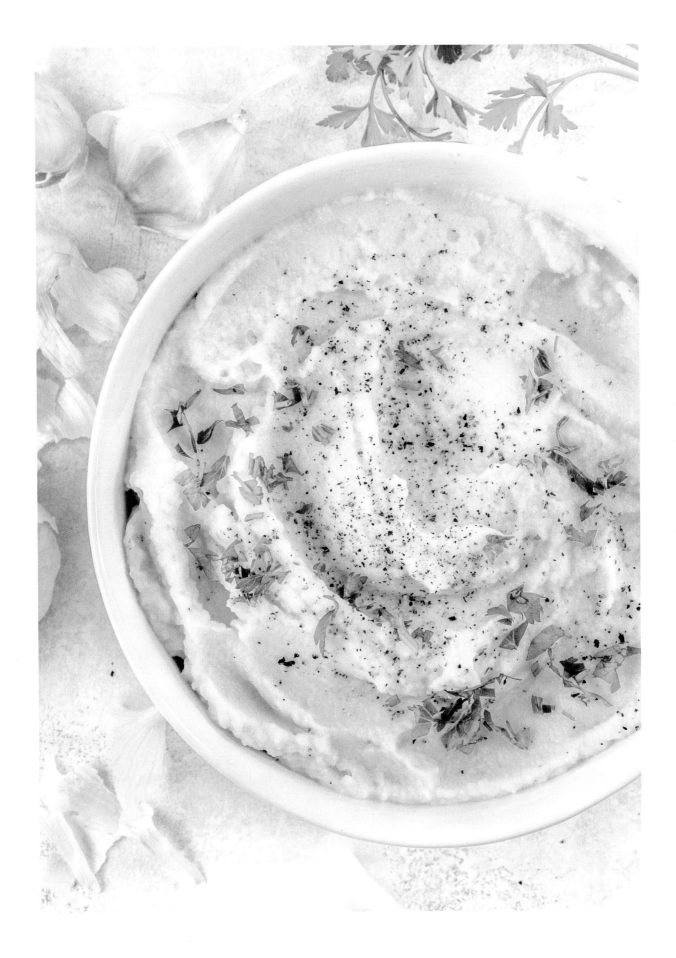

CHEDDAR CHIVE BISCUITS

Yield: 12 biscuits (1 per serving)

Prep Time: 10 minutes

Cook Time: 10 minutes

1½ cups blanched almond flour

1 tablespoon baking powder

½ teaspoon garlic powder

½ teaspoon salt

2 tablespoons chopped fresh chives

2 large eggs

½ cup sour cream

1 cup shredded cheddar cheese, divided

5 tablespoons unsalted butter, very cold

These fluffy, cheesy biscuits have only 1 gram of net carbs per serving. I love to serve them fresh out of the oven, broken in half and topped with a little butter.

1. Preheat the oven to 450°F. Coat a standard-size muffin pan with cooking spray.

2. In a large bowl, whisk together the almond flour, baking powder, garlic powder, salt, and chives.

3. Add the eggs, sour cream, and ½ cup of the cheese to the dry ingredients and stir to combine.

4. Using a cheese grater, grate the cold butter into the dough. Stir until well incorporated.

5. Using a spoon and a rubber spatula, distribute the dough equally among the wells of the muffin pan, filling each about three-quarters full. Slightly press the dough into the wells. Sprinkle the remaining ½ cup of cheese over the biscuits.

6. Bake for 10 minutes, or until a toothpick inserted into the center of a biscuit comes out clean. Let cool in the pan for 5 minutes, then carefully transfer the biscuits to a cooling rack. Serve while still warm or at room temperature. Store leftovers in the refrigerator for up to 3 days. Leftovers can be enjoyed at room temperature or cut in half and toasted.

PER SERVING:
CALORIES **241** · FAT **21g** · PROTEIN **9g** · TOTAL CARBS **3g** · FIBER **2g** · NET CARBS **1g**

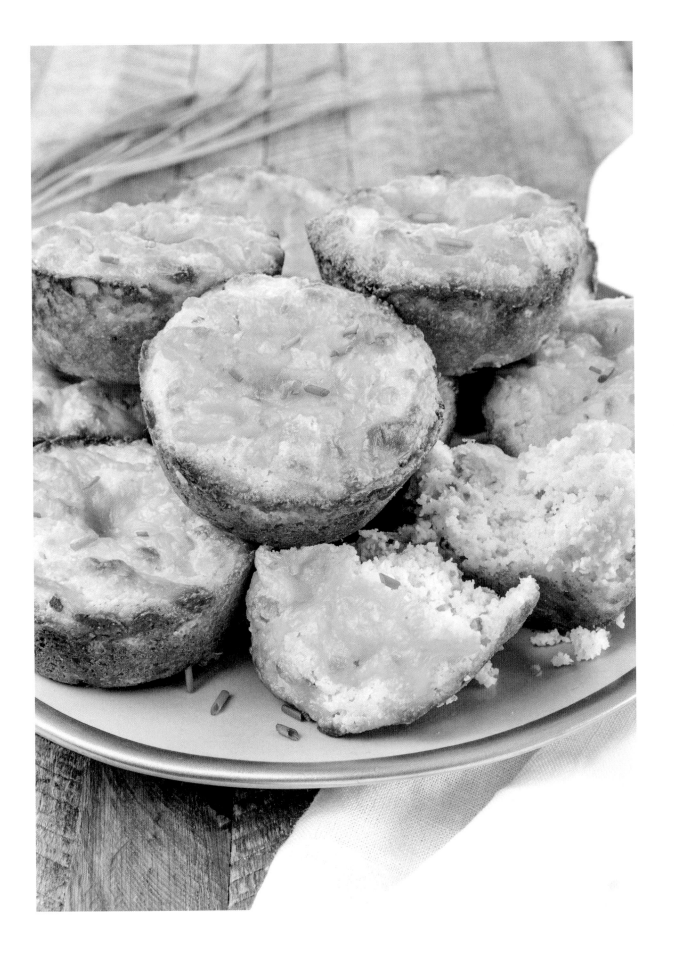

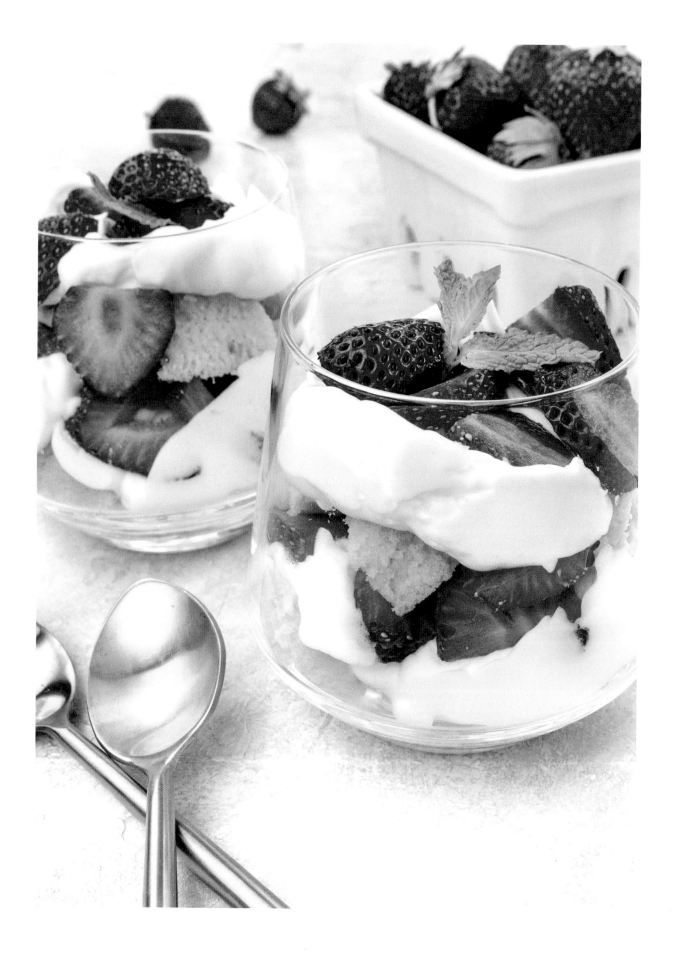

Desserts & Drinks

PEANUT BUTTER MOUSSE

Yield: 5 servings (½ cup per serving)

Prep Time: 10 minutes, plus 5 minutes to chill

½ cup heavy whipping cream

4 ounces cream cheese (½ cup), softened

½ cup natural peanut butter (salted)

½ teaspoon vanilla extract

½ cup Swerve confectioners'-style sweetener

2 tablespoons half-and-half

FOR GARNISH (OPTIONAL)

Roasted salted peanuts

Shaved sugar-free chocolate

This mousse is my go-to dessert to serve when friends or family come over for dinner. It's very easy to make and is ready in only 15 minutes, so you can spend your time visiting instead of in the kitchen!

1. Using an electric mixer, whip the cream in a mixing bowl until firm peaks form, 2 to 3 minutes. Place the bowl in the refrigerator.

2. In a separate large bowl, beat the cream cheese, peanut butter, and vanilla with an electric mixer until smooth, about 2 minutes. Add the sweetener and blend until smooth. Next, pour in the half-and-half and blend until smooth. Gently fold in the chilled whipped cream.

3. Refrigerate the mousse for 5 minutes, then transfer to individual serving dishes. If desired, top with peanuts and shaved sugar-free chocolate.

PER SERVING (WITHOUT GARNISH):
CALORIES **316** · FAT **30g** · PROTEIN **8g** · TOTAL CARBS **20g** · FIBER **2g** · ERYTHRITOL **14g** · NET CARBS **4g**

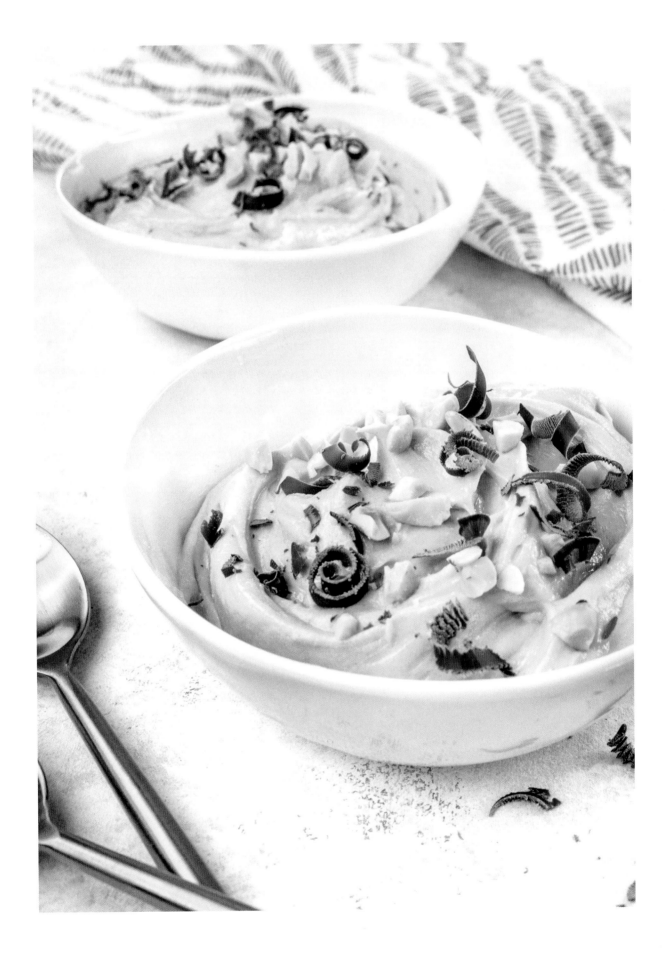

CHOCOLATE-COATED COOKIE DOUGH BITES

Yield: 18 cookie dough bites (2 per serving)

Prep Time: 20 minutes, plus 50 minutes to chill

½ cup (1 stick) unsalted butter, softened

3 tablespoons Swerve brown sugar

2 tablespoons Swerve confectioners'-style sweetener

½ teaspoon vanilla extract

½ teaspoon salt

⅔ cup blanched almond flour

1 cup stevia-sweetened dark chocolate chips, divided

1 tablespoon coconut oil

Let's be honest, we've all sneaked little bites of cookie dough while making cookies because it's so tasty! This recipe tastes just like chocolate chip cookie dough, but is safe to eat and keto-friendly because there are no raw eggs or sugar.

1. In a large mixing bowl, using an electric mixer on high speed, beat the butter and sweeteners until light and fluffy. Add the vanilla and salt and beat until incorporated, scraping the sides of the bowl as necessary.

2. Turn the mixer to low and slowly add the almond flour until well mixed.

3. Fold in ½ cup of the chocolate chips, then place the dough in the refrigerator for 15 minutes. While the dough is chilling, line a tray or plate(s) that will fit in your refrigerator or freezer with parchment paper.

4. Roll the chilled cookie dough into 18 equal-sized balls, about 2 inches in diameter, and place on the lined tray. Place the tray in the refrigerator for at least 1 hour or in the freezer for at least 30 minutes. The colder the dough balls are, the easier they are to work with.

5. In a microwave-safe bowl, melt the coconut oil and remaining ½ cup of chocolate chips in 30-second increments, stirring after each round of heating, until smooth.

6. Using a fork, dip the chilled cookie dough balls in the melted chocolate mixture, then put back on the lined tray. Place the tray in the freezer for 5 minutes, or until the chocolate has hardened. Store the balls in the refrigerator until ready to serve; they'll keep for up to 3 weeks.

PER SERVING:
CALORIES 207 · FAT 21g · PROTEIN 2g · TOTAL CARBS 22g · FIBER 7g · ERYTHRITOL 10g · NET CARBS 5g

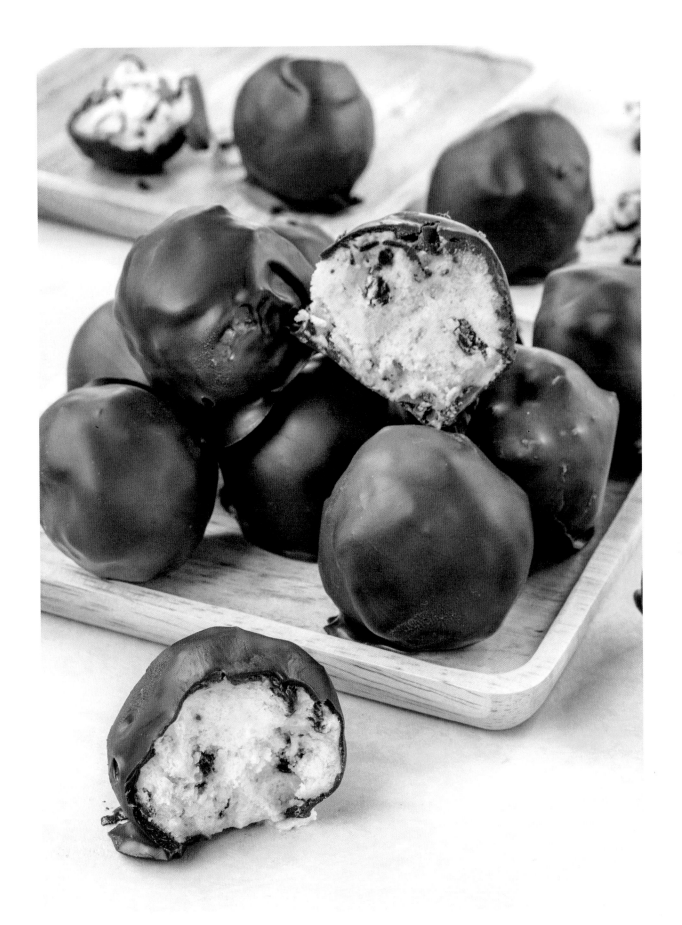

CANDIED BACON

Yield: 12 slices (1 per serving)

Prep Time: 5 minutes

Cook Time: 30 minutes

½ cup Swerve brown sugar

¼ teaspoon Chinese five-spice powder

⅛ to ¼ teaspoon red pepper flakes, depending on your heat preference

1 pound thick-cut bacon

In the heart of San Francisco, a brilliant restaurateur created something called "Millionaire's Bacon," which is a thick slice of baked bacon that is sweet, salty, and spicy all at the same time. The idea quickly spread through all the popular brunch spots in SF, with chefs doing spin-off versions. This is my easy and keto-friendly take.

1. Preheat the oven to 350°F. Line a rimmed baking sheet with parchment paper or a silicone baking mat.

2. In a small bowl, mix together the sweetener, Chinese five-spice, and red pepper flakes.

3. Arrange the bacon in a single layer on the prepared baking sheet, leaving no space between the slices. Sprinkle half of the brown sugar mixture on one side of the bacon, patting it down so that it sticks. Carefully flip each piece over and then do the same thing on the other side with the rest of the brown sugar mixture.

4. Bake until browned and glossy, 25 to 30 minutes. (Keep a close eye on the bacon during the last 5 to 10 minutes of cooking. Depending on the thickness of the bacon, it can burn easily.)

5. Transfer to a fresh sheet of parchment paper and let cool for 5 to 10 minutes before serving. The bacon will crisp up as it cools.

note Make sure to get thick-cut bacon to prevent burning.

PER SERVING:
CALORIES **168** · FAT **13g** · PROTEIN **13g** · TOTAL CARBS **9g** · FIBER **0g** · ERYTHRITOL **8g** · NET CARBS **1g**

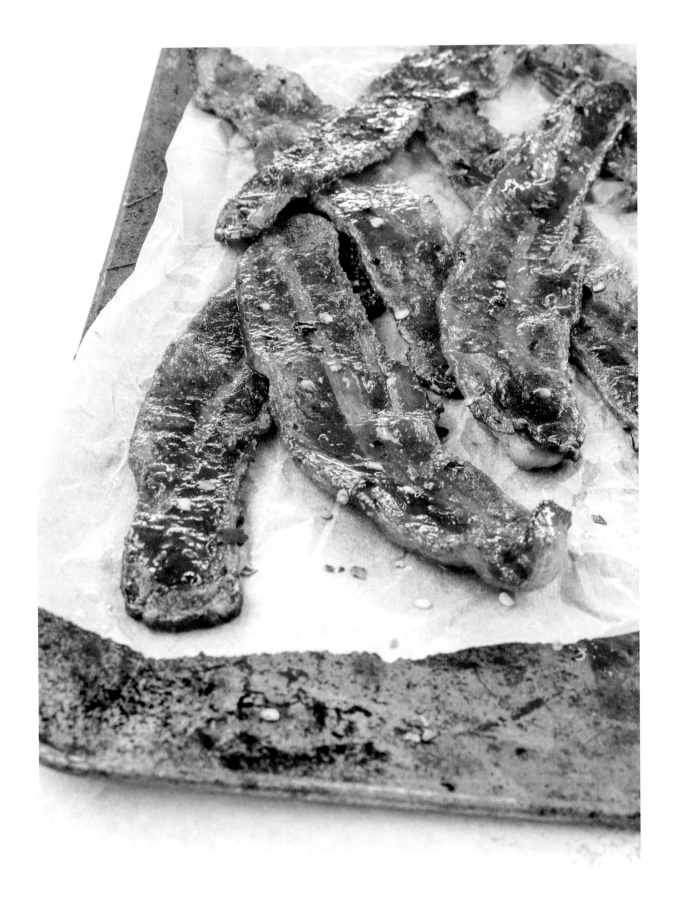

COCONUT MACAROONS

Yield: 14 cookies (1 per serving)

Prep Time: 10 minutes

Cook Time: 22 minutes

2 large egg whites

½ cup coconut milk

½ teaspoon vanilla extract

¼ cup Swerve confectioners'-style sweetener

1 tablespoon coconut flour

2 cups unsweetened shredded coconut

Pinch of salt

These cookies are the perfect dessert for the coconut lovers out there!

1. Preheat the oven to 350°F. Line a baking sheet with parchment paper.

2. Place the egg whites, coconut milk, vanilla, sweetener, and coconut flour in a large bowl. With an electric mixer, beat until thick and frothy, 2 to 3 minutes.

3. Add the shredded coconut to the egg white mixture and stir to combine.

4. Using a measuring spoon and your hands, pack about 2 tablespoons of the mixture into a ball and place on the prepared baking sheet. Repeat with the remaining coconut mixture, spacing the balls 1 to 2 inches apart.

5. Bake for 18 to 22 minutes, or until the macaroons are golden brown.

PER SERVING:

CALORIES **75** · FAT **7g** · PROTEIN **1g** · TOTAL CARBS **5g** · FIBER **1g** · ERYTHRITOL **2.5g** · NET CARBS **1.5g**

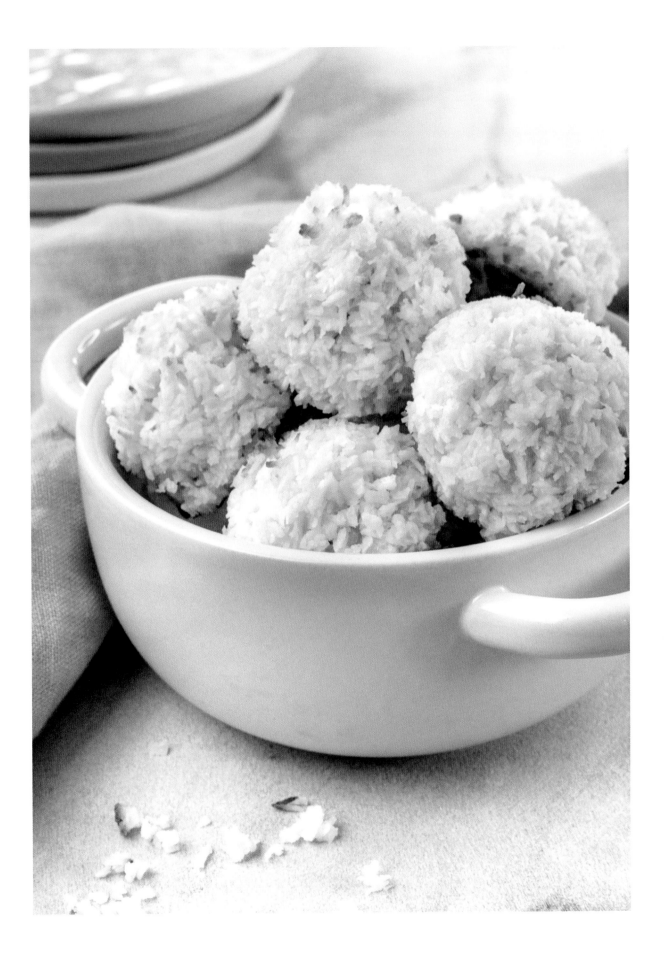

TINA'S CANDIED PECANS

Yield: 6 servings (8 to 10 pecan halves per serving)

Prep Time: 5 minutes

Cook Time: 8 minutes

⅓ cup Swerve brown sugar

¼ teaspoon ground cinnamon

¼ teaspoon salt

1 tablespoon water

1 cup raw pecan halves

One of my best friends, Tina, and I developed this recipe together for you! We love the combination of sweet and salty, and these candied pecans really hit the spot. Enjoy them as a snack or use them as a topper for desserts or salads, like I do in the Strawberry Spinach Salad recipe on page 250.

1. Line a rimmed baking sheet with parchment paper and set a wire rack on top.

2. In a medium saucepan over medium heat, heat the sweetener, cinnamon, salt, and water, stirring occasionally with a spatula, until the sauce starts to bubble. Allow it to bubble for 10 seconds, then add the pecans and toss to fully coat. Let it bubble for another 2 to 3 minutes, stirring periodically. Watch carefully so the sauce doesn't burn.

3. Using a slotted spatula, transfer the pecans to the wire rack, allowing the excess sauce to drip onto the parchment paper below. (If you don't have a wire cooling rack, when lifting the pecans from the pan with the slotted spatula, allow as much of the brown sugar sauce to drip back into the pan as possible.) Clean the saucepan immediately and allow the pecans to cool completely. Store in an airtight container at room temperature for up to 3 weeks.

PER SERVING:
CALORIES **134** · FAT **13g** · PROTEIN **2g** · TOTAL CARBS **13g** · FIBER **2g** · ERYTHRITOL **10.5g** · NET CARBS **0.5g**

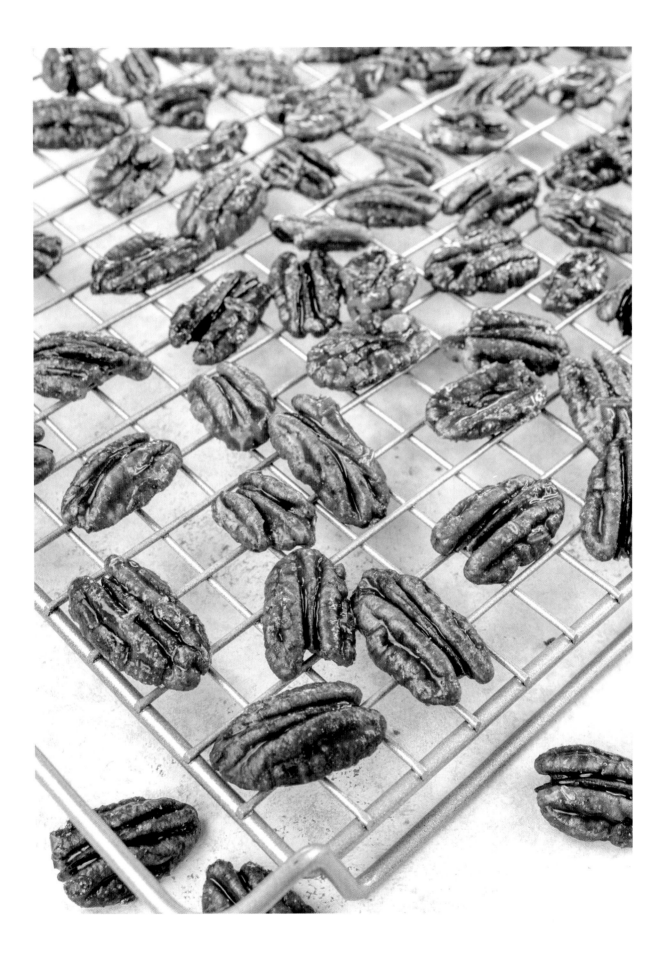

MINI PUMPKIN PIES

Yield: 12 mini pies (1 per serving)

Prep Time: 10 minutes

Cook Time: 45 minutes

CRUST

½ cup blanched almond flour

1½ tablespoons Swerve confectioners'-style sweetener

3 tablespoons chopped pecans

¼ teaspoon ground cinnamon

¼ teaspoon salt

2 tablespoons cold unsalted butter, chopped

PUMPKIN PIE FILLING

1 (15-ounce) can pumpkin puree

½ cup half-and-half

2 large eggs

⅔ cup Swerve confectioners'-style sweetener

1 tablespoon pumpkin pie seasoning

1 teaspoon vanilla extract

¼ teaspoon salt

Serving tip:
Top with Whipped Cream (page 292) and a sprinkle of ground cinnamon, if desired.

There are many reasons why I like to make individual-sized desserts: they are adorable, they cook much faster than an entire pie or cake, and they help with portion control so you know exactly how much you're eating. The nutty and buttery pecan crust in these mini pies pairs perfectly with the creamy pumpkin filling.

1. Preheat the oven to 350°F. Line a standard-size muffin pan with cupcake liners.

2. Make the crusts: Whisk together the dry ingredients, then add the butter and mix with your hands until incorporated and the pieces of butter are in small crumbles.

3. Put about 1 tablespoon of the crust mixture in each muffin well and press into the bottom of the liner. Par-bake until browned, 8 to 10 minutes. Remove from the oven and set aside.

4. While the crusts are baking, use an electric mixer to mix together the ingredients for the filling with an electric mixer until well blended. Pour the filling mixture evenly over the par-baked crusts, filling the wells almost to the top.

5. Bake for 30 to 35 minutes, or until a knife comes out clean when inserted into the center and the tops begin to crack.

6. Remove from the oven and place on a cooling rack. Allow to firm up for 10 minutes before removing the pies from the pan. Enjoy at room temperature or place in the refrigerator to chill before serving. Store leftovers in the fridge for up to a week.

PER SERVING:
CALORIES **76** · FAT **6g** · PROTEIN **2g** · TOTAL CARBS **13g** · FIBER **1g** · ERYTHRITOL **9g** · NET CARBS **3g**

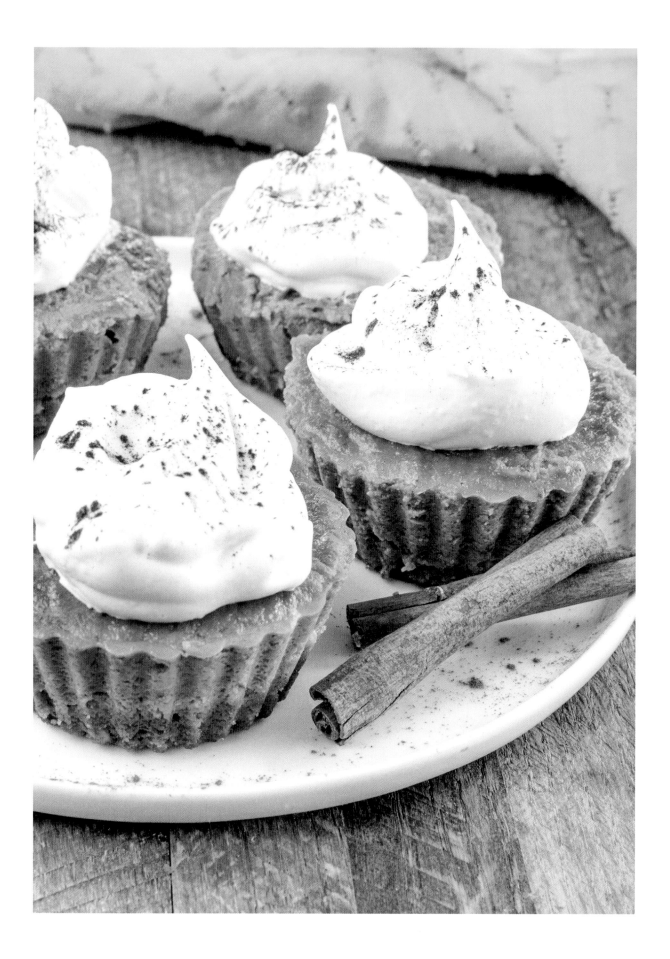

5-MINUTE STRAWBERRY SHORTCAKE PARFAIT FOR TWO

Yield: 2 servings

Prep Time: 5 minutes (not including time to make whipped cream)

Cook Time: 1½ minutes

MUG SHORTCAKE

⅓ cup blanched almond flour

1½ tablespoons Swerve confectioners'-style sweetener

1½ teaspoons coconut flour

¼ teaspoon baking powder

Pinch of salt

2 tablespoons unsalted butter, melted and cooled

1 large egg

¼ teaspoon vanilla extract

KETO WHIPPED CREAM

⅓ cup heavy whipping cream

2½ teaspoons Swerve confectioners'-style sweetener

½ teaspoon vanilla extract

4 large strawberries, sliced

Fresh mint leaves, for garnish (optional)

This simple summertime favorite takes only a few minutes to make, and it is the perfect treat to share with someone special.

1. Put all the dry ingredients for the shortcake in a 16-ounce microwave-safe mug and mix with a fork.

2. Add the melted butter, egg, and vanilla and use the fork to combine. Smooth the top and microwave for 1 minute to 1 minute 25 seconds, or until the cake is set and the center is no longer jiggly.

3. Carefully remove the mug from the microwave, then run a knife around the edge and flip the cake over onto a plate. Cube the cake and divide it into 4 equal portions.

4. Make the whipped cream: Using an electric mixer, whip the cream, sweetener, and vanilla for 3 to 4 minutes, until stiff peaks form.

5. To assemble the parfaits, have on hand two 12-ounce glasses. (I like to use stemless wine glasses.) In each glass, layer one portion of cubed cake, then 2½ tablespoons of whipped cream, and then 1 sliced strawberry. Repeat once more. Each glass should have 2 layers of each ingredient.

6. Garnish with fresh mint leaves, if desired.

PER SERVING: CALORIES **394** · FAT **37g** · PROTEIN **8g** · TOTAL CARBS **17g** · FIBER **3g** · ERYTHRITOL **10.5g** · NET CARBS **3.5g**

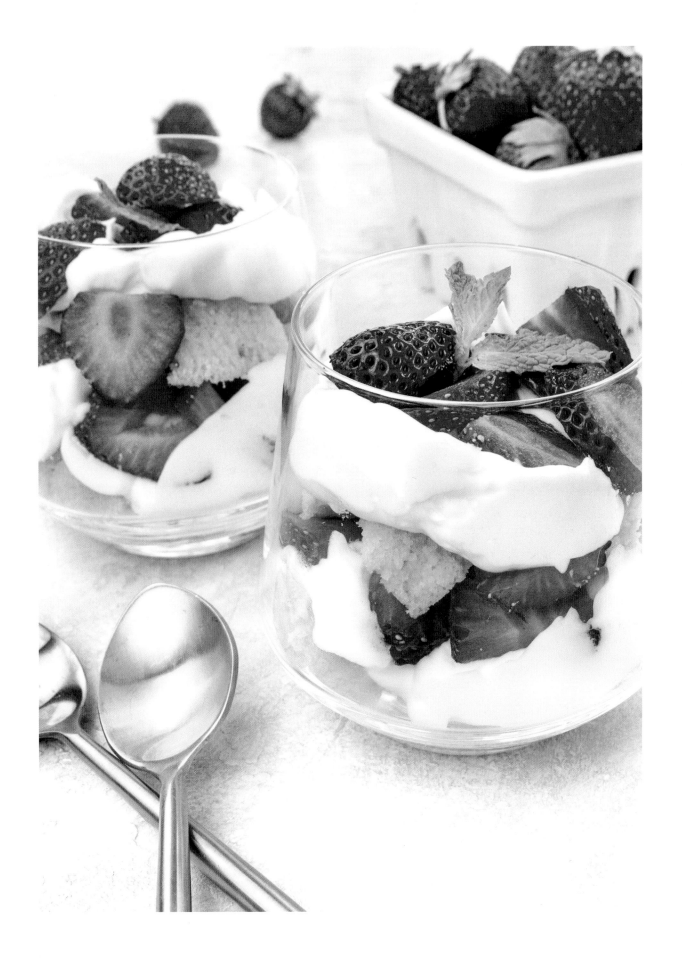

OLIVIA'S SNICKERDOODLES

Yield: 12 cookies (1 per serving)

Prep Time: 15 minutes

Cook Time: 12 minutes

CINNAMON SUGAR COATING

1 tablespoon Swerve confectioners'-style sweetener

1 teaspoon ground cinnamon

COOKIES

1 cup blanched almond flour

¼ cup coconut flour

½ teaspoon baking powder

¼ teaspoon salt

¼ teaspoon ground cinnamon

¼ cup plus 2 tablespoons Swerve granular sweetener

1 large egg

½ cup (1 stick) unsalted butter, softened

½ teaspoon vanilla extract

My daughter, Olivia, and I made about ten batches of these cookies before dialing in a recipe that we loved. While the cookies turned out great, the memories are my favorite part!

1. Preheat the oven to 325°F. Line a baking sheet with parchment paper.

2. Whisk together the ingredients for the cinnamon sugar coating in a small bowl, then set aside.

3. In a medium mixing bowl, whisk together the dry ingredients for the cookies. Add the egg, melted butter, and vanilla and use an electric mixer to blend the wet and dry ingredients.

4. Using a spoon, make 12 equal-size balls of dough, about 1¼ inches in diameter.

5. Roll the dough balls in the cinnamon sugar and place on the prepared baking sheet, about 2 inches apart. Use the bottom of a glass to press and slightly flatten each dough ball to about 3 inches in diameter by ⅜ inch thick.

6. Bake for 10 to 12 minutes, until golden brown. Allow the cookies to cool completely on the baking sheet before moving them; they will firm up as they cool. Store leftovers in a zip-top bag on the counter for up to 1 week.

PER SERVING:

CALORIES 98 · FAT 10g · PROTEIN 1g · TOTAL CARBS 7g · FIBER 1g · ERYTHRITOL 4.5g · NET CARBS 1.5g

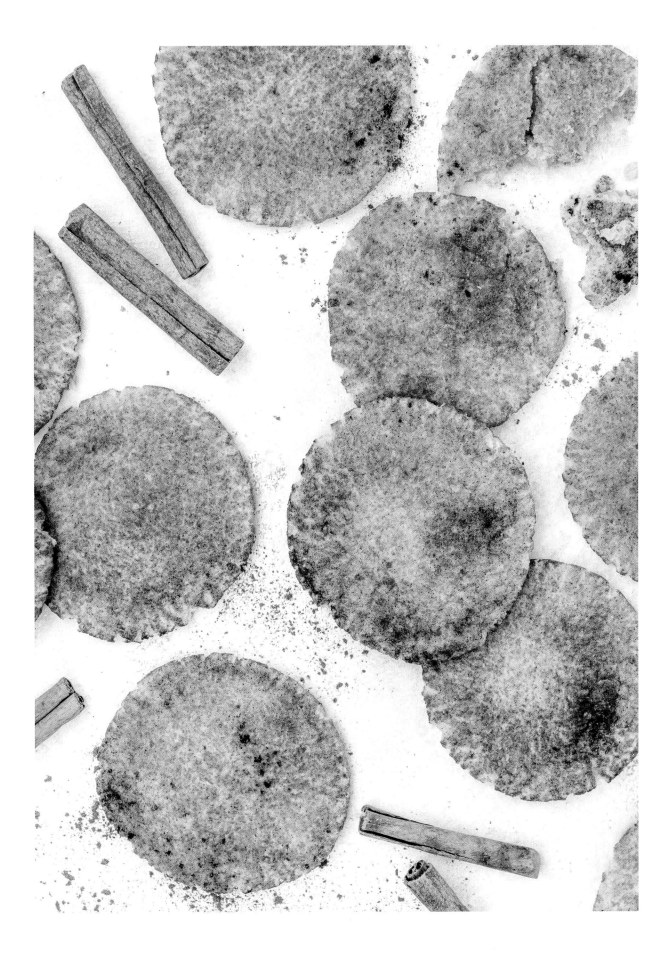

LEMON BARS

Yield: 9 bars (1 per serving)

Prep Time: 15 minutes

Cook Time: 39 minutes

CRUST

1 cup blanched almond flour

3 tablespoons Swerve confectioners'-style sweetener

½ teaspoon salt

2 tablespoons unsalted butter, softened

½ teaspoon vanilla extract

LEMON FILLING

Grated zest of 2 lemons

¾ cup fresh lemon juice (3 to 4 lemons)

3 large eggs

¾ cup Swerve confectioners'-style sweetener

¼ cup blanched almond flour

TOPPING (OPTIONAL)

1 tablespoon Swerve confectioners'-style sweetener

Of all the desserts my mom would make when I was growing up, her lemon bars were my favorite. I've tested countless versions, looking for a keto-friendly lemon bar that my mom would give a thumbs-up to. This is it!

1. Preheat the oven to 350°F. Line an 8-inch square baking dish or pan with parchment paper, leaving paper overhanging 2 sides of the pan for easy removal.

2. Make the crust: Whisk together the almond flour, sweetener, and salt, then add the butter and vanilla and use your hands to combine the ingredients until the mixture has a doughlike consistency.

3. Press the crust mixture evenly across the bottom of the prepared pan. Use a fork to poke holes throughout the crust. Par-bake for 10 to 14 minutes, or until lightly golden brown.

4. While the crust is baking, make the lemon filling: Put all the filling ingredients in a bowl and whisk until well combined and smooth.

5. Pour the filling over the par-baked crust and bake for 22 to 25 minutes, or until the filling is set. Remove from the oven and allow to cool completely.

6. Use the overhanging parchment paper to lift the bars out of the pan, then slice into squares. If desired, sift 1 tablespoon of confectioners'-style sweetener over the top for a classic powdered "sugar" topping. Enjoy chilled or at room temperature. Store leftovers in the refrigerator for up to 2 weeks.

PER SERVING:
CALORIES **74** · FAT **6g** · PROTEIN **3g** · TOTAL CARBS **17g** · FIBER **1g** · ERYTHRITOL **15g** · NET CARBS **1g**

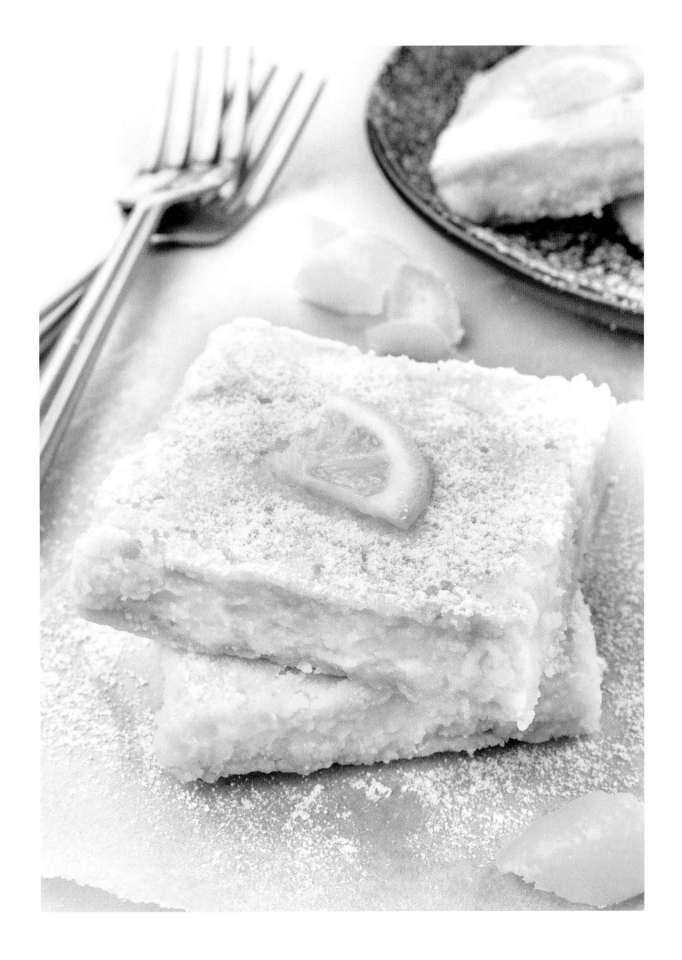

BOARDWALK CHOCOLATE-COVERED BACON

Yield: 6 slices (1 per serving)

Prep Time: 15 minutes, plus 15 minutes to chill

Cook Time: 16 minutes

6 slices thick-cut bacon

⅓ cup stevia-sweetened chocolate chips (semisweet or dark)

1½ teaspoons MCT oil or melted coconut oil

Just about an hour's drive down the coast from our house is the Santa Cruz Beach Boardwalk, which is full of rides, carnival games, and souvenir shops. It is also the home of chocolate-covered bacon. Although putting chocolate on bacon started out as a novelty, it's pretty well known that chocolate and bacon are epic together!

1. Preheat the oven to 400°F. Line a rimmed baking sheet with parchment paper.

2. Lay the bacon on the prepared baking sheet, being sure not to overlap the slices. Bake until crispy, 12 to 15 minutes, depending on the thickness of the bacon. Place the bacon on a paper towel–lined plate to absorb the excess fat.

3. In a medium microwave-safe bowl, melt the chocolate chips in the microwave for 30 seconds, then stir. If the chips aren't fully melted, return them to the microwave for another 15 to 20 seconds. Make sure all the chocolate is melted, but be careful not to burn the chocolate. Stir well, then add the MCT oil and stir again until fully combined and smooth.

4. Line a clean baking sheet or a large plate with parchment paper. Place a slice of crispy bacon on the lined baking sheet or plate. Using a spoon or your fingers, spread the chocolate evenly over the bacon slice until it's well coated, then flip the bacon over and repeat on the other side.

5. Place the chocolate-covered bacon in the freezer for 15 minutes to allow the chocolate to harden, then enjoy! Store leftovers in the fridge for up to 1 week.

PER SERVING:
CALORIES 113 · FAT 9g · PROTEIN 5g · TOTAL CARBS 6g · FIBER 3g · ERYTHRITOL 2.5g · NET CARBS 0.5g

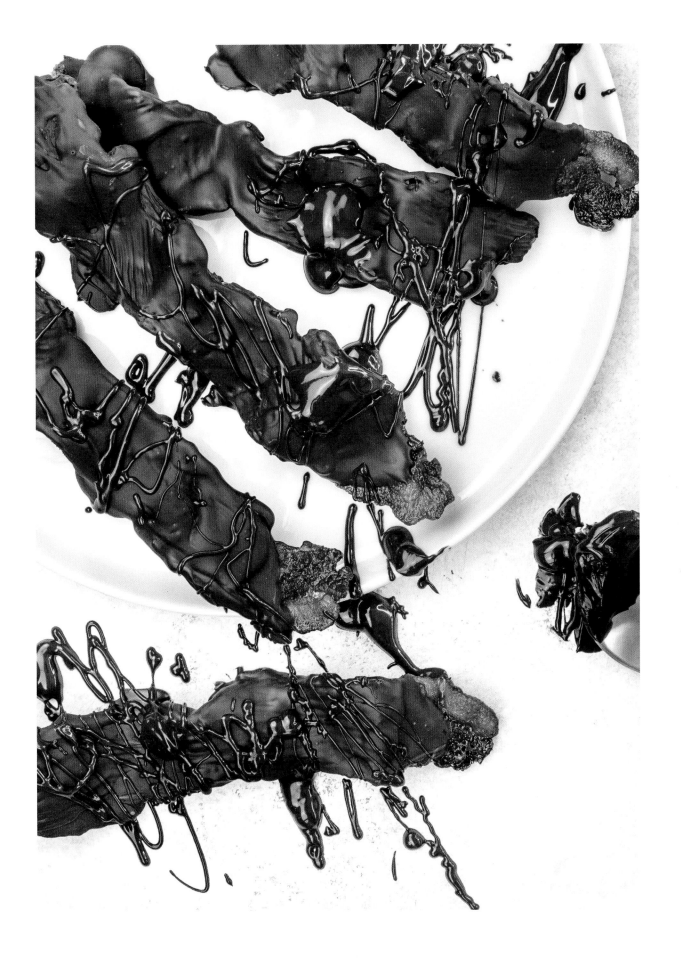

WHIPPED CREAM

Yield: 6 servings (about 3½ tablespoons per serving)

Prep Time: 4 minutes

⅔ cup heavy whipping cream

1 tablespoon plus 1 teaspoon Swerve confectioners'-style sweetener

1 teaspoon vanilla extract

Place all the ingredients in a medium mixing bowl and whip with an electric mixer until stiff peaks form, 3 to 4 minutes. Whipped cream can be made ahead and kept in an airtight container in the refrigerator; use within 2 to 3 days.

PER SERVING:
CALORIES **90** · FAT **9g** · PROTEIN **0g** · TOTAL CARBS **4g** · FIBER **0g** · ERYTHRITOL **2g** · NET CARBS **2g**

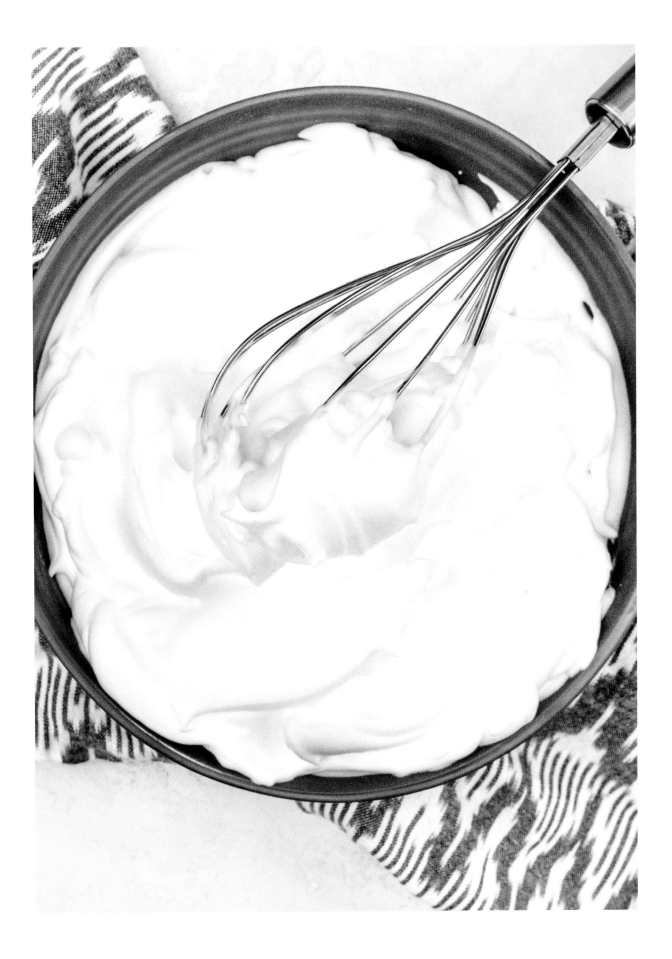

CAFÉ MOCHA

Yield: One 10-ounce serving

Prep Time: 2 minutes (not including time to brew coffee)

2 tablespoons heavy whipping cream

2 tablespoons Swerve confectioners'-style sweetener, or sweetener of choice to taste

1 tablespoon unsweetened cocoa powder

1 cup brewed hot coffee

Coffee and chocolate, what more could you want?

In a 12-ounce mug, whisk together the cream, sweetener, and cocoa powder to make a paste. Slowly pour in the hot coffee while whisking to combine.

note A handheld milk frother works really well for mixing everything together!

Variation: Iced Mocha. Replace the hot coffee with cold brew coffee. Serve in a tall glass filled with ice.

Serving tip:
Top with Whipped Cream (page 292) and a sprinkle of ground cinnamon, if desired.

PER SERVING:
CALORIES 119 · FAT 12g · PROTEIN 2g · TOTAL CARBS 22g · FIBER 2g · ERYTHRITOL 18g · NET CARBS 2g

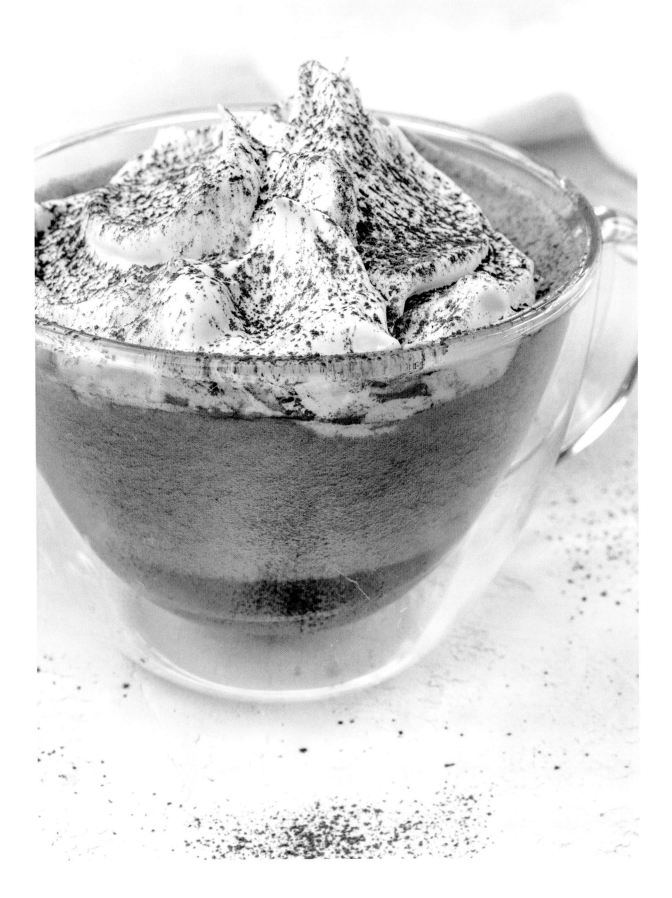

CHAI TEA LATTE

Yield: One 12-ounce serving

Prep Time: 2 minutes

Cook Time: 5 minutes

1 chai tea bag

1 cup boiling water

⅓ cup unsweetened vanilla-flavored almond milk

2 tablespoons half-and-half

⅛ teaspoon vanilla extract

1 teaspoon Swerve granular or confectioners'-style sweetener, or sweetener of choice to taste

Pinch of ground cinnamon, for sprinkling

This simple latte is a nice balance of spice and sweetness and is perfect for a chilly day or cozy night at home.

1. Place the tea bag in a 12-ounce mug. Pour the boiling water over the tea bag and allow to steep for 4 to 5 minutes.

2. Put the almond milk, half-and-half, and vanilla in a microwave-safe glass, then add the sweetener and stir. Heat the almond milk mixture in the microwave for 30 to 45 seconds or until hot. Use a frother or blender to froth the milk.

3. Remove the tea bag from the mug, pour in the frothed almond milk mixture, and gently stir. Sprinkle with the cinnamon and serve.

PER SERVING:
CALORIES **51** · FAT **4g** · PROTEIN **1g** · TOTAL CARBS **4g** · FIBER **0g** · ERYTHRITOL **3g** · NET CARBS **1g**

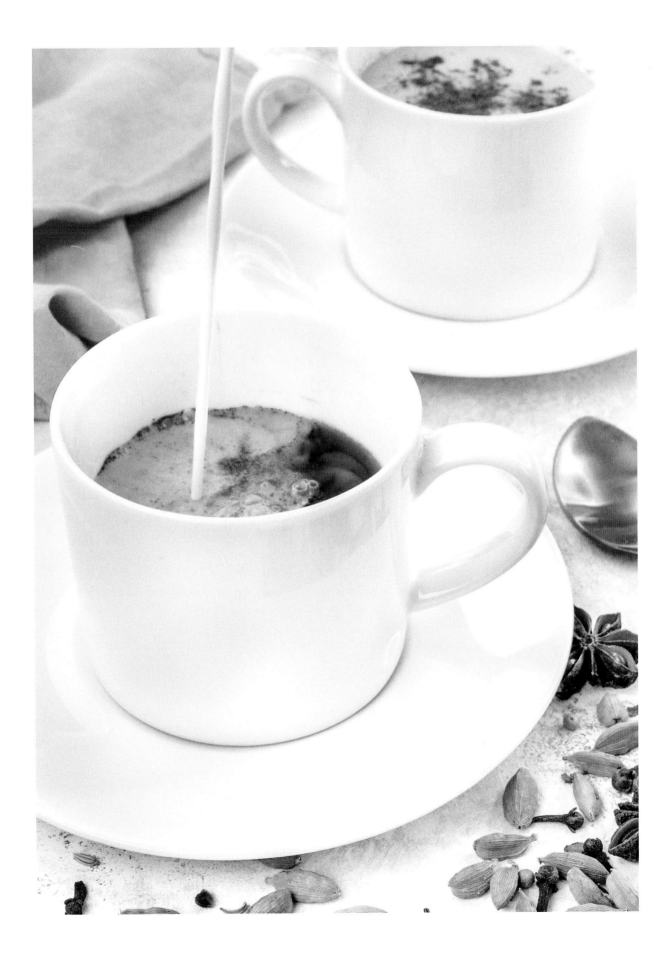

BLUEBERRY COLLAGEN SMOOTHIE

⏱ 30 · 🥛 · ⊘

Yield: Two 10-ounce servings

Prep Time: 5 minutes

½ cup frozen blueberries

1½ cups unsweetened vanilla-flavored almond milk

1 scoop vanilla-flavored or plain MCT powder (optional; see notes)

1 to 2 teaspoons Swerve confectioners'-style sweetener, or sweetener of choice to taste

1 scoop collagen peptides

4 to 6 ice cubes

Smoothies are a great meal option to take on the go, especially if you have a small personal blender at home. This blueberry vanilla smoothie is delicious and nutritious!

Place all the ingredients in a blender and blend until smooth. Use 1 teaspoon sweetener for a less sweet smoothie and 2 teaspoons for a sweeter smoothie.

notes If you're new to MCT powder, I recommend easing into it, starting with a teaspoon at a time; it can cause stomach upset if you don't work up to using larger amounts. I used vanilla-flavored MCT powder to make this smoothie. If you use plain MCT powder or omit it altogether, I recommend you add a few drops of vanilla extract to the smoothie.

Collagen peptides come in powdered form and are known to help skin, hair, bones, and joints, as well as help with muscle repair. It dissolves easily into both hot and cold liquids, and it can even be used in baked goods. The unflavored option is great to put in anything because it really does not have a taste at all.

PER SERVING (WITH 2 TSP. SWEETENER):
CALORIES 97 · FAT 6g · PROTEIN 5.5g · TOTAL CARBS 10g · FIBER 3g · ERYTHRITOL 3g · NET CARBS 4g

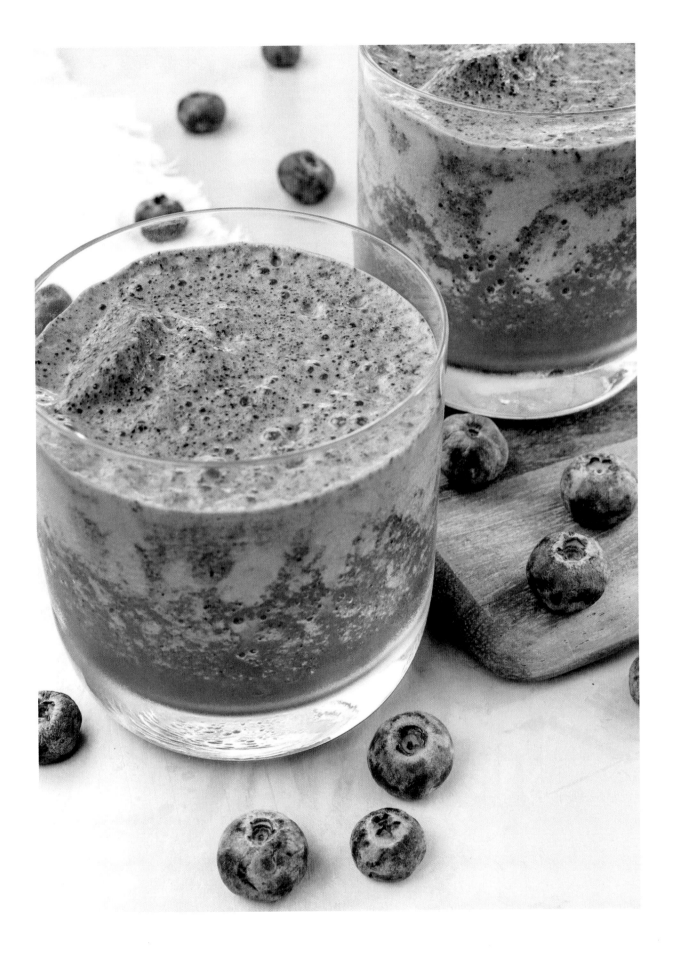

CHOCOLATE-DIPPED STRAWBERRY SMOOTHIE

Yield: One 10-ounce serving

Prep Time: 5 minutes

¾ cup unsweetened almond milk

¼ cup heavy whipping cream

2 tablespoons unsweetened cocoa powder

2 tablespoons Swerve confectioners'-style sweetener

4 medium strawberries, cut into quarters

1 cup ice

Chocolate and strawberries are one of my favorite combinations. This smoothie is a simple way to whip up a decadent and delicious treat.

Place all the ingredients in a blender and blend until smooth.

PER SERVING:
CALORIES **265** · FAT **24g** · PROTEIN **4g** · TOTAL CARBS **30g** · FIBER **6g** · ERYTHRITOL **18g** · NET CARBS **6g**

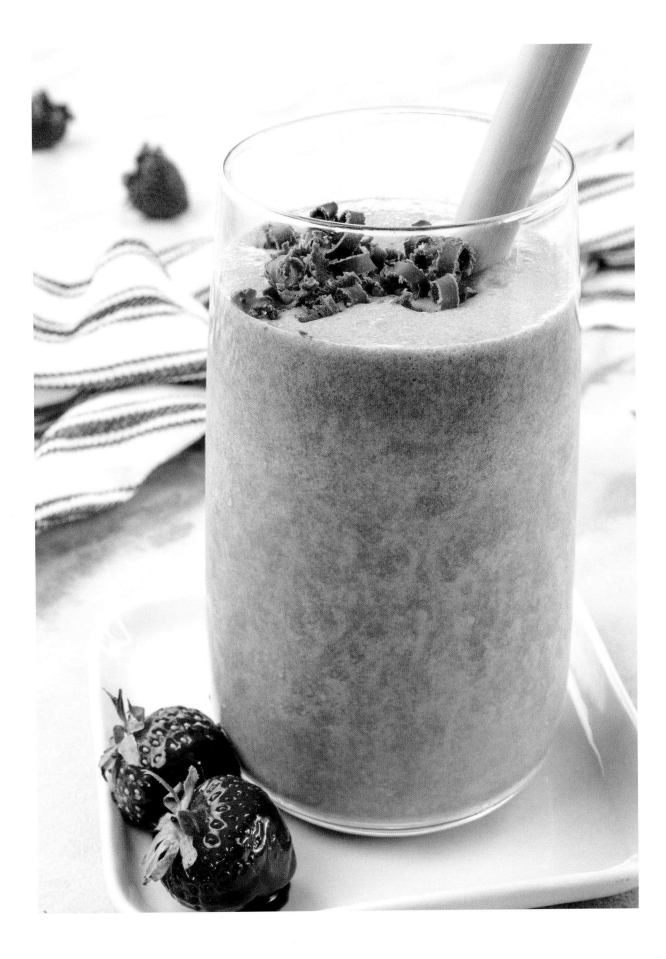

LEMONADE

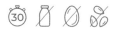

Yield: Five 8-ounce servings

Prep Time: 5 minutes

½ cup fresh lemon juice (4 to 5 lemons)

4½ cups water

2 to 3 tablespoons Swerve confectioners'-style sweetener, or sweetener of choice to taste

Lemonade is the quintessential summertime drink, but did you know that there are almost 25 grams of sugar in one glass of traditional lemonade? Enjoy this refreshing summertime classic with only about 2.5 grams of net carbs per glass.

Mix all the ingredients in a 1½-quart jug. Adjust the sweetener to taste, adding more if you like a less tart lemonade. To serve, fill a 10-ounce or larger glass with ice and pour in 1 cup of lemonade.

PER SERVING (WITH 3 T. SWEETENER):
CALORIES 8 · FAT 0g · PROTEIN 0g · TOTAL CARBS 8g · FIBER 0g · ERYTHRITOL 5.4g · NET CARBS 2.6g

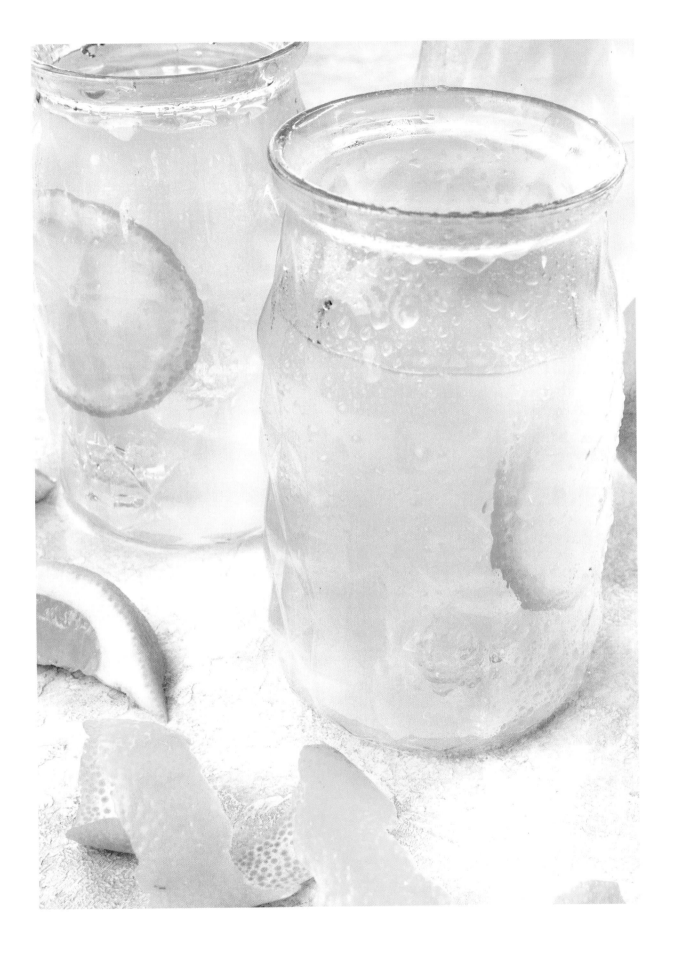

VIRGIN MOJITO

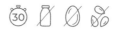

Yield: One 6- to 8-ounce serving

Prep Time: 5 minutes

2 tablespoons packed fresh mint leaves

1 to 2 teaspoons Swerve confectioners'-style sweetener, or sweetener of choice to taste

2 lime wedges

Ice cubes

Club soda

A refreshing and delicious drink that you can enjoy year-round! I love the little flecks of mint paired with the tart lime juice. You can also multiply this recipe and make a pitcher if you are serving several people.

In a highball glass, muddle the mint leaves and sweetener. Squeeze in the lime wedges and then drop the wedges into the glass. Fill with ice and top with club soda. Stir before serving.

note If you like tart drinks, 1 teaspoon of sweetener should be enough for you; if you like things on the sweeter side, use 2 teaspoons. Taste the drink after stirring it. Depending on how acidic your lime wedges are, you may want to add a touch more sweetener.

PER SERVING (WITH 2 TSP. SWEETENER):
CALORIES **6** · FAT **0g** · PROTEIN **0g** · TOTAL CARBS **7g** · FIBER **0g** · ERYTHRITOL **6g** · NET CARBS **1g**

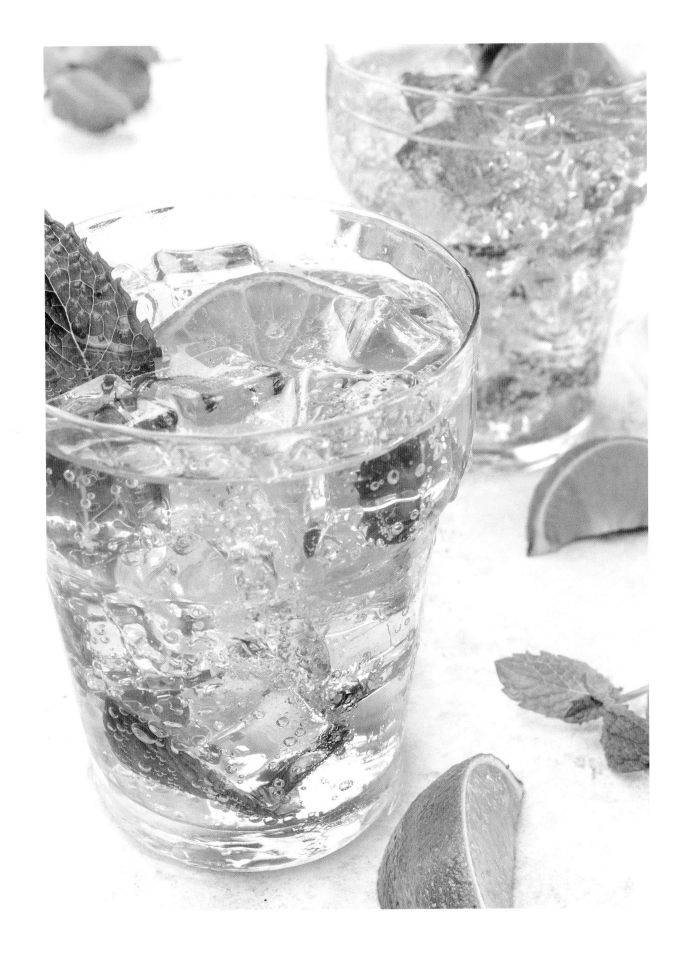

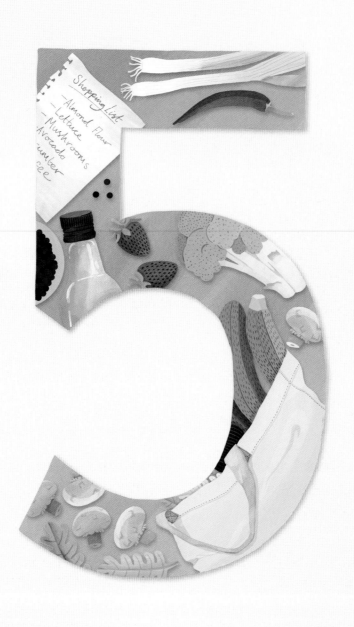

chapter 5:
30-DAY MEAL PLAN

Many people find meal plans to be a helpful tool because they like to have a place to start or enjoy following a prewritten menu. In this section, you will find a 30-day meal plan that is simple and approachable. For example, the plan makes use of leftovers (some of which carry over to the following week) and includes tips for prepping meals and components in advance, as well as weekly shopping lists. I recommend that you do your shopping on Sunday (or the day before the start of your work week) so that you're ready for the week ahead. Feel free to swap any meals with one of the non-recipe options on page 66 if you're short on time or don't feel like following a recipe, or to add an easy side from page 67 if you'd like a heartier meal. Many of us enjoy taking a night off to order in or go out to dinner with family and friends, so don't feel the need to cook or eat at home every single night. (See pages 69 to 71 for more on making smart choices when dining out.) If you are feeling hungry between meals, feel free to have a keto-friendly snack. (See page 65 for recommended snack foods.) If you'd like to have a sweet treat after a meal, feel free to do that as well. There are many dessert recipes in this book, starting on page 272, as well as countless recipes online!

Because everyone has different caloric and macro goals, the recipe serving sizes are only recommendations; you may eat more or less than one serving of each meal in the plan, using the nutrition information provided with the recipes along with your current hunger level as a guide. Remember, this is just a framework, so feel free to make adjustments to best fit your lifestyle, goals, and tastes!

If you prefer not to follow the meal plan, that is A-OK, too. Feel free to skip this section and do what works for you!

note You may need to make some adjustments to the plan depending on the number of people you are feeding. As written, the plan is designed to feed up to two people with leftovers. If you are serving three or more, you may need to double some recipes; on the other hand, if you are the only person eating these meals, you may find that the plan yields more food than you can reasonably consume. I have included the number of servings each recipe makes so that you can plan accordingly.

Keep These Items Stocked for Use Throughout the Meal Plans

PANTRY/CONDIMENTS

☐ apple cider vinegar

☐ avocado oil

☐ coconut oil

☐ cooking spray (olive oil or coconut oil)

☐ mayonnaise

☐ olive oil

☐ soy sauce or coconut aminos

☐ toasted sesame oil

SPICES/BAKING

☐ baking powder

☐ curry powder

☐ dried dill weed

☐ dried oregano leaves

☐ dried parsley

☐ fine sea salt

☐ garlic powder

☐ ground black pepper

☐ ground cinnamon

☐ ground cumin

☐ paprika

☐ pumpkin pie spice

☐ sugar-free maple syrup

☐ Swerve brown sugar

☐ Swerve confectioners'-style sweetener

☐ Swerve granular sweetener

☐ vanilla extract

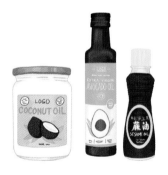

You can find downloadable copies of the weekly shopping lists and more at ketokarma.com/printables

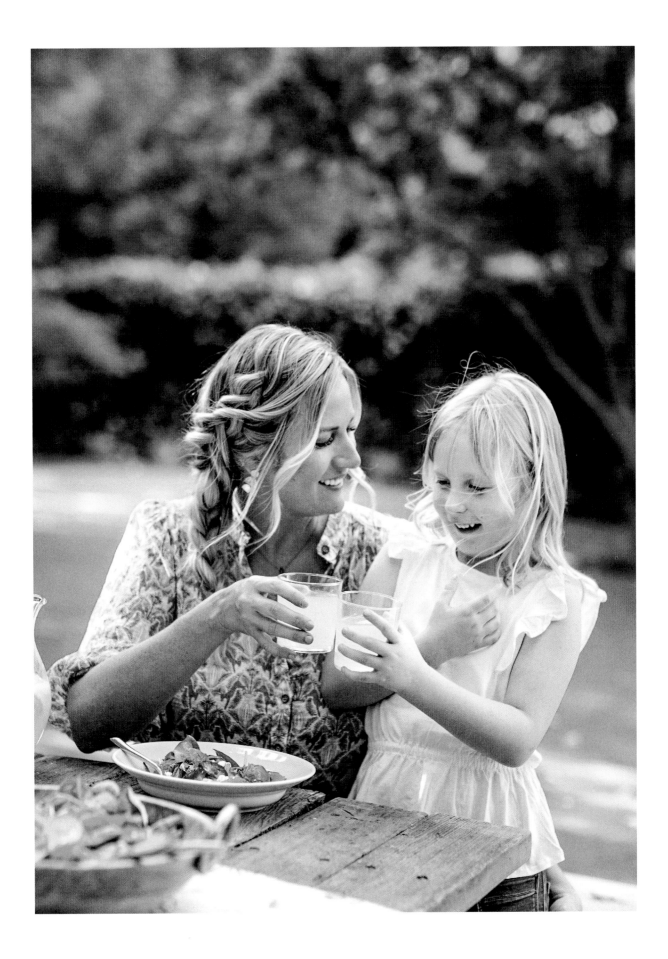

WEEK 1 MEAL PLAN

(#) = number of servings

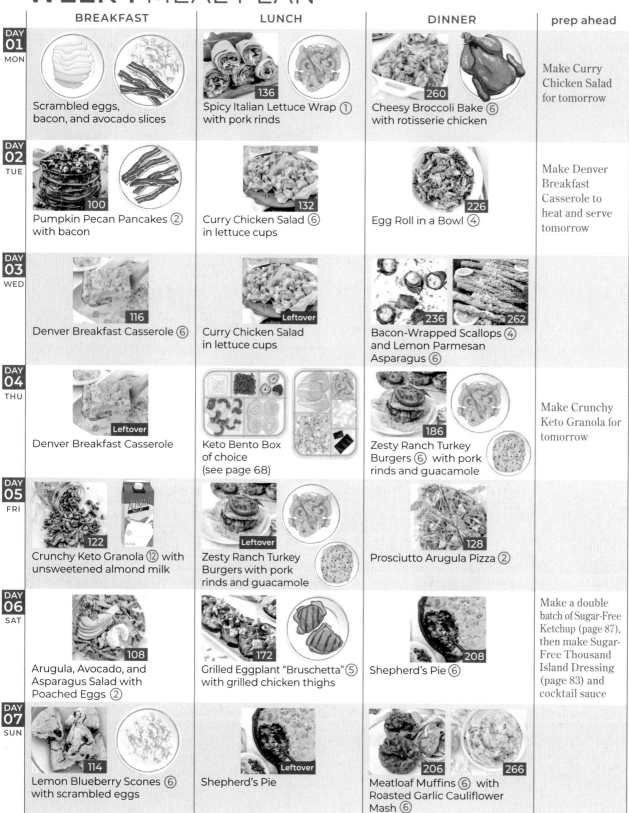

	BREAKFAST	LUNCH	DINNER	prep ahead
DAY 01 MON	Scrambled eggs, bacon, and avocado slices	Spicy Italian Lettuce Wrap ① with pork rinds — 136	Cheesy Broccoli Bake ⑥ with rotisserie chicken — 260	Make Curry Chicken Salad for tomorrow
DAY 02 TUE	Pumpkin Pecan Pancakes ② with bacon — 100	Curry Chicken Salad ⑥ in lettuce cups — 132	Egg Roll in a Bowl ④ — 226	Make Denver Breakfast Casserole to heat and serve tomorrow
DAY 03 WED	Denver Breakfast Casserole ⑥ — 116	Curry Chicken Salad in lettuce cups — Leftover	Bacon-Wrapped Scallops ④ — 236 and Lemon Parmesan Asparagus ⑥ — 262	
DAY 04 THU	Denver Breakfast Casserole — Leftover	Keto Bento Box of choice (see page 68)	Zesty Ranch Turkey Burgers ⑥ with pork rinds and guacamole — 186	Make Crunchy Keto Granola for tomorrow
DAY 05 FRI	Crunchy Keto Granola ⑫ with unsweetened almond milk — 122	Zesty Ranch Turkey Burgers with pork rinds and guacamole — Leftover	Prosciutto Arugula Pizza ② — 128	
DAY 06 SAT	Arugula, Avocado, and Asparagus Salad with Poached Eggs ② — 108	Grilled Eggplant "Bruschetta" ⑤ with grilled chicken thighs — 172	Shepherd's Pie ⑥ — 208	Make a double batch of Sugar-Free Ketchup (page 87), then make Sugar-Free Thousand Island Dressing (page 83) and cocktail sauce
DAY 07 SUN	Lemon Blueberry Scones ⑥ with scrambled eggs — 114	Shepherd's Pie — Leftover	Meatloaf Muffins ⑥ with Roasted Garlic Cauliflower Mash ⑥ — 206 / 266	

WEEK 1 SHOPPING LIST

PRODUCE:

- ☐ **arugula**, 3 cups
- ☐ **asparagus**, 2 pounds (about 30 spears)
- ☐ **avocados**, 2
- ☐ **baby arugula**, 1 cup
- ☐ **basil**, 2 tablespoons chopped
- ☐ **blueberries**, 2 ounces (about ⅓ cup)
- ☐ **broccoli florets**, 1 pound (about 2 medium heads)
- ☐ **butter lettuce**, 1 head
- ☐ **cauliflower**, 2 large heads
- ☐ **celery**, 4 stalks
- ☐ **cilantro**, 1 tablespoon chopped
- ☐ **coleslaw mix**, 1 (14-ounce) bag
- ☐ **eggplant**, 1 medium
- ☐ **garlic**, 2 bulbs
- ☐ **green bell pepper**, 1
- ☐ **green onions**, 1 bunch
- ☐ **guacamole**, premade
- ☐ **iceberg lettuce**, 1 head
- ☐ **lemons**, 3
- ☐ **Roma tomato**, 1 medium
- ☐ **thyme leaves**, 1 tablespoon chopped
- ☐ **tomato**, 1
- ☐ **yellow onion**, 1
- ☐ **zucchini**, 1 small

Also buy the ingredients for the **Keto Bento Box** of your choice (see page 68). If making **Keto Yum Yum Sauce** (page 89) for the Egg Roll in a Bowl and/or **Sugar-Free Thousand Island Dressing** (page 83) for the Cheeseburger Salad, add those ingredients to your shopping list as well.

MEAT:

- ☐ **bacon**, 2 packages
- ☐ **bacon, thick-cut**, 6 slices
- ☐ **Black Forest ham**, 4 slices
- ☐ **chicken thighs**, 2
- ☐ **ground beef**, 1 pound
- ☐ **ground bison or beef**, 1 pound
- ☐ **ground pork**, 1 pound
- ☐ **ground turkey (preferably dark meat)**, 2 pounds
- ☐ **ham**, 8 ounces
- ☐ **prosciutto**, 4 ounces
- ☐ **rotisserie chickens**, 2
- ☐ **salami**, 12 slices
- ☐ **sea scallops**, 16 large (about 1 pound)

DAIRY AND EGGS:

- ☐ **butter, unsalted**, 4 tablespoons (½ stick)
- ☐ **cheddar cheese, shredded**, 4 cups
- ☐ **cream cheese**, 2 ounces
- ☐ **eggs**, 3 dozen
- ☐ **feta cheese, crumbled**, ½ cup
- ☐ **half-and-half**, 2 tablespoons
- ☐ **heavy whipping cream**, ½ cup
- ☐ **mozzarella cheese, low-moisture, shredded**, ⅔ cup
- ☐ **mozzarella cheese, shredded**, ½ cup
- ☐ **Parmesan cheese, grated**, 1¼ cups
- ☐ **Parmesan cheese, shaved**, ½ cup
- ☐ **pepper Jack cheese, shredded**, 2 cups (if you can't find it preshredded, you can buy a block and shred it yourself, or substitute Monterey Jack or cheddar)
- ☐ **provolone cheese**, 2 slices
- ☐ **ricotta, whole-milk**, ¼ cup
- ☐ **sour cream**, ½ cup

PANTRY AND CONDIMENTS:

- ☐ **almond milk, unsweetened**, 1 carton
- ☐ **almonds, slivered**, 1½ cups
- ☐ **beef broth or red wine**, ¼ cup
- ☐ **chia seeds**, ¼ cup
- ☐ **crushed tomatoes**, ½ cup
- ☐ **Dijon mustard**, ½ teaspoon
- ☐ **ketchup, sugar-free**, ¾ cup (if making homemade, see page 87 for ingredients)
- ☐ **peanuts, roasted salted**, 1 cup
- ☐ **pecans, raw**, 1 cup + 3 tablespoons
- ☐ **pepperoncini**, 2
- ☐ **pork rinds**, 1 large bag
- ☐ **pumpkin puree**, ¼ cup
- ☐ **pumpkin seeds**, 1 cup
- ☐ **Sriracha sauce or Yum Yum Sauce** (page 89) (optional, for Egg Roll in a Bowl)
- ☐ **tomato paste**, 2 tablespoons
- ☐ **unsweetened shredded coconut**, ½ cup

BAKING AND SPICES:

- ☐ **almond flour, blanched**, 2¾ cups
- ☐ **flaxseed meal**, ½ cup
- ☐ **ginger powder**, 1 teaspoon
- ☐ **ranch herb mix**, 2 tablespoons (if making homemade, see page 85 for ingredients)
- ☐ **sesame seeds**, 1 tablespoon
- ☐ **turmeric powder**, 1 teaspoon

WEEK 2 MEAL PLAN

(#) = number of servings

	BREAKFAST	LUNCH	DINNER	prep ahead
DAY 08 MON	Lemon Blueberry Scones with scrambled eggs (Leftover)	Meatloaf Muffins with side salad (Leftover)	Shrimp Scampi with Zucchini Noodles (4)	Assemble On-the-Go Cobb Salads for tomorrow
DAY 09 TUE	Blueberry Collagen Smoothie (2) with macadamia nuts	On-the-Go Cobb Salads (5)	Reuben Casserole (8) with side salad	Make Marinara Sauce (page 82) for Stuffed Bell Peppers for tomorrow
DAY 10 WED	Pumpkin Pecan Pancakes (2) and bacon	Reuben Casserole (Leftover)	Stuffed Bell Peppers (8) and side salad	
DAY 11 THU	Crunchy Keto Granola with unsweetened almond milk (Leftover)	Stuffed Bell Peppers (Leftover)	Crispy Baked Chicken Thighs (6) and Three-Cheese Zucchini au Gratin (4)	
DAY 12 FRI	Scrambled eggs, bacon, and sliced avocado	Crispy Baked Chicken Thighs and Three-Cheese Zucchini au Gratin (Leftover) (Leftover)	Mike's Spinach Salad with Warm Bacon Dressing (2)	Make Everything Bagels for tomorrow
DAY 13 SAT	Toasted Everything Bagels (6) with cream cheese	Shrimp Cocktail (5) with side salad	Beef and Broccoli (4)	
DAY 14 SUN	Three-Cheese Soufflés (4) with baby arugula	Turkey or ham sandwiches on Everything Bagels (Leftover)	Chicken Satay Skewers with Peanut Sauce (4) and a double batch of Thai Cucumber Salad (2)	

WEEK 2 SHOPPING LIST

PRODUCE:

☐ **avocado,** 1

☐ **baby arugula,** 1 bag

☐ **baby spinach,** 6 ounces

☐ **bell peppers (any color),** 4

☐ **blueberries, frozen,** ½ cup

☐ **broccoli florets,** 6 cups

☐ **cauliflower, riced,** 1 cup

☐ **cherry tomatoes,** 15

☐ **cilantro,** 1 bunch

☐ **cucumbers,** 2 large and 2 mini

☐ **garlic,** 1 bulb

☐ **ginger, grated,** 2½ teaspoons

☐ **green onions,** 3

☐ **lemons,** 2

☐ **lime,** 1

☐ **parsley,** 1 bunch

☐ **portobello mushroom,** 1

☐ **red onion,** 1

☐ **romaine lettuce,** 1 head

☐ **shallot,** 1

☐ **side salad,** ingredients for 4 meals

☐ **yellow onion,** 1

☐ **zucchini,** 4 large

MEAT:

☐ **bacon,** 1 package

☐ **bacon, thick-cut,** 4 slices

☐ **chicken tenders,** 1¼ pounds

☐ **chicken thighs, boneless, skinless,** 6 (3 to 4 ounces each)

☐ **deli ham,** 1 package

☐ **deli turkey,** 1 package

☐ **flank steak,** 1 pound

☐ **ground beef,** 1 pound

☐ **Italian sausage, bulk,** 8 ounces

☐ **shrimp, large,** 1¼ pounds cooked and 1 pound raw

DAIRY AND EGGS:

☐ **butter, unsalted,** 6 tablespoons

☐ **cheddar cheese, shredded,** 2¼ cups

☐ **cream cheese,** 4 ounces

☐ **eggs,** 3 dozen

☐ **goat cheese, crumbled,** ½ cup

☐ **Gruyère cheese, shredded,** ¼ cup

☐ **half-and-half,** ¾ cup

☐ **heavy whipping cream,** 1 tablespoon

☐ **Italian cheese blend, shredded,** 8 ounces

☐ **mozzarella cheese, low-moisture, shredded,** 3 cups

☐ **Parmesan cheese, grated,** 4 cups

☐ **sour cream,** 1 cup

☐ **Swiss cheese,** shredded or sliced, 8 ounces

☐ **whipped cream cheese,** ⅓ cup

BAKING AND SPICES:

☐ **almond flour, blanched,** 2 cups

☐ **caraway seeds,** 1 teaspoon *(optional, for Reuben Casserole)*

☐ **cream of tartar,** ½ teaspoon

☐ **everything bagel seasoning,** 2 tablespoons

☐ **flaxseed meal,** ¼ cup

☐ **powdered stevia,** 4 (1-gram) packets

☐ **red pepper flakes,** ½ teaspoon *(optional, for Shrimp Scampi)*

☐ **sesame seeds,** 2 teaspoons

If making **Sugar-Free Thousand Island Dressing** (page 83) for the Reuben Casserole, add those ingredients to your shopping list as well.

PANTRY AND CONDIMENTS:

☐ **almond milk, unsweetened,** for serving with Crunchy Keto Granola

☐ **almond milk, vanilla-flavored, unsweetened,** 1½ cups

☐ **beef broth,** ¼ cup

☐ **coconut milk, full-fat,** ⅔ cup

☐ **collagen peptides,** 1 scoop

☐ **Dijon mustard,** 1½ teaspoons

☐ **fish sauce,** 1 tablespoon

☐ **ketchup, sugar-free,** 1 cup *(if making homemade, see page 87 for ingredients)*

☐ **macadamia nuts,** 2 ounces

☐ **marinara sauce, no sugar added,** 2 cups *(if making homemade, see page 82 for ingredients)*

☐ **MCT powder, vanilla-flavored or plain,** 1 scoop *(optional, for Blueberry Collagen Smoothie)*

☐ **pecans, raw,** 3 tablespoons chopped

☐ **peanut butter, salted,** ¼ cup

☐ **peanuts,** for garnishing Chicken Satay Skewers with Peanut Sauce and Thai Cucumber Salad

☐ **pork rinds,** 1½ ounces

☐ **prepared horseradish,** ¼ cup

☐ **pumpkin puree,** ¼ cup

☐ **ranch dressing,** ½ cup + 2 tablespoons *(if making homemade, see page 86 for ingredients)*

☐ **red wine vinegar,** 2 tablespoons

☐ **sauerkraut,** 1 pound

☐ **Sriracha sauce,** 1 to 2 teaspoons *(optional, for Chicken Satay Skewers with Peanut Sauce)*

☐ **white vinegar,** ½ cup

☐ **white wine, dry,** ¼ cup

WEEK 3 MEAL PLAN

(#) = number of servings

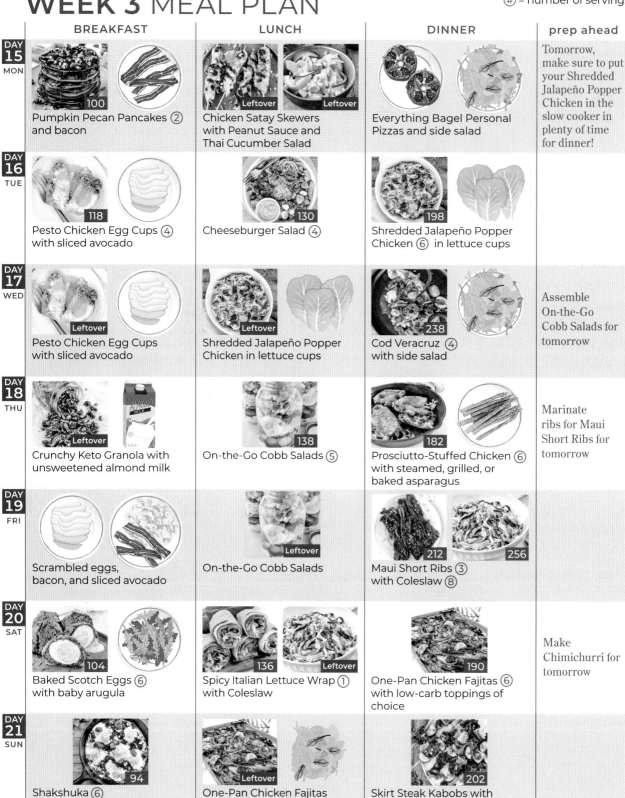

	BREAKFAST	LUNCH	DINNER	prep ahead
DAY 15 MON	Pumpkin Pecan Pancakes (2) and bacon	Chicken Satay Skewers with Peanut Sauce and Thai Cucumber Salad (Leftover)	Everything Bagel Personal Pizzas and side salad	Tomorrow, make sure to put your Shredded Jalapeño Popper Chicken in the slow cooker in plenty of time for dinner!
DAY 16 TUE	Pesto Chicken Egg Cups (4) with sliced avocado	Cheeseburger Salad (4)	Shredded Jalapeño Popper Chicken (6) in lettuce cups	
DAY 17 WED	Pesto Chicken Egg Cups with sliced avocado (Leftover)	Shredded Jalapeño Popper Chicken in lettuce cups (Leftover)	Cod Veracruz (4) with side salad	Assemble On-the-Go Cobb Salads for tomorrow
DAY 18 THU	Crunchy Keto Granola with unsweetened almond milk (Leftover)	On-the-Go Cobb Salads (5)	Prosciutto-Stuffed Chicken (6) with steamed, grilled, or baked asparagus	Marinate ribs for Maui Short Ribs for tomorrow
DAY 19 FRI	Scrambled eggs, bacon, and sliced avocado	On-the-Go Cobb Salads (Leftover)	Maui Short Ribs (3) with Coleslaw (8)	
DAY 20 SAT	Baked Scotch Eggs (6) with baby arugula	Spicy Italian Lettuce Wrap (1) with Coleslaw (Leftover)	One-Pan Chicken Fajitas (6) with low-carb toppings of choice	Make Chimichurri for tomorrow
DAY 21 SUN	Shakshuka (6)	One-Pan Chicken Fajitas chopped and made into a salad with spring mix (Leftover)	Skirt Steak Kabobs with Chimichurri (4)	

WEEK 3 SHOPPING LIST

PRODUCE:

- ☐ **asparagus,** 12 stalks
- ☐ **avocados,** 3
- ☐ **baby arugula,** 1 bag
- ☐ **baby spinach,** 1 cup chopped
- ☐ **butter lettuce,** 1 head
- ☐ **carrot,** 1 large
- ☐ **cherry tomatoes,** 15
- ☐ **cilantro,** 1 bunch
- ☐ **cremini mushrooms,** 5
- ☐ **cucumbers,** 2 mini
- ☐ **garlic,** 2 bulbs
- ☐ **ginger,** 2 tablespoons grated
- ☐ **green bell pepper,** 1
- ☐ **green cabbage,** 1 head
- ☐ **green onion,** 1
- ☐ **iceberg lettuce,** 1 head
- ☐ **jalapeño pepper,** 1
- ☐ **limes,** 2
- ☐ **parsley,** 1 bunch
- ☐ **red bell peppers,** 2
- ☐ **red cabbage,** ½ head
- ☐ **red chili pepper,** 1
- ☐ **red onions,** 2
- ☐ **Roma tomato,** 1
- ☐ **romaine lettuce,** 2 heads
- ☐ **side salad ingredients** for 2 meals
- ☐ **spring mix,** 1 bag
- ☐ **tomato,** 1
- ☐ **yellow onions,** 2 medium
- ☐ **zucchini,** 1 medium to large

Also purchase the fajita toppings and pizza toppings of your choice. If making **Sugar-Free Thousand Island Dressing** (page 83) for the Cheeseburger Salad, add those ingredients to your shopping list as well.

MEAT:

- ☐ **bacon,** 2 packages
- ☐ **Black Forest ham,** 4 slices
- ☐ **chicken breasts, boneless, skinless,** 3¼ pounds
- ☐ **chicken thighs, deboned, with skin on,** 6 (3 to 4 ounces each)
- ☐ **cod fillets,** 4 (4 to 6 ounces each)
- ☐ **deli meat (turkey or ham),** 10 slices
- ☐ **deli sliced chicken breast,** 4 slices
- ☐ **flanken short ribs,** 6 (½ inch thick)
- ☐ **ground beef,** 1 pound
- ☐ **pork sausage, bulk,** 1 pound
- ☐ **prosciutto,** 6 ounces
- ☐ **salami,** 12 slices
- ☐ **skirt steak,** 1 pound

DAIRY AND EGGS:

- ☐ **cheddar cheese, shredded,** 3¼ cups
- ☐ **cream cheese,** 1 (8-ounce) package + 2 ounces
- ☐ **eggs,** 2 dozen
- ☐ **feta cheese, crumbled,** ¾ cup
- ☐ **Gruyère cheese, shredded,** ½ cup
- ☐ **Parmesan cheese, grated,** ¾ cup
- ☐ **provolone cheese,** 2 slices

PANTRY AND CONDIMENTS:

- ☐ **almond milk, unsweetened,** for serving with Crunchy Keto Granola
- ☐ **capers,** 1 tablespoon
- ☐ **dill pickle,** 1
- ☐ **jalapeños, diced,** 1 (4-ounce) can
- ☐ **marinara sauce, no sugar added** *(if making homemade, see page 82 for ingredients)*
- ☐ **olives, mixed, pitted and halved,** ½ cup
- ☐ **pecans, raw,** 3 tablespoons chopped
- ☐ **pepperoncini,** 2
- ☐ **pesto,** 4 teaspoons
- ☐ **pumpkin puree,** ¼ cup
- ☐ **ranch dressing,** ½ cup + 2 tablespoons *(if making homemade, see page 86 for ingredients)*
- ☐ **red wine vinegar,** 2 tablespoons
- ☐ **tomatoes, diced,** 2 (14½-ounce) cans

BAKING AND SPICES:

- ☐ **almond flour, blanched,** ¾ cup
- ☐ **chili powder,** 1 tablespoon
- ☐ **coarse salt,** 1¼ teaspoons
- ☐ **Italian or poultry seasoning,** 2 teaspoons
- ☐ **poppy seeds,** 1 teaspoon *(optional, for Coleslaw)*
- ☐ **red pepper flakes,** 1½ teaspoons
- ☐ **smoked paprika,** 1 teaspoon

WEEK 4 MEAL PLAN

(#) = number of servings

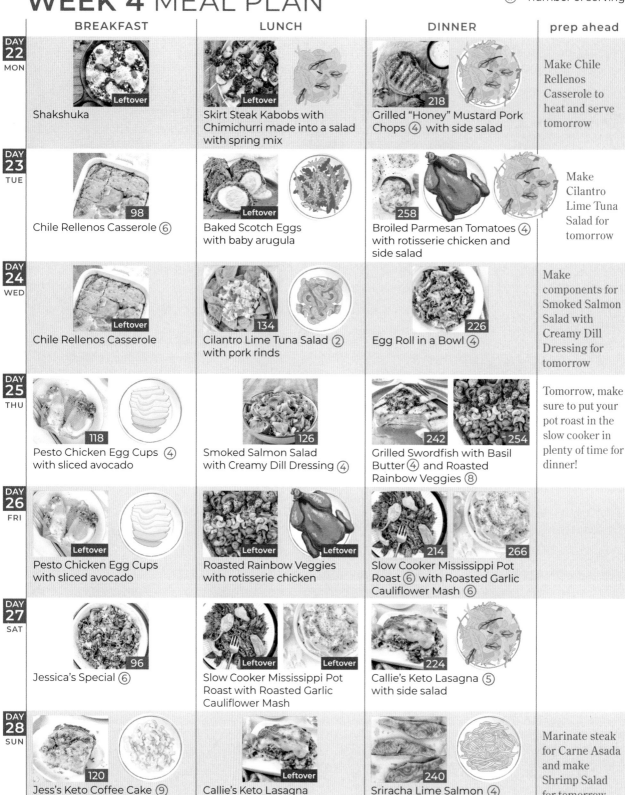

	BREAKFAST	LUNCH	DINNER	prep ahead
DAY 22 MON	Shakshuka (Leftover)	Skirt Steak Kabobs with Chimichurri made into a salad with spring mix (Leftover)	218 Grilled "Honey" Mustard Pork Chops (4) with side salad	Make Chile Rellenos Casserole to heat and serve tomorrow
DAY 23 TUE	98 Chile Rellenos Casserole (6)	Baked Scotch Eggs with baby arugula (Leftover)	258 Broiled Parmesan Tomatoes (4) with rotisserie chicken and side salad	Make Cilantro Lime Tuna Salad for tomorrow
DAY 24 WED	Chile Rellenos Casserole (Leftover)	134 Cilantro Lime Tuna Salad (2) with pork rinds	226 Egg Roll in a Bowl (4)	Make components for Smoked Salmon Salad with Creamy Dill Dressing for tomorrow
DAY 25 THU	118 Pesto Chicken Egg Cups (4) with sliced avocado	126 Smoked Salmon Salad with Creamy Dill Dressing (4)	242 Grilled Swordfish with Basil Butter (4) and Roasted Rainbow Veggies (8) 254	Tomorrow, make sure to put your pot roast in the slow cooker in plenty of time for dinner!
DAY 26 FRI	Pesto Chicken Egg Cups with sliced avocado (Leftover)	Roasted Rainbow Veggies with rotisserie chicken (Leftover)	214 Slow Cooker Mississippi Pot Roast (6) with Roasted Garlic Cauliflower Mash (6) 266	
DAY 27 SAT	96 Jessica's Special (6)	Slow Cooker Mississippi Pot Roast with Roasted Garlic Cauliflower Mash (Leftover)	224 Callie's Keto Lasagna (5) with side salad	
DAY 28 SUN	120 Jess's Keto Coffee Cake (9) with scrambled eggs	Callie's Keto Lasagna (Leftover)	240 Sriracha Lime Salmon (4) with zucchini noodles	Marinate steak for Carne Asada and make Shrimp Salad for tomorrow

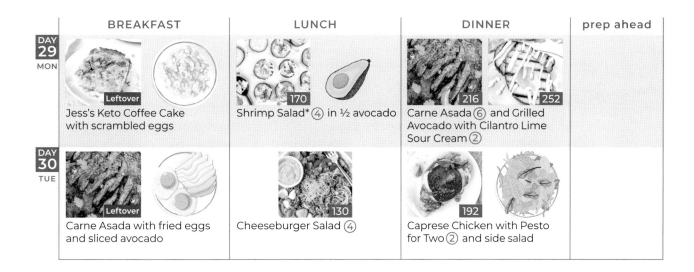

	BREAKFAST	LUNCH	DINNER	prep ahead
DAY 29 MON	Jess's Keto Coffee Cake with scrambled eggs	Shrimp Salad* ④ in ½ avocado · 170	Carne Asada ⑥ and Grilled Avocado with Cilantro Lime Sour Cream ② · 216 · 252	
DAY 30 TUE	Carne Asada with fried eggs and sliced avocado	Cheeseburger Salad ④ · 130	Caprese Chicken with Pesto for Two ② and side salad · 192	

*The Shrimp Salad Cucumber Rounds recipe on
page 170 makes about 1 cup of shrimp salad, which
is enough to stuff four avocado halves using about
¼ cup per avocado half.

WEEK 4 SHOPPING LIST

PRODUCE:

- [ ] **avocados,** 6
- [ ] **baby arugula,** 1 bag
- [ ] **baby spinach,** 5 ounces
- [ ] **basil,** 1 bunch
- [ ] **broccoli,** 1 large head
- [ ] **button mushrooms,** 7 ounces
- [ ] **cauliflower,** 1 large head
- [ ] **celery,** 2 stalks
- [ ] **cherry tomatoes,** 8
- [ ] **chives,** 1 tablespoon chopped
- [ ] **cilantro,** 1 bunch
- [ ] **coleslaw mix,** 1 (14-ounce) bag
- [ ] **cremini mushrooms,** 8 ounces
- [ ] **dill, fresh,** 1 tablespoon + 1 teaspoon chopped
- [ ] **English cucumber,** 1
- [ ] **garlic,** 2 bulbs
- [ ] **green onions,** 1 bunch
- [ ] **jalapeño pepper,** 1
- [ ] **lemons,** 2
- [ ] **limes,** 4
- [ ] **mixed greens,** 1 bag
- [ ] **orange bell pepper,** 1
- [ ] **radishes,** 20
- [ ] **red onions,** 2 medium
- [ ] **Roma tomatoes,** 4
- [ ] **romaine lettuce,** 1 head
- [ ] **side salad,** ingredients for 4 meals
- [ ] **spring mix,** 1 bag
- [ ] **yellow squash,** 2 small
- [ ] **zucchini,** 2 medium and 2 large

If making **Keto Yum Yum Sauce** (page 89) for the Egg Roll in a Bowl and/or **Sugar-Free Thousand Island Dressing** (page 83) for the Cheeseburger Salad, add those ingredients to your shopping list as well.

MEAT:

- [ ] **chicken breasts, boneless, skinless,** 2 (about 5 ounces each)
- [ ] **chuck roast,** 1 (3 pounds)
- [ ] **deli chicken breast,** 4 slices
- [ ] **ground beef,** 1 pound
- [ ] **ground pork,** 1 pound
- [ ] **ground turkey,** 1 pound
- [ ] **Italian sausage, mild, bulk,** 1 pound
- [ ] **pork chops, bone-in,** 4 (1 inch thick)
- [ ] **pork sausage, bulk,** 1 pound
- [ ] **rotisserie chicken,** 1 large
- [ ] **salmon fillets,** 4 (4 to 6 ounces each)
- [ ] **shrimp,** 8 ounces frozen precooked
- [ ] **skirt steak,** 2 pounds
- [ ] **smoked salmon,** 6 ounces
- [ ] **swordfish steaks,** 4 (5 to 6 ounces each)
- [ ] **tuna, packed in water,** 1 (5-ounce) can

DAIRY AND EGGS:

- [ ] **butter, salted,** ¼ cup (½ stick)
- [ ] **butter, unsalted,** 3 sticks
- [ ] **cheddar cheese, shredded,** 3 cups
- [ ] **crème fraîche or sour cream,** ½ cup
- [ ] **eggs,** 3 dozen
- [ ] **feta cheese, crumbled,** ¼ cup
- [ ] **half-and-half,** 1¼ cups
- [ ] **mozzarella cheese, fresh,** 3 ounces
- [ ] **mozzarella cheese, shredded,** 1 cup
- [ ] **Parmesan cheese, grated,** 1⅔ cups
- [ ] **ricotta, whole milk,** 1 cup + 2 tablespoons
- [ ] **sour cream,** ¼ cup

PANTRY AND CONDIMENTS:

- [ ] **almond milk, unsweetened,** ¼ cup
- [ ] **beef broth,** ½ cup
- [ ] **capers,** 1 tablespoon
- [ ] **Dijon mustard,** 1 tablespoon
- [ ] **dill pickle,** 1
- [ ] **green chilies, whole,** 1 (27-ounce) can
- [ ] **hot sauce,** 1 teaspoon *(optional, for Chile Rellenos Casserole)*
- [ ] **marinara sauce, no-sugar-added,** 1½ cups *(to make homemade, see page 82 for ingredients)*
- [ ] **pepperoncini,** 1 large jar
- [ ] **pesto,** 3 tablespoons + 1 teaspoon
- [ ] **pork rinds,** 1 large bag
- [ ] **prepared yellow mustard,** 2 tablespoons
- [ ] **Sriracha sauce,** 1½ teaspoons

BAKING AND SPICES:

- [ ] **almond flour, blanched,** 2½ cups
- [ ] **cayenne pepper,** 1 pinch *(optional, for Jessica's Special)*
- [ ] **dried minced onions,** 1 tablespoon
- [ ] **ginger powder,** 1 teaspoon
- [ ] **Italian seasoning**
- [ ] **Old Bay seasoning,** ½ teaspoon *(optional, for Shrimp Salad)*
- [ ] **sesame seeds,** 1 tablespoon

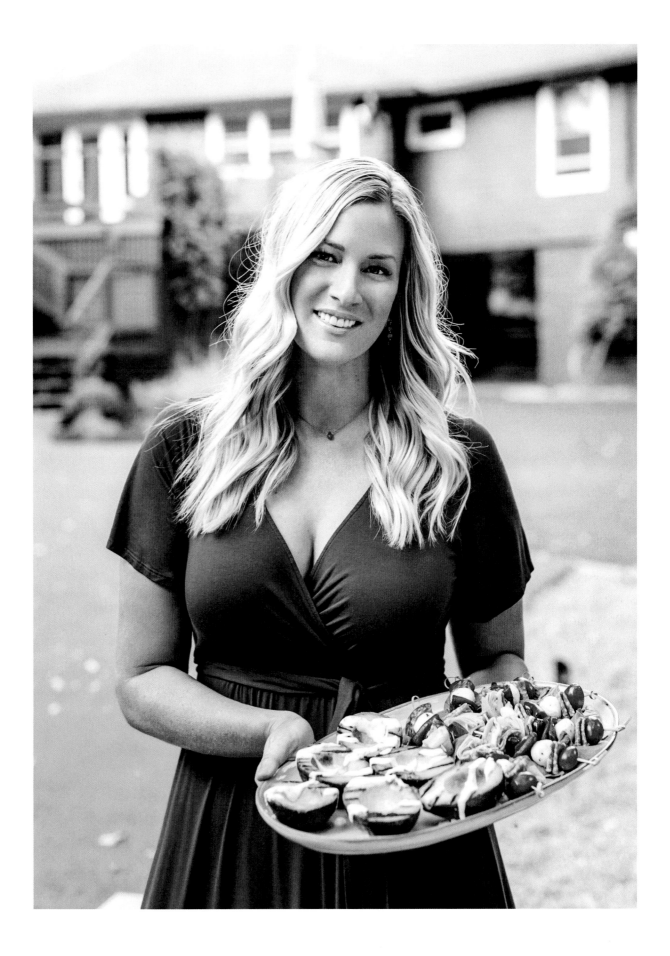

CLOSING LETTER

You are worthy *now,* not when.

We all have goals and desires. Change is often a good thing, and it's human nature to want to evolve and improve, but in our society, there's a lot of pressure to look and act a certain way. All too often, we tell ourselves that once we are _____ [fill in the blank with words like *thinner, more successful, financially stable,* etc.], then we will be happy. But the truth is, you are worthy of love, happiness, and belonging as you are, right now.

I will be the first to say that I had to learn this lesson the hard way. I remember thinking that if I could just lose weight, then everything would be better. While I was so thankful to have lost the weight and felt so much better physically, I still found that self-worth or self-love seemed just out of reach, and my inner critic was thriving.

Your worth isn't dependent on you fitting back into the jeans you wore in college or getting promoted at work. I want you to know that as you are, at this very moment, you are enough. SIMULTANEOUSLY, you can strive for more in your quest to become exactly who you want to be.

The goal is to separate your worth from your goals in a healthy way by loving yourself during every phase of your journey. Stop being so hard on yourself, but don't settle, and don't ever count yourself out. If you truly desire positive change, the key is to give yourself the same level of love, compassion, care, and grace that you would extend to your child, your spouse, or your best friend. This way, your worth is a constant instead of being held hostage by a particular variable or goal.

As someone who has struggled with low self-esteem for most of my life, I'll freely admit that truly loving yourself is easier said than done. It can be so much easier for us to see good and the beauty in others than it is to see those same qualities in ourselves, and living and operating from a place of worthiness takes ongoing practice.

Most of us have been down the long, hard road of second-guessing ourselves, feeling inferior, and letting fear guide our lives. It's time to break those chains by realizing your strength and your ability to be exactly who you want to be.

For those of you who have felt broken, hopeless, or damaged beyond repair, I want to share something with you that helped me recognize my struggles, my pain, and my worth in a new light.

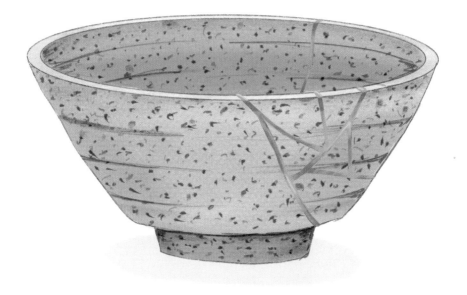

This illustration depicts a bowl that has been repaired using a process called Kintsugi. *Kintsugi* ("golden joinery"), also known as *Kintsukuroi*, is the Japanese art of repairing broken pottery by using lacquer dusted or mixed with powdered gold. Items that are broken are not discarded or devalued; instead, they are put back together, and the cracks are mended with gold. This process of repair does two amazing things. First, it embraces the history of the piece and encourages us to see the beauty in imperfection, and in the ability to heal that is present in all of us. Second, because the cracks are repaired with gold, the piece is not only more beautiful after being mended, but more valuable, too. This reminds us that the pain and struggles in life—those things that create "cracks" inside us—do not reduce our value; they shape us into exactly who we are today. Therefore, we should view whatever damage we have incurred with empathy, compassion, vulnerability, and purpose, because often pain is a catalyst for growth and leads us down new, more positive paths in life.

I want you to know that regardless of what you've been through, you are strong, you are beautiful, you are valuable, you are worthy, and you are never beyond repair. I encourage you to share your story, to be vulnerable, to always be a work in progress, and to allow yourself to heal from the inside out.

All my love,

Suzanne

ACKNOWLEDGMENTS

Mick: Thank you for being by my side for the last fourteen years. I wouldn't want to be on this journey with anyone else but you. Thank you for loving me and supporting my dreams no matter how big or small. I love you, always and forever.

Olivia: When I count my blessings, I count you twice. Thank you for bringing so much joy, love, humor, and snuggles into my life. You are my world, and I am so proud of you!

Mom: Writing this book was so emotional, but it was so special and healing that we were able to talk about so many of our own struggles with self-worth during my time in Florida. Thank you for being so open and vulnerable. I am so thankful for all your guidance, advice, and support. I love you so much.

Dad: I truly don't have the words to tell you how much you mean to me. I cherish our time together so much—every phone call, every FaceTime, every visit. Thank you for always being more than willing to hop on a plane and be the world's best Pop Pop as well as my rock. I love you so much!

John and Cher: I love you both very much. Thank you for your love and support. I truly cherish our time together and love that we live so close to one another.

Emily: To my second mom and Oliva's Oma, I love you so much. Thank you for your endless love and encouragement. I feel so thankful to have you in my life.

Jess and Dan: Where do I begin? Thank you for being friends who really feel more like family. Thank you for the countless laughs, texts, walks around the circle, hot tub conversations, Kim K cheers, advice, love, support, and once-in-a-lifetime dinners. I am so thankful for your friendship, and I love you so much!

Callie and Robert: Is it okay if I just talk about how much I love you guys and how amazing your wedding was?! Can we go back to Italy and do it again? Seriously, though, I love you both so much. Thank you for almost twenty years of friendship. How the heck did we get so old?

Tina and Steve: To my favorite mermaid and "old guy," I love you both so much. Living so far away never seems to get easier, but I cherish every moment we spend together. In loving memory of Callie Brown, the coolest and sweetest pug to ever live.

Melissa and Matt: Thank you for your endless support and encouragement. We miss you already, but I'm so thankful for phone calls and FaceTime. Love you guys!

Megan S.: I am so thankful that my journey led me to meet you. I am so proud of everything you are accomplishing. You are the real deal, and I'm honored to be your friend.

Jenny P.: Words truly can't describe how amazing, selfless, compassionate, and caring you are. I am so thankful for your friendship and support. I love you!

Mike, Karin, and Devin: I love you guys so much and miss you more and more each year! Devin, thank you for being Olivia's BFF and playmate.

Beverly M.: Thank you for your guidance, wisdom, and care. You have truly helped me change my life, outlook, and perspective. You have such a beautiful gift of helping others. Thank you for sharing it with me.

Ryan Lowery: You are living proof that positivity always wins. Thank you for inspiring me and the rest of the world to live with gratitude and positivity. I am so thankful for your endless support, kindness, and friendship.

Brené Brown: Thank you for sharing your work, your heart, and your wisdom so vulnerably with the world. You have touched my heart and life, and for that I am so grateful. Thank you for your support and encouragement.

VB Team and Designers: A special thank you for the countless hours spent pouring your talent, care, and passion into every page to make this book a reality. I am BEYOND thankful to be a part of the Victory Belt family!

Susan: Thank you for your friendship, kindness, inside jokes, honesty, and love. You make the world a better place by being in it. Thank you for keeping my sanity in check! I love and appreciate you so much!

Lance: Thank you for believing in me, especially in moments when I struggled. You are hands down the most amazing and positive cheerleader. Thank you for everything you do!

Erich: Your enthusiasm for making this world a better and healthier place is contagious. Thank you for the amazing impact you have made and continue to make in this world.

Pam and Holly: Thank you for your kindness, suggestions, passion, and meticulous attention to detail. I appreciate you both more than I can say, and I'm glad you two were not around to grade my homework in college. All jokes aside, THANK YOU!

Jennifer Skog and Chelsea Foster: My dream team for all things style, photography, and design. Thank you both for sharing your gifts and talents to make this book come to life. I love and admire both of you! Thank you for this amazing cover!

Betsy and Jessie: Thank you for the most beautiful food styling I've ever seen. It was so much fun to photograph all of these gorgeous dishes with you. Thank you for sharing your gifts, talents, and tricks with me!

Jessica Morgan: You are truly beautiful inside and out, and I'm so thankful and honored to work with you. Thank you for being the most amazing teammate!

Instagram/Facebook/Blog Family: To the kind, vulnerable, supportive, and loving keto community, thank you all for showing up, being seen, supporting one another, and being brave. All of you inspire me, and you are proof that kindness and love always win and that no one ever has to face the world alone.

RECOMMENDATIONS AND RESOURCES

Books

Here are some of my favorite books about life, mindset, and mental health:

- *Becoming* by Michelle Obama
- *Better Than Before* by Gretchen Rubin
- *Big Magic* by Elizabeth Gilbert
- *Braving the Wilderness* by Brené Brown
- *Dare to Lead* by Brené Brown
- *Daring Greatly* by Brené Brown
- *The Gifts of Imperfection* by Brené Brown
- *GRIT* by Angela Duckworth
- *The Happiness Project* by Gretchen Rubin
- *Mindset* by Carol Dweck
- *Tribe of Mentors* by Tim Ferriss
- *Why We Get Fat: And What to Do About It* by Gary Taubes

Documentaries and Recorded Talks

Here are some of my favorite documentaries and recorded talks:

- **"The Call to Courage":** Brené Brown (Netflix).
- **"Demonization and Deception in Cholesterol Research":** Dr. David Diamond (YouTube).
- **Fat: A Documentary (2019):** FAT tells the farfetched but completely true history of how people in the United States became so unhealthy.
- **Fed Up (2014):** A film about the dangers of sugar and how it has contributed to the obesity epidemic in the United States.
- **Health Theory:** A weekly interview show hosted by Quest Nutrition cofounder Tom Bilyeu. Each episode offers tactical steps one can take to improve their well-being and achieve their goals from the world's top health experts.

- **Impact Theory:** A weekly interview show that explores the mindsets of the world's highest achievers to uncover their secrets to success.

- **The Magic Pill (2017):** Doctors, scientists, and chefs around the globe combat illness with dietary changes, believing fat should be embraced as a source of fuel.

- **"The Power of Vulnerability":** Brené Brown (TED Talk).

- **"Reversing Type 2 Diabetes Starts with Ignoring the Guidelines":** Dr. Sarah Hallberg (TED Talk).

- **That Sugar Film (2014):** An Australian documentary showing one man's journey as he changes his diet to one that is high in sugar, all while eating "healthy" foods that are often lower in fat but have added sugar.

- **Women of Impact: Empowering You and All Women to Recognize That You Really Can Become the Hero of Your Own Life:** An ongoing series hosted by Lisa Bilyeu.

Keto-Related Nonprofit Foundations and Conferences

- **The Charlie Foundation (charliefoundation.org):** Diet therapies for people with epilepsy.

- **Low-Carb Denver (lowcarbconferences.com):** An annual keto conference featuring the latest science and nutritional approaches including low-carb, keto, carnivore, and intermittent fasting.

- **MaxLove Project (maxloveproject.org):** Helping SuperKids Thrive Against the Odds—a nonprofit that provides education about keto to fight cancer.

- **The Metabolic Health Summit (metabolichealthsummit.com):** An annual keto conference that is open to the public to learn all about keto.

Keto Mastery Certification Course

With the rise of the keto movement, plenty of people want more information—not only to help themselves, but to help friends and family, too. Keto Mastery is an online certification program designed by my two friends Dr. Ryan Lowery and Dr. Jacob Wilson, the authors of *The Ketogenic Bible*. Their goal is to encourage coaches, doctors, practitioners, and everyday individuals to take a deep dive into the keto lifestyle in order to understand and apply keto principles. Keto Mastery is a digital course with more than 50 interactive lectures and videos from scientists, thought leaders, and individuals who have had success with the keto lifestyle. You can find information at ketogenic.com/mastery/.

MEASUREMENT AND TEMPERATURE CONVERSION CHART

CUP TO TABLESPOONS TO TEASPOONS TO MILLILITERS

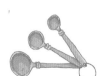

1 cup	=	16 Tbsp.	=	48 tsp.	=	240 ml
¾ cup	=	12 Tbsp.	=	36 tsp.	=	180 ml
⅔ cup	=	11 Tbsp.	=	32 tsp.	=	160 ml
½ cup	=	8 Tbsp.	=	24 tsp.	=	120 ml
⅓ cup	=	5 Tbsp.	=	16 tsp.	=	80 ml
¼ cup	=	4 Tbsp.	=	12 tsp.	=	60 ml

1 tablespoon = 15 ml

1 teaspoon = 5 ml

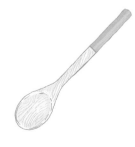

CUP TO FLUID OUNCES

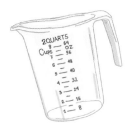

1 cup	=	8 fl. oz.
¾ cup	=	6 fl. oz.
⅔ cup	=	5 fl. oz.
½ cup	=	4 fl. oz.
⅓ cup	=	3 fl. oz.
¼ cup	=	2 fl. oz.

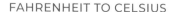
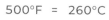
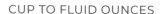

FAHRENHEIT TO CELSIUS

500°F	=	260°C
475°F	=	245°C
450°F	=	235°C
425°F	=	220°C
400°F	=	205°C
375°F	=	190°C
350°F	=	180°C
325°F	=	160°C
300°F	=	150°C
275°F	=	135°C
250°F	=	120°C
225°F	=	107°C

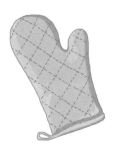

PRINTABLE WORKSHEETS

On the next few pages, you will find examples of several worksheets that you can use at home for accountability, journaling, and meal planning. Visit ketokarma.com/printables to download and print these free worksheets.

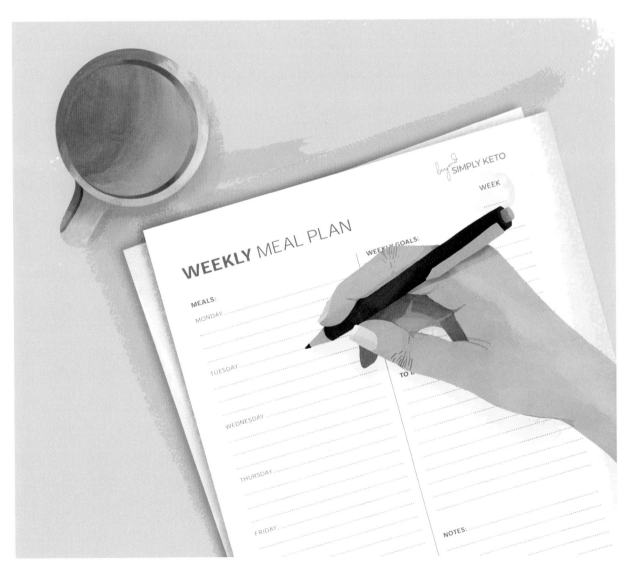

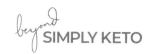

30-DAY KETO ACCOUNTABILITY

DAY
01

DAY
02

DAY
03

DAY
04

DAY
05

DAY
06

DAY
07

DAY
08

DAY
09

DAY
10

DAY
11

DAY
12

DAY
13

DAY
14

DAY
15

DAY
16

DAY
17

DAY
18

DAY
19

DAY
20

DAY
21

DAY
22

DAY
23

DAY
24

DAY
25

DAY
26

DAY
27

DAY
28

DAY
29

DAY
30

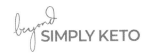

30-DAY ACCOUNTABILITY with weight

STARTING WEIGHT: ....

STARTING INCHES: ....

DAY 01 **DAY 02** **DAY 03** **DAY 04** **DAY 05**

DAY 06 **DAY 07** **DAY 08** **DAY 09** **DAY 10**

LBS. LOST: ....

INCHES LOST: ....

DAY 11 **DAY 12** **DAY 13** **DAY 14** **DAY 15**

DAY 16 **DAY 17** **DAY 18** **DAY 19** **DAY 20**

LBS. LOST: ....

INCHES LOST: ....

DAY 21 **DAY 22** **DAY 23** **DAY 24** **DAY 25**

DAY 26 **DAY 27** **DAY 28** **DAY 29** **DAY 30**

LBS. LOST: ....

INCHES LOST: ....

TOTAL WEIGHT LOST: ....

TOTAL INCHES LOST: ....

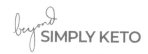

SELF-CARE WEEKLY JOURNAL

WEEK

....

WEEKLY POSITIVE AFFIRMATION:

I am ....

(strong, enough, smart, kind, beautiful, etc.) Work on replacing negative self-talk with positive and supportive words. Start each day by looking in the mirror and repeating this statement to yourself. If a critical inner voice chimes in, replace those thoughts with this affirmation.

3 THINGS I'M GRATEFUL FOR THIS WEEK:

1. ....

....

2. ....

....

3. ....

....

MY GOALS FOR THIS WEEK ARE:

1. ....

....

2. ....

....

3. ....

....

SELF-CARE PLAN FOR THE WEEK:

These tasks can take as little as 5 to 10 minutes or however long you have. Self-care looks different for each of us. Quick things can include a 20-minute walk, a bath, a guided meditation, deep breathing exercises, etc. If you have more time, try having lunch with a friend or family member, seeing a counselor, taking a 45-minute walk, going for a swim, getting a massage, or cleaning the house.

SUNDAY..

....

MONDAY..

....

TUESDAY..

....

WEDNESDAY..

....

THURSDAY..

....

FRIDAY..

....

SATURDAY..

....

SELF-CARE:
- [ ] SUNDAY
- [ ] MONDAY
- [ ] TUESDAY
- [ ] WEDNESDAY
- [ ] THURSDAY
- [ ] FRIDAY
- [ ] SATURDAY

SLEEP:
- [ ] SUNDAY
- [ ] MONDAY
- [ ] TUESDAY
- [ ] WEDNESDAY
- [ ] THURSDAY
- [ ] FRIDAY
- [ ] SATURDAY

WATER:
- [ ] SUNDAY
- [ ] MONDAY
- [ ] TUESDAY
- [ ] WEDNESDAY
- [ ] THURSDAY
- [ ] FRIDAY
- [ ] SATURDAY

EXERCISE:
- [ ] SUNDAY
- [ ] MONDAY
- [ ] TUESDAY
- [ ] WEDNESDAY
- [ ] THURSDAY
- [ ] FRIDAY
- [ ] SATURDAY

....
- [ ] SUNDAY
- [ ] MONDAY
- [ ] TUESDAY
- [ ] WEDNESDAY
- [ ] THURSDAY
- [ ] FRIDAY
- [ ] SATURDAY

....
- [ ] SUNDAY
- [ ] MONDAY
- [ ] TUESDAY
- [ ] WEDNESDAY
- [ ] THURSDAY
- [ ] FRIDAY
- [ ] SATURDAY

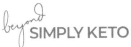

DAILY JOURNAL

DAY
....

MEALS AND SNACKS:

BREAKFAST:...

....

....

....

LUNCH:...

....

....

....

DINNER:...

....

....

SNACK:...

....

....

....

SLEEP:

....

....

....

WATER: ☐ ☐ ☐ ☐ ☐ ☐ ☐ ☐ ☐

EXERCISE: ....

.... STEPS:..............

....

.... WEIGHT:..............

OTHER NOTES: ....

....

....

....

GRATITUDE: ....

....

....

....

MOOD & EMOTIONS: ....

....

....

....

SELF-CARE NOTES: ....

....

....

....

WEEKLY MEAL PLAN

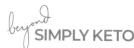

WEEK

MEALS:

MONDAY..

TUESDAY..

WEDNESDAY..

THURSDAY..

FRIDAY...

SATURDAY..

SUNDAY...

WEEKLY GOALS:

TO DO:...

NOTES:...

OVERVIEW:...

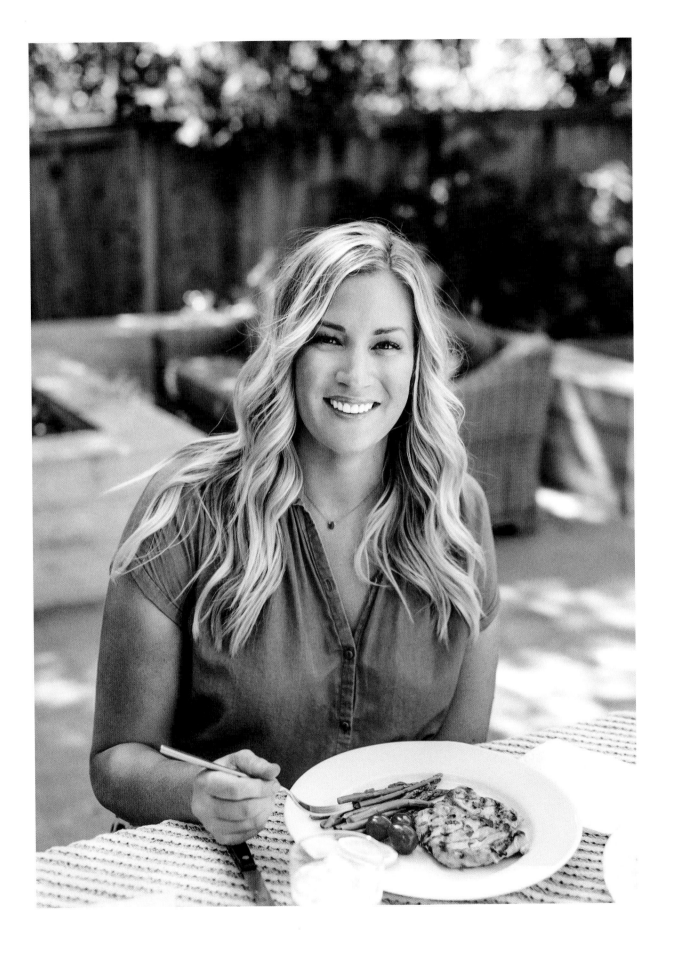

RECIPE INDEX

basics

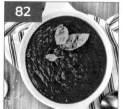
82 Marinara Sauce

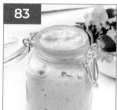
83 Sugar-Free Thousand Island Dressing

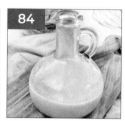
84 Simple Vinaigrette

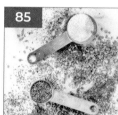
85 Ranch Herb Mix

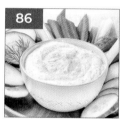
86 Ranch Dip/Dressing

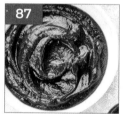
87 Sugar-Free Ketchup

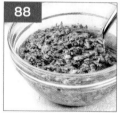
88 Chimichurri

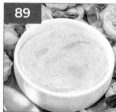
89 Keto Yum Yum Sauce

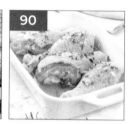
90 Rosemary Lemon Marinade

breakfast

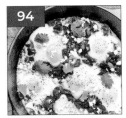

94

Shakshuka

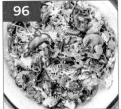

96

Jessica's Special

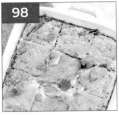

98

Chile Rellenos Casserole

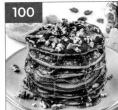

100

Pumpkin Pecan Pancakes

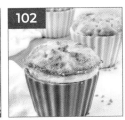

102

Three-Cheese Soufflés

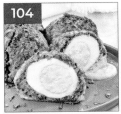

104

Baked Scotch Eggs

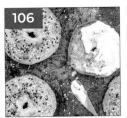

106

Everything Bagels

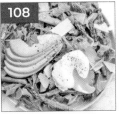

108

Arugula, Avocado, and Asparagus Salad with Poached Eggs

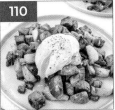

110

Corned Beef Hash with Radishes

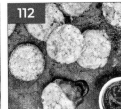

112

Cauli Hash Browns

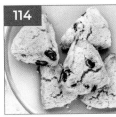

114

Lemon Blueberry Scones

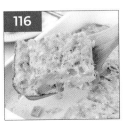

116

Denver Breakfast Casserole

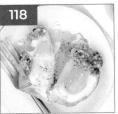

118

Pesto Chicken Egg Cups

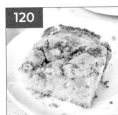

120

Jess's Keto Coffee Cake

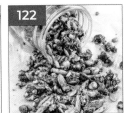

122

Crunchy Keto Granola

lunch & light meals

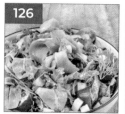

126
Smoked Salmon Salad with Creamy Dill Dressing

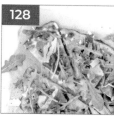

128
Prosciutto Arugula Pizza

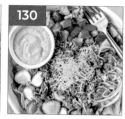

130
Cheeseburger Salad

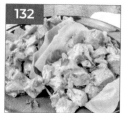

132
Curry Chicken Salad

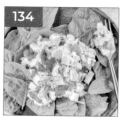

134
Cilantro Lime Tuna Salad

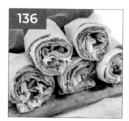

136
Spicy Italian Lettuce Wrap

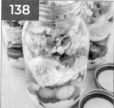

138
On-the-Go Cobb Salads

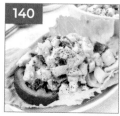

140
Egg Salad Wraps

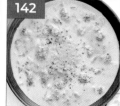

142
Broccoli Cheddar Soup

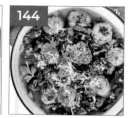

144
Italian Wedding Soup

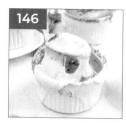

146
French Onion Soup

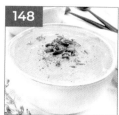

148
Cream of Mushroom Soup

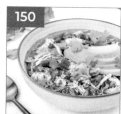

150
Shredded Chicken Taco Soup

appetizers & snacks

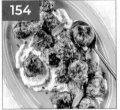
154
Lamb Feta Meatballs with Mint Yogurt Sauce

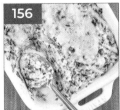
156
Spinach Artichoke Dip

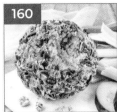
158
Salt and Vinegar Wings

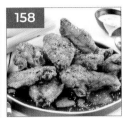
160
Loaded Bacon Cheese Ball

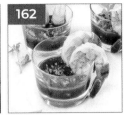
162
Shrimp Cocktail

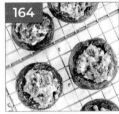
164
Sausage-Stuffed Mushrooms

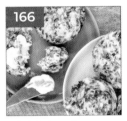
166
Mini Spinach Soufflés

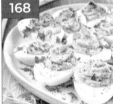
168
Herbed Deviled Eggs

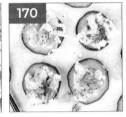
170
Shrimp Salad Cucumber Rounds

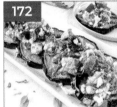
172
Grilled Eggplant "Bruschetta"

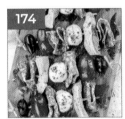
174
Antipasto Skewers

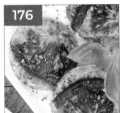
176
Caprese Pizza Crisps

chicken & turkey

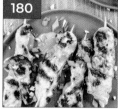
180
Chicken Satay Skewers with Peanut Sauce

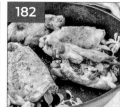
182
Prosciutto-Stuffed Chicken

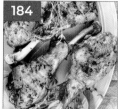
184
Roasted Turkey Legs

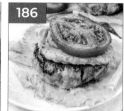
186
Zesty Ranch Turkey Burgers

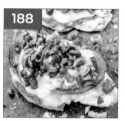
188
Muffuletta Chicken

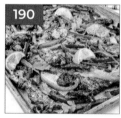
190
One-Pan Chicken Fajitas

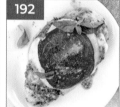
192
Caprese Chicken with Pesto for Two

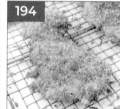
194
Crispy Baked Chicken Thighs

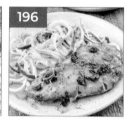
196
Creamy Sun-Dried Tomato and Basil Chicken

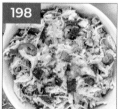
198
Shredded Jalapeño Popper Chicken

beef & pork

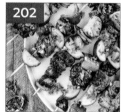
202
Skirt Steak Kabobs with Chimichurri

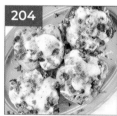
204
Stuffed Bell Peppers

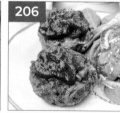
206
Meatloaf Muffins

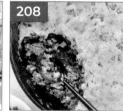
208
Shepherd's Pie

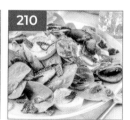
210
Mike's Spinach Salad with Warm Bacon Dressing

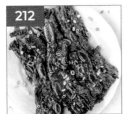
212

Maui Short Ribs

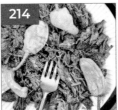
214

Slow Cooker Mississippi Pot Roast

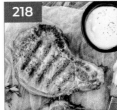
216

Carne Asada

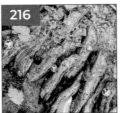
218

Grilled "Honey" Mustard Pork Chops

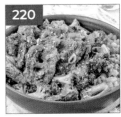
220

Beef and Broccoli

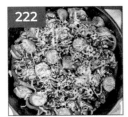
222

Italian Sausage with Peppers

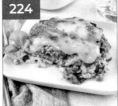
224

Callie's Keto Lasagna

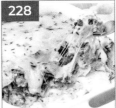
226

Egg Roll in a Bowl

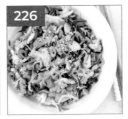
228

Reuben Casserole

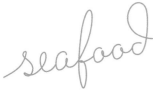
seafood

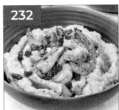
232

Cajun Shrimp and "Grits"

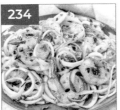
234

Shrimp Scampi with Zucchini Noodles

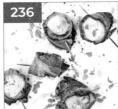
236

Bacon-Wrapped Scallops

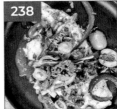
238

Cod Veracruz

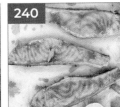
240

Sriracha Lime Salmon

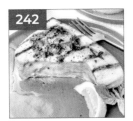
242

Grilled Swordfish with Basil Butter

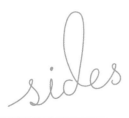

sides

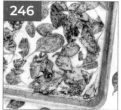

246

Baked Spinach Chips

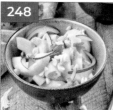

248

Thai Cucumber Salad

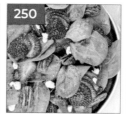

250

Strawberry Spinach Salad with Candied Pecans

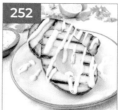

252

Grilled Avocado with Cilantro Lime Sour Cream

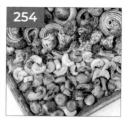

254

Roasted Rainbow Veggies

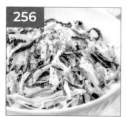

256

Coleslaw

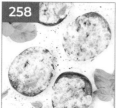

258

Broiled Parmesan Tomatoes

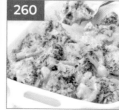

260

Cheesy Broccoli Bake

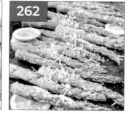

262

Lemon Parmesan Asparagus

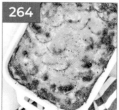

264

Three-Cheese Zucchini au Gratin

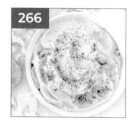

266

Roasted Garlic Cauliflower Mash

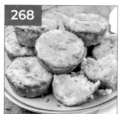

268

Cheddar Chive Biscuits

Desserts & Drinks

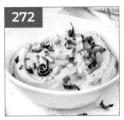
272
Peanut Butter Mousse

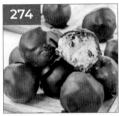
274
Chocolate-Coated Cookie Dough Bites

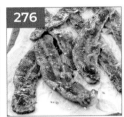
276
Candied Bacon

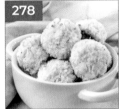
278
Coconut Macaroons

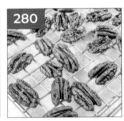
280
Tina's Candied Pecans

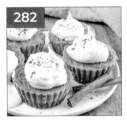
282
Mini Pumpkin Pies

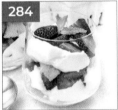
284
5-Minute Strawberry Shortcake Parfait for Two

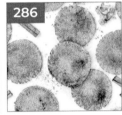
286
Olivia's Snickerdoodles

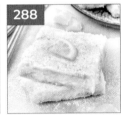
288
Lemon Bars

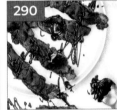
290
Boardwalk Chocolate-Covered Bacon

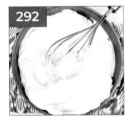
292
Whipped Cream

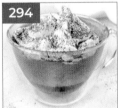
294
Café Mocha

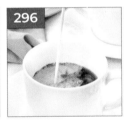
296
Chai Tea Latte

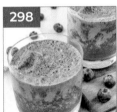
298
Blueberry Collagen Smoothie

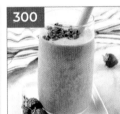
300
Chocolate-Dipped Strawberry Smoothie

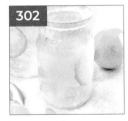
302
Lemonade

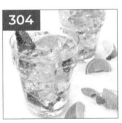
304
Virgin Mojito

ALLERGEN INDEX

RECIPES	PAGE	⏱30	🥛	⊘	🌾
Marinara Sauce	82		✓	✓	✓
Sugar-Free Thousand Island Dressing	83	✓	✓	✓	✓
Simple Vinaigrette	84	✓	✓	✓	✓
Ranch Herb Mix	85	✓	✓	✓	✓
Ranch Dip/Dressing	86				✓
Sugar-Free Ketchup	87	✓	✓	✓	✓
Chimichurri	88	✓	✓	✓	✓
Keto Yum Yum Sauce	89				✓
Rosemary Lemon Marinade	90	✓	✓	✓	✓
Shakshuka	94				✓
Jessica's Special	96	✓			✓
Chile Rellenos Casserole	98				✓
Pumpkin Pecan Pancakes	100	✓			
Three-Cheese Soufflés	102				✓
Baked Scotch Eggs	104				
Everything Bagels	106	✓			
Arugula, Avocado, and Asparagus Salad with Poached Eggs	108	✓			✓
Corned Beef Hash with Radishes	110				✓
Cauli Hash Browns	112				✓
Lemon Blueberry Scones	114				
Denver Breakfast Casserole	116				✓
Pesto Chicken Egg Cups	118	✓			
Jess's Keto Coffee Cake	120				
Crunchy Keto Granola	122	✓	✓		
Smoked Salmon Salad with Creamy Dill Dressing	126	✓		✓	✓
Prosciutto Arugula Pizza	128	✓			
Cheeseburger Salad	130	✓		✓	✓
Curry Chicken Salad	132		✓		
Cilantro Lime Tuna Salad	134	✓	✓		✓
Spicy Italian Lettuce Wrap	136	✓			✓
On-the-Go Cobb Salads	138	✓			✓
Egg Salad Wraps	140	✓	✓		✓
Broccoli Cheddar Soup	142			✓	✓
Italian Wedding Soup	144				
French Onion Soup	146			✓	✓
Cream of Mushroom Soup	148			✓	✓
Shredded Chicken Taco Soup	150		✓	✓	✓
Lamb Feta Meatballs with Mint Yogurt Sauce	154				
Spinach Artichoke Dip	156			✓	✓
Salt and Vinegar Wings	158			✓	✓
Loaded Bacon Cheese Ball	160			✓	
Shrimp Cocktail	162	✓	✓	✓	✓
Sausage-Stuffed Mushrooms	164			✓	✓
Mini Spinach Soufflés	166	✓			
Herbed Deviled Eggs	168				✓
Shrimp Salad Cucumber Rounds	170		✓		✓
Grilled Eggplant "Bruschetta"	172	✓		✓	✓
Antipasto Skewers	174	✓		✓	✓
Caprese Pizza Crisps	176	✓		✓	✓
Chicken Satay Skewers with Peanut Sauce	180		✓	✓	
Prosciutto-Stuffed Chicken	182			✓	✓
Roasted Turkey Legs	184			✓	✓
Zesty Ranch Turkey Burgers	186	✓		✓	✓
Muffuletta Chicken	188			✓	✓

RECIPES	PAGE	⏱30	🥛	⦸	🥜
One-Pan Chicken Fajitas	190		✓	✓	✓
Caprese Chicken with Pesto for Two	192	✓		✓	
Crispy Baked Chicken Thighs	194	✓			✓
Creamy Sun-Dried Tomato and Basil Chicken	196	✓		✓	✓
Shredded Jalapeño Popper Chicken	198			✓	✓
Skirt Steak Kabobs with Chimichurri	202	✓	✓	✓	✓
Stuffed Bell Peppers	204			✓	✓
Meatloaf Muffins	206				
Shepherd's Pie	208				✓
Mike's Spinach Salad with Warm Bacon Dressing	210	✓	✓		✓
Maui Short Ribs	212		✓	✓	✓
Slow Cooker Mississippi Pot Roast	214			✓	✓
Carne Asada	216		✓	✓	✓
Grilled "Honey" Mustard Pork Chops	218		✓		✓
Beef and Broccoli	220		✓	✓	✓
Italian Sausage with Peppers	222			✓	✓
Callie's Keto Lasagna	224				✓
Egg Roll in a Bowl	226	✓	✓		✓
Reuben Casserole	228				✓
Cajun Shrimp and "Grits"	232			✓	✓
Shrimp Scampi with Zucchini Noodles	234	✓		✓	✓
Bacon-Wrapped Scallops	236	✓	✓	✓	✓
Cod Veracruz	238	✓	✓	✓	✓
Sriracha Lime Salmon	240	✓	✓	✓	✓
Grilled Swordfish with Basil Butter	242	✓		✓	✓
Baked Spinach Chips	246	✓	✓	✓	✓
Thai Cucumber Salad	248	✓	✓	✓	
Strawberry Spinach Salad with Candied Pecans	250	✓		✓	
Grilled Avocado with Cilantro Lime Sour Cream	252			✓	✓
Roasted Rainbow Veggies	254		✓	✓	✓
Coleslaw	256	✓	✓		✓
Broiled Parmesan Tomatoes	258	✓			✓
Cheesy Broccoli Bake	260	✓		✓	✓
Lemon Parmesan Asparagus	262	✓		✓	✓
Three-Cheese Zucchini au Gratin	264			✓	✓
Roasted Garlic Cauliflower Mash	266		✓	✓	
Cheddar Chive Biscuits	268	✓			
Peanut Butter Mousse	272	✓		✓	
Chocolate-Coated Cookie Dough Bites	274			✓	
Candied Bacon	276		✓	✓	✓
Coconut Macaroons	278		✓		✓
Tina's Candied Pecans	280	✓	✓	✓	
Mini Pumpkin Pies	282				
5-Minute Strawberry Shortcake Parfait for Two	284	✓			
Olivia's Snickerdoodles	286	✓			
Lemon Bars	288				
Boardwalk Chocolate-Covered Bacon	290		✓	✓	✓
Whipped Cream	292	✓		✓	✓
Café Mocha	294	✓		✓	✓
Chai Tea Latte	296	✓		✓	
Blueberry Collagen Smoothie	298	✓	✓	✓	
Chocolate-Dipped Strawberry Smoothie	300	✓		✓	
Lemonade	302	✓	✓	✓	✓
Virgin Mojito	304	✓	✓	✓	✓

GENERAL INDEX